D1822936

THE ANESTHETIC PLAN: FROM PHYSIOLOGIC PRINCIPLES TO CLINICAL STRATEGIES

THE ANESTHETIC PLAN: FROM PHYSIOLOGIC PRINCIPLES TO CLINICAL STRATEGIES

Stanley Muravchick, M.D., Ph.D.
Associate Professor of Anesthesia
Hospital of the University of Pennsylvania
Philadelphia, Pennsylvania

Mosby
Year Book

St. Louis   Baltimore   Boston   Chicago   London   Philadelphia   Sydney   Toronto

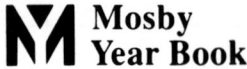

Mosby
Year Book

Dedicated to Publishing Excellence

Sponsoring Editor: Susan M. Gay
Associate Managing Editor, Manuscript Services: Deborah Thorp
Production Coordinator: Nancy C. Baker
Proofroom Supervisor: Barbara M. Kelly

Copyright © 1991 by Mosby-Year Book, Inc.
A Year Book Medical Publishers imprint of Mosby-Year Book, Inc.

Mosby-Year Book, Inc.
11830 Westline Industrial Drive
St. Louis, MO 63146

All rights reserved. No part of this publication may be reproduced, stored in a retrieval system, or transmitted, in any form or by any means, electronic, mechanical, photocopying, recording, or otherwise, without prior written permission from the publisher. Printed in the United States of America.

Permission to photocopy or reproduce solely for internal or personal use is permitted for libraries or other users registered with the Copyright Clearance Center, provided that the base fee of $4.00 per chapter plus $.10 per page is paid directly to the Copyright Clearance Center, 21 Congress Street, Salem, MA 01970. This consent does not extend to other kinds of copying, such as copying for general distribution, for advertising or promotional purposes, for creating new collected works, or for resale.

1 2 3 4 5 6 7 8 9 0 V C 95 94 93 92 91

Library of Congress Cataloging-in-Publication Data
Muravchick, Stanley.
    The anesthetic plan : from physiologic principles to clinical
strategies / Stanley Muravchick.
        p.   cm.
    Includes bibliographical references.
    Includes index.
    ISBN 0-8151-6241-3
    1. Anesthesiology. 2. Anesthetics—Toxicology. 3. Anesthesia—
Complications and sequelae. I. Title.
    [DNLM: 1. Anesthetics—adverse effects. 2. Anesthetics—
pharmacology. 3. Intraoperative Complications—chemically induced.
4. Risk Factors. QV 81 M972a]
RD82.M87 1991   90-6586
617.9'6041—dc20   CIP
DNLM/DLC
for Library of Congress

This book is dedicated to my mother, Rebecca, and to the memory of my father, Harry: they taught me to love scholarship and to respect knowledge, values that led me to this undertaking; and to my wife, Dr. Arlene Olson, and my daughter, Rose: they gave me the gentle encouragement and consistent support that sustained my enthusiasm during three difficult years.

PREFACE

This book is a direct result of questions asked of me by my residents, many of which I was simply unable to answer immediately. It also became apparent to me that many fundamental physiologic mechanisms and pharmacologic relationships are not adequately described in standard textbooks, even though I believe them to be essential for the formulation of a rational anesthetic plan. Clinical experience, of course, can be a wonderful teacher, but the lessons are often obscure and misinterpreted until they are refashioned in the context of current scientific concepts of applied physiology and pharmacology. That is the objective of this book; in an environment as complex as that of the operating room, a little bit of knowledge can truly be a dangerous thing.

Throughout the first half of this century, anesthesiology was largely an empirical discipline taught by a process of apprenticeship. One learned directly from the clinical master; when things went wrong without apparent reason, the patient was assumed to "have taken a bad anesthetic." Some anesthetic protocols usually worked well, but others did not and were eventually discarded. Although still young enough to have a distinct genealogy, the specialty has expanded its scientific knowledge base exponentially since the end of World War II. With rapid application and acceptance of complex physiologic monitoring into daily practice, the transformation of anesthesiology into a controlled, daily exercise of the principles of applied physiology and pharmacology is nearly complete.

Virtually every anesthetic plan can be derived directly from our understanding of how these drugs alter end-organ and integrated organ-system functions, our recognition of the various expressions of anesthetic toxicity, and epidemiologic data regarding the demographic, technical, and judgmental factors that influence perioperative risk and anesthetic outcome. These are the primary issues to which this book is addressed, although this is obviously not a complete textbook of anesthesia. Nor does it have the authority or critical detail needed to satisfy serious researchers or career academicians. The references chosen are meant to be representative and not comprehensive. Wherever possible,

I have referred to widely distributed journals rather than to obscure texts, subspecialty publications, or symposia proceedings.

The reader is expected to be conversant with general medical terminology; it is also assumed that the prerequisite of a reasonably sound medical education has been met. All of the figures, to the best of my knowledge, are original in general visual presentation or in specific detail or context, although the reader undoubtedly may find similar representations elsewhere. Their purpose is to convey concisely the complex relationships difficult to describe completely in text. Some artistic license has been exercised to illustrate and integrate widely accepted concepts, although the most idiosyncratic or obscure data are referenced. The various tables summarize and condense the "conventional wisdom" for different topics, but the reader is cautioned that time may prove some of it to be seriously flawed.

In summary, this book is an overview of the essential interrelationships that make anesthesiology comprehensible, predictable, and intellectually satisfying for intelligent and well-trained practitioners. It is a companion to the textbooks of basic and clinical science and of subspecialty medicine needed for comprehensive understanding. *The Anesthetic Plan: From Physiologic Principles to Clinical Strategies* is to a three-volume, multi-authored textbook of anesthesiology what a blueprint is to a completed edifice: a schematic for the essential conceptual relationships as I see them.

Stanley Muravchick, M.D., Ph.D.

ACKNOWLEDGMENTS

The technical and secretarial skills of Joan Aster Walls, Jocelyn Jenik-Black, and Joan Meranze were indispensable. My original editor at Mosby-Year Book, Inc., Nancy Puckett, and my colleagues here in the Department of Anesthesia at the Hospital of the University of Pennsylvania gave me advice, direction, and expertise, all of which were much needed, and sincerely appreciated.

Stanley Muravchick, M.D., Ph.D.

CONTENTS

1

Formulating a Plan

No plan for anesthetic management can guarantee a satisfactory perioperative course, although appropriate selection of anesthetic techniques and agents should, at the very least, minimize patient discomfort and facilitate surgery. Can an appropriate anesthetic plan reduce perioperative morbidity or influence anesthetic-related mortality? To establish this hypothesis definitively would require subjecting a large number of patients, in a randomized fashion, to various anesthetic protocols. Contemporary standards for clinical evaluation, choice of anesthetic agents, and the details of intraoperative management would thus have to be deliberately ignored, and a study of this sort could not be ethically, morally, or legally condoned. It may never be possible to prove conclusively, therefore, that a sound anesthetic plan and an optimal perioperative course are related in cause-and-effect fashion, but two indirect lines of evidence, one epidemiologic and the other empirical, support this hypothesis.

First, there has been a progressive decline in anesthetic-related morbidity and mortality (Chapter 11) coincident with the dramatic growth of the knowledge base for applied physiology and pharmacology that forms the foundation for virtually all modern concepts in anesthesiology. Second, the traditional "contraindications" to general anesthesia such as extremes of age or debilitating disease, once invoked because some patients were believed to be intrinsically unfit to "endure" general anesthesia, have virtually disappeared. This chapter describes a general, fundamental approach to patient assessment and a preliminary approach to general concepts important in the design of an anesthetic plan. Specific considerations and risk factors related to disease of individual organ systems will be discussed in subsequent chapters.

PREANESTHETIC ASSESSMENT

Traditional Approach

The time-honored, traditional medical "workup" requires a detailed medical history followed, in sequence, by a physical examination of the patient and subsequent review of laboratory data.[1] It serves well for purposes of screening and general diagnosis, but it is unwieldy and inefficient as a system for preoperative anesthetic evaluation because it is constructed to consider all possible diagnoses, and, in particular, those with multiple organ system involvement.[2] Diagnosis rests on a stack of informational strata, each of which represents a technique of inquiry applied across all major organ systems (Fig 1–1).

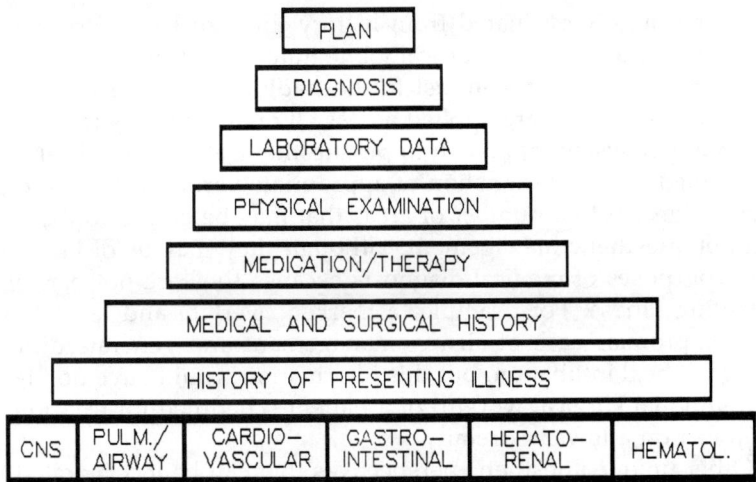

FIG 1–1.
Traditional stratified or "horizontal" medical approach to preoperative evaluation, shown schematically. It is designed to consolidate signs, symptoms, laboratory and physical findings, and other data derived from a variety of organ systems into a unifying diagnostic entity and plan for medical therapy.

This "horizontal" approach initially gives each major organ system equal weight. Excluding no details, it ultimately defines a particular organ system as the locus of one or a number of potential disease processes, which must then be distinguished by a process of differential diagnosis. The chronology and the symptoms and signs of the admitting diagnosis derived from this technique of evaluation may be highly relevant to the formulation of a plan for anesthetic management: fever accompanied by 24 hours of nausea and vomiting may lead not only to a diagnosis of appendicitis but will also significantly alter anesthetic management. On the other hand, the natural history of the discovery of an asymptomatic colonic lesion, in and of itself, rarely influences the anesthetic plan for elective hemicolectomy.

Vertical Integration

An organ system approach to preoperative anesthetic assessment differs from the traditional, horizontally integrated concept by focusing on the current functional level and the degree of functional reserve retained by each major organ system. In this approach, defining the underlying disease process itself is less important than the assessment of the functional level of the major organ systems. Since each organ system is thoroughly evaluated from history through laboratory data, in sequence, the analysis is "vertically integrated" up through techniques of inquiry (Fig 1–2), in contrast to the traditional approach, in which techniques of inquiry are applied across all organ systems in turn.

An organ system approach to preanesthetic assessment is also easily modified by the designation of appropriate vertical columns to give special attention to a number of areas that may be critical to the mechanism of anesthetic management, although they may be of little interest for purposes of medical diagnosis because they are not part of the presenting illness. For example, a marked overbite and large tongue may compromise ease of airway management and generate difficulty during tracheal intubation, but this information would have no place in the traditional surgical workup of a patient scheduled for excision of a melanoma on a lower extremity.

Other unique anesthetic perspectives that can be incorporated into an organ system approach include general body habitus, ease of vascular access, and physical or psychologic factors that influence the relative risk of regurgitation or reflux of gastric contents. A vertical ap-

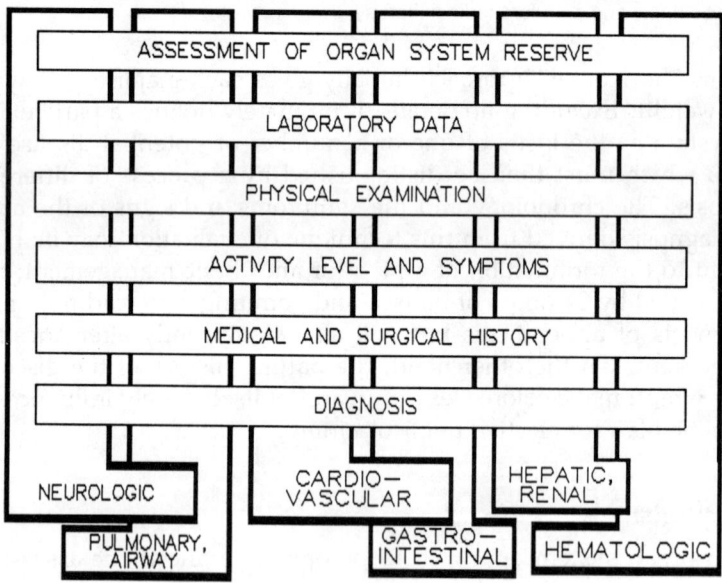

FIG 1–2.
Organ system approach to preanesthetic assessment of physical status, shown schematically. Function and functional reserve of critical organ systems and physical factors that may modify the design of the anesthetic plan are evaluated by a process of vertical integration of all available data for each organ system.

proach also applies the details of a history of specific adverse reactions to prior anesthetics to the appropriate organ system. Rarely do any, and virtually never do all, of these factors become a focal point in the horizontally integrated, traditional approach to medical assessment. They can, however, be given appropriate priority in an organ system approach to preanesthetic assessment.

Application of the organ system approach begins with a general, overall analysis of the patient's activity level and vigor; it then determines, system by system, evidence of dysfunction and the need for current therapy.[3] In this approach, some diagnostic perspective for the possibilities of common etiology may be sacrificed to provide a clear identification of those organ systems that make up the "weak link" in the chain of vital organ system interdependence.

This form of assessment cannot, however, be successfully utilized without the application of clinical judgment: there must be a relative weighting of the available data for each organ system, as well as subjective assessment of the degree to which the dysfunction compromises not just basal levels of function but also functional reserve. Clinical experience is also required to permit a judgment to be made as to whether the dysfunction is *compensated* or *decompensated* (i.e., whether the findings and symptomatology are proportional to the severity of the underlying disease or whether the dysfunction is masked or minimized by compensatory changes in other organ systems). Is the patient as sick, or sicker, than he would appear "on paper?"

Physical Status

Because the "vertical" approach to preanesthetic assessment requires organization of available data and subsequent integration of this information with the anesthesiologist's own estimate of functional level, it leads directly and efficiently to formulation of an American Society of Anesthesiologists (ASA) physical status classification. Formally defined (Table 1–1) and adopted in 1963,[4] assignment of ASA physical status is now a required component of every preanesthetic assessment. It is an act of clinical judgment based exclusively on identification of organ system disease and evaluation of the extent to which that disease impairs normal function or incapacitates the patient.

ASA physical status assignment does not, and should not, consider age per se, the nature of surgery required, or the duration of preexisting disease. It is a clinician's tool for preanesthetic assessment of the presence of pathology that compromises organ system function and functional reserve. Originally conceived by Saklad[5] more than 40

TABLE 1–1.

Original Definition of ASA Physical Status Categories

Class 1	A normally healthy patient
Class 2	A patient with mild systemic disease
Class 3	A patient with moderate to severe disease that is not incapacitating
Class 4	A patient with incapacitating disease that is a constant threat to life
Class 5	A moribund patient who is not expected to survive 24 hours with or without operation

years ago to facilitate statistical evaluation of anesthetic risk, it was subsequently refined and popularized to assist in the determination of the role of anesthesia in perioperative mortality.[6] Although some inconsistency is unavoidable,[7] this system is now universally accepted in anesthesia and widely utilized in other specialties as well because it has fulfilled the original expectation that it would correlate with the perioperative mortality[8, 9] (Fig 1–3).

There is also evidence to support the obvious corollary that preoperative diagnosis and treatment of some forms of organ system dysfunction can improve postoperative outcome.[10] Other attempts at defining more specific multifactorial risk indices[11] have done little more than reconfirm what has long been clinically evident: that the extent of preoperative organ system impairment determines both perioperative mortality[12] and the incidence and severity of postoperative complications.[13] In contemporary anesthetic practice, therefore, regardless of the type of surgery or hospital facility, healthy patients having elective surgery should do well unless they become the victims of human error.[14, 15] Patients with disease severe enough to limit activity, however, are subject to a progressively higher incidence of perioperative complications and death.[6, 13, 16, 17]

Organ System Functional Reserve

The chapters that follow discuss the interactions between individual anesthetic agents and specific organ systems. The general principles of compensation and decompensation, however, are applicable to all organ systems. Virtually without exception, every form of general or regional anesthesia is associated with cardiovascular or respiratory depression, interruption of sympathetic nervous system activity, or a combination of these effects. In the absence of disease, no compensation is needed, and even an organ system depressed by anesthetic agents would have not only adequate basal function but also sufficient

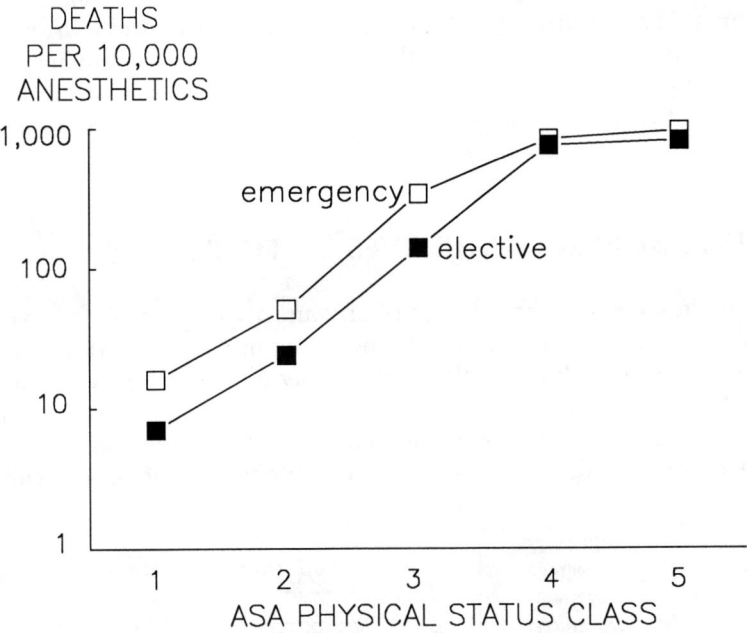

FIG 1–3.
Perioperative mortality (within 48 hours of surgery) is related directly to ASA physical status. These data are circa 1970. (Adapted from Vacanti CF, VanHouten RJ, Hill RC: *Anesth Analg* 1970; 49:564–566.)

additional capacity (functional reserve) to accommodate large fluid and electrolyte loads, increased work of breathing, pain, and other forms of stress.

In the presence of mild to moderate organ system dysfunction, functional reserve is reduced, but increased demand may still be met easily if the function of an organ system can be augmented by supportive mechanisms such as increased sympathetic nervous system activity. These patients have compensated disease: activity and even laboratory studies may be within normal limits if patients are in situations of submaximal stress. As disease becomes more severe, however, function is further impaired and compensatory mechanisms may become inadequate, compromising activity or the adequacy of metabolic function. Under these circumstances, the organ system is decompensated. The additional depressant effect of anesthetics on organ systems and tissues is then profound enough to interrupt compensatory mechanisms, producing the acute decompensation and loss of homeostasis that make anesthetized patients "unstable." With multiple organ system dysfunction, in particular, the fragile equilibrium maintained under conditions of minimal demand may collapse entirely under the weight of the pharmacologic, surgical, and pathophysiologic assault of the perioperative experience.

INITIAL DESIGN OF THE ANESTHETIC PLAN

The initial step in the design of any anesthetic plan is a simple determination of whether an anesthetic is required (Fig 1–4). Some patients on the operating room schedule may need the undivided attention of an anesthesiologist, but they may not necessarily need an anesthetic. Paraplegics with complete spinal cord transection, for example, often require urethral sphincterotomy or debridement of a decubitus

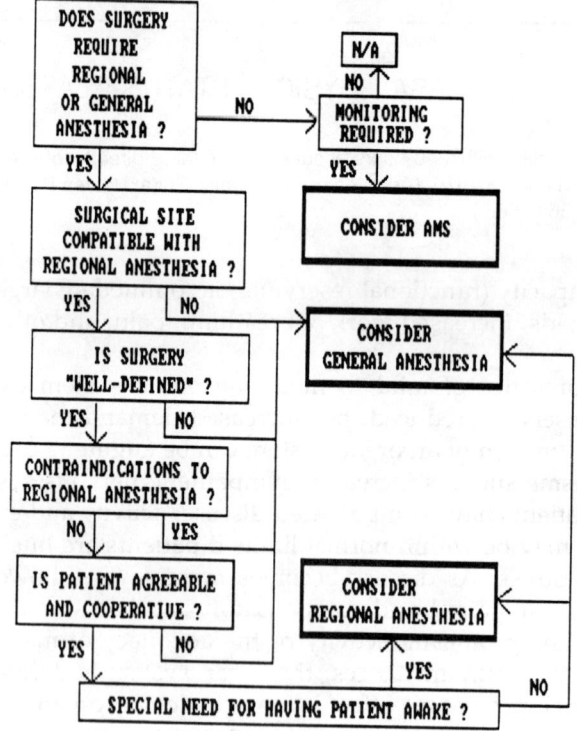

FIG 1–4.

Decision-making schematic for initial design of the plan for anesthetic management. *AMS* = anesthesia monitoring and sedation; *N/A* = no action required.

ulcer, yet they may have complete absence of sensation at the operative site. The goal of intraoperative management for these patients is not anesthesia, but rather the control or elimination of acute hypertension due to autonomic hyperreflexia (Chapter 4). Similarly, many debilitated or extremely high-risk patients may have their need for analgesia met adequately solely by infiltration of local anesthetics or application of topical anesthetics to the operative field.

None of these options should be dismissed out of hand. They require a considered estimate of the intensity and duration of discomfort to be experienced by the patient, a value judgment regarding the relative risk of providing systemic sedation or anxiolysis to minimize psychologic stress, and an assessment of the need for (and exact nature of) continuous monitoring of vital functions. Thus while neither of these situations represents the delivery of a "proper" anesthetic to the patient, neither are these AMS (anesthetic monitoring and sedation) or MAC (monitored anesthesia care) situations trivial.

REGIONAL ANESTHESIA

Regional anesthesia evolved long after general anesthesia had become routine.[18] Alexander Wood did not invent the syringe until 1853, and Halsted's first description of the clinical value of cocaine as a regional anesthetic was not published until 1884. The German surgeon August Bier deserves credit for the first intentional spinal anesthetic,[19] even though his name is more widely associated with the intravenous regional technique ("Bier block") that he described 10 years later, in 1908.[20] There followed, however, a 40-year period of intense and sometimes fruitful interest in regional anesthesia: the description and reports of the use of virtually every variety of intermittent and continuous approach to subarachnoid and epidural anesthesia appeared in specialty journals by 1942, almost always with implicit or explicit assertions of safety superior to that of general anesthetic techniques, but without objective supporting data.[21]

Successful regional anesthesia interrupts afferent (pain) pathways at the spinal root (subarachnoid or epidural analgesia), at the nerve plexus (plexus block anesthesia), or further distal along the course of the peripheral nerve (nerve or field block). However, the anatomy of the spinal cord and the distribution of peripheral nerves do not always provide safe and intimate access to major nerve conduction pathways by direct, percutaneous routes. Thus, from an anatomic perspective, site of surgery is the major determinant of the suitability of an anesthetic plan built around a choice of regional anesthetic techniques. After access to either the subarachnoid or the epidural space has been gained, subsequent distribution of local anesthetic solutions is easily accomplished by adjusting total anesthetic dose and modifying patient position and anesthetic specific gravity,[22, 23] or by adjustments to the volume of the injected anesthetic, respectively.[24, 25]

Respiratory Paralysis

The cephalad spread of the neural blockade produced by major regional techniques has been a matter of concern for more than 50 years because of two practical considerations: the obvious requirement that motor blockade be reliably limited so as not to extend to the innervation of the respiratory diaphragm (fifth through third cervical segments) and the acute cardiovascular effects of sympatholysis (neural blockade of the second lumbar and higher segments). Fortunately, the local anesthetic solutions in widest use interrupt transmission along sensory fibers at concentrations lower than those that cause full motor paralysis, producing a "differential" neural blockade[26] that can also be of diagnostic as well as of purely practical value.[27] Clinically useful dosage guidelines therefore can reliably provide mid- to upper-thoracic levels of sensory blockade while still affording a margin of safety for motor blockade. With the possible exception of patients with severe pulmonary disease who utilize intercostal muscles as accessory mechanisms for adequate ventilation, therefore, the risk of respiratory paralysis in patients having spinal or epidural anesthesia is essentially "all or none."[28, 29]

Sympatholysis

In contrast, sympatholysis of some degree is an inevitable consequence of the injection of local anesthetics into the subarachnoid or epidural space unless extremes of position and low-dose, low-volume anesthetic solutions are employed. A "saddle" pattern of subarachnoid neural blockade or a caudal epidural technique restricts the effects of local anesthetic to the sacral nerve roots. These options are obviously available only if compatible with the site of surgery. The extent of the sympatholysis produced by the subarachnoid or epidural injection of local anesthetics and the dependence of that patient on high levels of continuing sympathetic outflow combine to determine the severity of subsequent organ system compromise. In many cases any degree of sympathetic blockade may produce gross decompensation, while in others even a total "pharmacologic sympathectomy" may be adequately tolerated. Thus, for epidural and subarachnoid block, access to appropriate nerve roots is a purely technical, and usually a trivial, issue; quality and *controllability* of the subsequent polyneural blockade ultimately determine satisfactory outcome.

Access to Peripheral Nerves

When forms of regional anesthesia other than subarachnoid or epidural anesthesia are selected, *access*, not controllability, is usually the limiting factor. With the exception of the intravenous regional technique, which is confined to the extremities by the requirement for a tourniquet, clinical success almost always reflects the ease with which the appropriate plexus or peripheral nerve can be found and local anesthetics injected in their proximity. Control of the spread of the injected local anesthetic solution is a minor factor, addressed simply as part of "good" technique. Therefore, varieties of regional anesthesia that provide unambiguous and consistent anatomic landmarks, yet do not make extreme demands on patient cooperation (e.g., block of the brachial plexus), are the most commonly taught and the most widely utilized forms of regional anesthesia. Local custom and habits acquired during training are additional factors, but the ease with which a peripheral plexus, nerve, or field block can be accomplished remains the major determinant of the frequency of its clinical application.

Other Factors

Considerations other than access and controllability may also influence the selection of regional anesthesia. An appreciation of the time required for completion of the surgical procedure is essential, since duration of surgery may dictate the choice of local anesthetic (Table 1–2)

TABLE 1–2.
Duration of Local Anesthetics When Used
as Equipotent Epidural Solutions

Chloroprocaine	1–1.5 hr
Lidocaine	1–2 hr
Mepivacaine	1–2 hr
Bupivacaine	2–4 hr
Etidocaine	2–4 hr

or the need to utilize a catheter for continuous or repeated injection. In addition, surgery lasting more than 3 hours, especially if it requires that the patient be in other than the supine position, may become physically or psychologically exhausting. The use of large amounts of sedative or anxiolytic drugs would negate one of the major objectives of the regional anesthetic approach: to minimize the amount and the number of pharmacologic agents utilized.

A similar problem may be encountered when the procedure is emotionally traumatic (e.g., orchiectomy or amputation). Thus, when the scope of surgery is appropriate and unambiguous and its duration predictable, a plan for regional anesthesia that will satisfy the patient, the surgeon, and the anesthesiologist requires only the skillful application of standardized techniques to achieve success. No matter how flawlessly executed, a regional technique that subsequently becomes inadequate in duration, intensity, or sensory level because of a change in (or an erroneous evaluation of) surgical strategy not only will result in tangible emotional and physical stress for all concerned but also will require the addition of a second anesthetic technique, with all of its attendant risks, complications, discomfort, and cost.

Contraindications

Despite a brief post–World War II period of eclipse brought about by well-publicized,[30] but unfounded,[31] fears of residual paralysis after spinal anesthesia, regional anesthesia is currently practiced with few absolute contraindications.[19, 32, 33] Nevertheless, every thoughtful practitioner reviews a short list of criteria for exclusion before offering a patient this option (Table 1–3). Conventional wisdom avoids opportunities for planned or accidental lumbar puncture in patients with elevated intracranial pressure, even though this maneuver is frequently part of the patient's diagnostic evaluation; drainage of cerebrospinal fluid may, in fact, be an adjunct to a surgical procedure. Patients with pathologic or iatrogenic bleeding disorders are also frequently considered unsuitable for regional anesthetic techniques, although there persists a controversy regarding the use of regional techniques in patients who will subsequently receive heparin.

Fear of initiating meningitis keeps many from performing subarachnoid or epidural anesthesia in patients with sepsis, a "contraindication" that may, however, exist largely in theory because of the difficulties in distinguishing between febrile illness, bacteremia, and true sepsis, especially at the time of surgery. Infection, inflammation, or neoplasm of the soft tissues through which the probing needles re-

TABLE 1–3.

Why Regional Anesthesia Is Not Routinely Selected for Appropriate Surgical Procedures

Absolute contraindications	
All regionals	Patient refusal, infection at site of injection
Spinal/epidural	Hypovolemic shock, sepsis, increased intracranial pressure, bleeding disorder, progressive central nervous system diseases
Unacceptable side effects	
All regionals	Pain, hematoma, paresthesias from needle placement
Spinal/epidural	Headaches, backache, urinary retention
Major potential complications	
All regionals	Central nervous system and cardiac toxicity from local anesthetics
Spinal/epidural	Hypotension from sympathectomy, need for volume infusion, total spinal with respiratory compromise, meningitis, epidural hematoma
Practical considerations	
All regionals	Inadequate time/equipment/personnel to perform block, fear of failure, fear of lawsuit for residual neuropathy, lack of patient cooperation
Spinal/epidural	Technical difficulty in patients with obesity or prior lumbar surgery, need for early ambulation

quired for regional anesthesia are to be advanced may also convince the anesthesiologist to offer only general anesthesia. A history of chronic backache, headache, or lumbar spinal surgery is sufficient for some to exclude the option of regional anesthesia, but the objective data actually contradict this position.[34]

Also of some concern is the effect of local areas of tissue acidosis, which may impede the spread of the pharmacologically active form of the local anesthetic molecule, impairing the quality of plexus anesthesia. On more solid physiologic ground is avoidance of subarachnoid or epidural block in patients with gross circulating hypovolemia due to dehydration or hemorrhage,[35] or its use in patients with aortic valvular stenosis, functional cardiac outflow tract obstruction, or other syndromes of fixed cardiac output. In these patients a fragile state of compensated disease is maintained only by sustained, high levels of sympathetic tone; acute pharmacologic sympathectomy may have catastrophic hemodynamic consequences (Chapters 4 and 6).

Any plan for regional anesthesia is, of course, conditional on patient acceptance. Efforts to forcibly impose a regional technique would not only be unethical but also would constitute legal trespass. A completely successful regional anesthetic experience, however, requires more than submission to the will of the anesthesiologist and the surgeon. It requires trust and confidence without which even the most technically superb form of neural blockade provides only a tenuously adequate perioperative experience. Patients, of course, need relief of surgical and postoperative pain, but they may also prefer amnesia or anxiolysis to cope with the sense of loss of control.

Regional anesthesia therefore requires not only manual skills but also the ability to quickly gain the trust and respect of the patient. In no other area of anesthetic practice is the difference in the personalities of anesthesiologists so obvious as in their willingness to provide (and their consistency of success in achieving) regional anesthesia for a variety of surgical procedures. Otherwise the choice of a specific form of regional anesthesia is largely a matter of excluding those techniques that are unsuitable because of the site of surgery, or other procedural

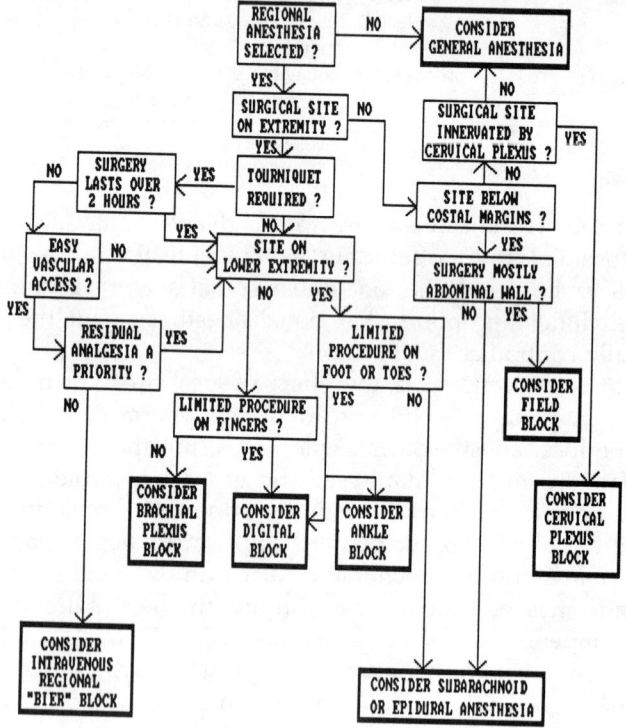

FIG 1–5.

Decision-making schematic for choice of regional anesthetic technique. Options are determined largely by the anatomic site of surgery and the duration of the surgical procedure.

factors, or the desire to incorporate both intraoperative and postoperative analgesia into a single approach (Fig 1–5).

GENERAL ANESTHESIA

Historical Perspective

The terms *general anesthesia* and *inhalational anesthesia* are, to many, virtually synonymous. This association reflects the historical role of inhalational agents as the first surgical anesthetics[36-38] and their continuing usage, which has spanned the entire era of "modern" surgery without interruption (Fig 1–6). The value of this contribution to the development of surgery and its importance as the first major accomplishment of American medicine cannot be overstated. Surgical mortality was more than 20% in preanesthetic 19th century England, and need for operation was considered equivalent to a sentence of purgatory, the operating theater described as a "chamber of horrors."

It was clear almost immediately, however, that widespread use of

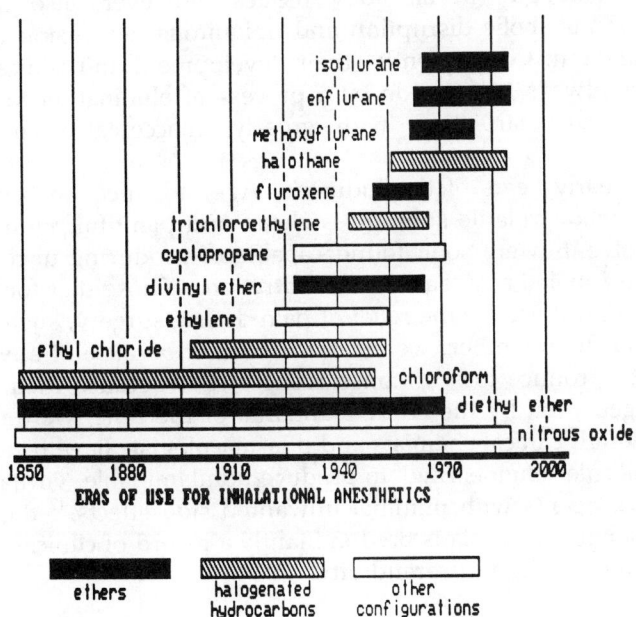

FIG 1–6.
Eras of use for inhalational anesthetics of various chemical configurations. Introduction of the electrocautery largely precluded the use of flammable, nonhalogenated anesthetic agents by 1975. For further discussion, see Fineberg et al.[68]

anesthetics to achieve "blessed oblivion" and more deliberate, precise surgery was to be accomplished at a considerable cost in terms of anesthetic-related mortality. In 1848, one year after its introduction as a general anesthetic in England, chloroform was prophetically and precisely characterized as "subtle poison." Three months later it caused the death of Hannah Greener, a young woman with an ingrown toenail who became the first documented victim of an anesthetic that was selected solely because it was less pungent, and thus more pleasant, than diethyl ether.[36] The first anesthetic-related death from diethyl ether was eventually reported, too, 20 years after the introduction of this drug into practice, as was death from nitrous oxide, an agent once generally regarded as so safe that it was widely and openly used for recreational intoxication.[39] In fact, in the first century of anesthetic administration in the United Kingdom, there were almost 25,000 anesthesia related deaths.[40]

Inhalational agents were, and remain, simple to administer. They provide all needed components of anesthesia, including relaxation of skeletal muscle, thereby facilitating surgical procedures. Their high degree of solubility in all body tissues, however, also produces generalized metabolic disruption and ubiquitous depression of organ system function. Consequently, their development and clinical evaluation have always been made by a process of elimination to exclude those molecular structures with grossly unacceptable characteristics.[41]

In the early years of the Industrial Age, advances in commercial chemistry made volatile substances cheap and plentiful. Hundreds of organic solvents were soon found capable of producing unconsciousness when inhaled at adequate concentrations. Those that found their way into clinical use for the relief of pain during surgery, such as chloroform and diethyl ether, were serviceable not because of any unique capacity to produce loss of consciousness, but because their side effects, judged even by the crude standards of the time, were manageable. Although clinical chemists and pharmacologists have recently utilized "molecular engineering" to produce nonflammable, virtually inert inhalational agents with minimal unwanted side effects,[42] the history of inhalational anesthesia is predominantly a record of clinical observation, trial and error, and serendipity.

Inhalational Anesthesia

Inhalational agents provide an intrinsic safety factor when they are used as part of a plan that includes spontaneous ventilation: with increasing depth of anesthesia, the respiratory depressant properties of these anesthetics make the further uptake of anesthesia a self-limiting phenomenon. This reduces the likelihood of inadvertent overdosage. These anesthetics can also be used safely even when the ability of the patient to detoxify and eliminate metabolic end-products is compromised, since exhalation, not biotransformation, terminates their anesthetic effects.

In exchange for this predictability and the reliable simplicity of the processes of uptake and elimination, inhalational anesthesia is qualitatively rigid: the structural and chemical properties of the anesthetic molecule itself, not the technique of administration, determine the relative proportions of sedation, amnesia, analgesia, muscle relaxation, and reflex depression present when the patient is fully anesthetized. Inhalational anesthesia lacks an intrinsic mechanism for adjusting the relative intensity of any of these effects, although some subtle changes may be produced by varying the depth of anesthesia. In a colloquial sense, inhalational anesthesia is a "one-size-fits-all" approach to the clinical pharmacology of general anesthesia.

Intravenous Anesthesia

Intravenous anesthetic agents, on the other hand, have highly localized effects on nervous system function, usually mediated by stereospecific receptors at the cell surface, or at subcellular sites. The limited nature of the effect of each drug on total nervous system function therefore requires the routine application of anesthetic polypharmacy, a clinical strategy more complex, but more flexible, than that possible with inhalational agents. General anesthesia with intravenous agents encourages a "custom-tailored" approach to general anesthesia: hypnosis may be altered independently of analgesia, or amnesia may be made more profound without influencing the degree of muscle relaxation, if that is desired.

There were only scattered experiments with intravenous anesthesia before the beginning of the 20th century, many with parenteral solutions of ether.[43] Short-acting barbiturates did not become widely available until 1932. General familiarity and availability of drugs and techniques for producing and monitoring intraoperative neuromuscular blockade, an achievement that made intravenous anesthesia compatible with modern surgical techniques, evolved over the subsequent period of 40 years.[18]

Increased inherent risk of overdosage and prolonged duration of anesthetic effect counterbalance the remarkable flexibility and adaptability of the intravenous approach to general anesthesia.[44] It has always been characterized as "fatally easy" to administer; even within the framework of modern anesthetic history it has been called "an ideal method of euthanasia."[45] Comprehensive knowledge of clinical pharmacology is required for its consistently successful application. Pharmacokinetic variability occasionally produces gross prolongation of anesthesia or delayed emergence, and additional monitoring, consistent vascular access, and appropriate facilities and personnel may be needed for recovery.

The advocates of inhalational anesthesia accept stereotyped modes of anesthetic induction, maintenance, and emergence in exchange for simplicity and economy of preparation and a reliable duration of anesthetic effect. Those who practice intravenous anesthesia, on the other hand, forego simplicity and predictability in order to gain the greatest possible flexibility in manipulating the intensity of the components of general anesthesia. These twin principles of *simplicity* and *specificity*, like inhalational and intravenous anesthesia, coexist in modern practice. Each can be used to best, or to least, advantage, but both have a proper place in the contemporary anesthetic armamentarium. The sections that follow provide a brief guide for making these choices when developing an anesthetic plan.

CLINICAL STRATEGIES FOR ANESTHETIC MAINTENANCE

The first step in formulating an anesthetic plan is to select an approach to anesthetic maintenance. Inhalational agents provide the most basic and simple mode of general anesthesia. The preeminent side effect of each of the three potent inhalational anesthetics currently available (halothane, enflurane, and isoflurane) is essentially the same: depression of arterial blood pressure by a multiplicity of mechanisms, in each case combining some degree of myocardial depression with alteration of vascular tone.[46] If a decision has been made to utilize general anesthesia, therefore, the next step in design of an anesthetic plan is to determine whether any of these agents would exacerbate preexisting myocardial failure, hypotension, or circulating hypovolemia. In the absence of these relative contraindications, the diffuse disruption of reflexive and local cardiac, vascular, bronchomotor, and biliary smooth muscle function produced by inhalational agents can be used to unique and special advantage to control arterial hypertension, or to prevent spasm of the biliary tract or the bronchi (Fig 1–7).

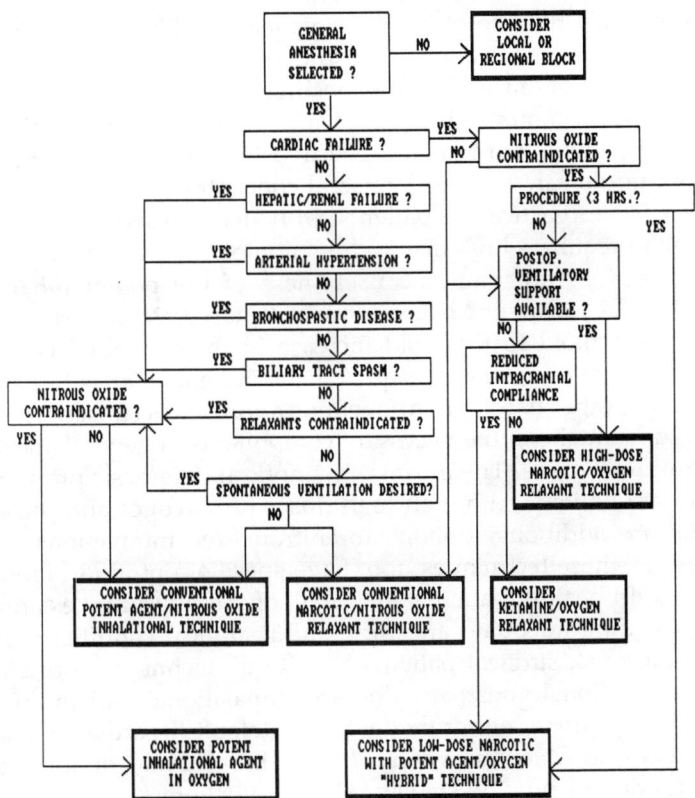

FIG 1–7.

Decision-making schematic for choice of general anesthetic agents. Options are determined largely by specific organ system dysfunction or reduced organ system functional reserve. In some cases, specific contraindications to the use of nitrous oxide determine the choice of anesthetic technique.

Similarly, the ability of inhalational agents to reduce resting skeletal muscle tone, to varying degrees, may have special value in myasthenic patients, in whom neuromuscular blocking drugs are frequently avoided (Chapter 5). Finally, because of their guaranteed route and rate of excretion through exhalation, inhalational anesthetics may be appropriate for patients with hepatic or renal failure, since the metabolic pathways for biotransformation and excretion of injected drugs are often compromised. If consistently short duration of anesthetic effect is essential and the residual effects of the metabolic by-products of sedative or narcotic drugs are to be avoided, as is the case for surgical outpatients, inhalational agents may be the anesthetics of choice.

Occasionally the use of adjunctive agents can be a major factor in choosing an anesthetic regimen. Although nitrous oxide has been a ubiquitous component of routine anesthetic practice with both inhalational and intravenous techniques,[47] it is contraindicated in the management of patients with air trapped in a hollow viscus, in the chest, brain, or middle ear.[48] Clinically useful concentrations of nitrous oxide may also be impractical in patients with decompensated pulmonary disease who require a high inspired fraction of oxygen. Omission of nitrous oxide does not limit the usefulness of the potent inhalational agents, but, by virtue of MAC additivity (Chapter 2), this strategy necessitates a twofold to threefold increase in their inspired concentrations in order to achieve an adequate level of general anesthesia.

If, on the other hand, an intravenous approach is chosen, it may be difficult to maintain all the necessary components of general anesthesia without nitrous oxide. The intrinsic hypnotic and amnesic properties of narcotics are limited. Although high doses of narcotics and the use of ketamine are additional options for nitrous-free intravenous general anesthesia,[49] these techniques, too, have specific contraindications and limitations. In healthy patients, any or all of these techniques are capable of providing adequate anesthesia and surgical conditions. In the very ill, high-risk surgical patient, a "hybrid" technique consisting of combined fractional anesthetic doses of inhalational and intravenous agents is appropriate, either by design or default, in order to maintain stable metabolic functions where "pure" inhalational or intravenous techniques do not provide stability of vital functions.[50]

ANESTHETIC INDUCTION

In the context of the anesthetic plan, the word *induction* is a synonym for "taking in," or "beginning," a subsequent association. Contrary to the implications of common misusage, anesthesia is not "induced," nor do patients have to be coaxed into unconsciousness. Patients undergo an "induction" into the anesthetic state. In the absence of special considerations such as a difficult airway or a high risk of regurgitation, the choice of agents for this aspect of anesthetic management should be a logical continuation of the thinking used to select the maintenance technique.

Although its efficacy and efficiency have made it commonplace in clinical practice, a routine contemporary anesthetic induction sequence (thiopental-succinylcholine-tracheal intubation) may not necessarily represent the most appropriate, nor least stressful, mode of anesthetic induction for patients with ischemic heart disease.[51, 52] The widespread use of topical or intravenous lidocaine, narcotics, or antihypertensive agents as adjuncts to "smooth out" the vital signs during induction is indirect acknowledgment of the inability of thiopental to suppress the sympathoadrenal response to laryngoscopy and intubation (Chapter 4).

Similarly, anesthetic induction with large doses of narcotics or benzodiazepines in patients for whom inhalational anesthesia has been selected in order to minimize the likelihood of delayed emergence after minor surgery clearly makes little sense. If a potent inhalational agent is selected for anesthetic maintenance in order to minimize bronchospasm in an asthmatic patient, a slow inhalation induction with use of progressively higher inspired concentrations of the same agent, with adequate time provided for equilibrium between alveolar and brain anesthetic concentrations before stimulation of the tracheobronchial tree, would be a logical extension of that anesthetic plan.

The timing of agents selected for an intravenous induction sequence is also an important determinant of its smoothness and consistency. When given as a fast intravenous bolus, thiopental and succinylcholine are well matched for the time they require to achieve peak effect. Systemic narcotics, however, even those of very short onset such as fentanyl, must be given before thiopental in a rapid induction sequence if the peak of their narcotic effect is required during a laryngoscopy facilitated by a bolus injection of succinylcholine.

If succinylcholine is replaced by a nondepolarizing neuromuscular blocking drug, however, a more sustained hypnotic effect is needed during induction to ensure that all three of the basic anesthetic requirements for elective intubation (relaxation, oxygenation, and adequate depth of anesthesia) have been met. Similarly, if significant depth of inhalational anesthesia is part of the induction plan, a bolus injection of succinylcholine given at time of loss of consciousness will do little to facilitate tracheal intubation 10 or 15 minutes later, when end-tidal anesthetic concentrations have reached those levels associated with suppression of sympathoadrenal responses to laryngoscopy.[53]

EMERGENCE AND POSTOPERATIVE ANALGESIA

Many an otherwise elegant anesthetic plan has been ruined in the last 10 minutes by unanticipated or undesirable emergence phenomena. The diffuse and complex effects of inhalational anesthetics on all aspects of central nervous system function inevitably produce a postoperative "malaise" that includes the generalized cortical depression characteristic of any drug-induced encephalopathy, as well as various disinhibition phenomena. Neurologic examination of patients during recovery from anesthesia[54] suggests that there is surprisingly little consistency in the timing or form of the inevitable, transient neurologic dysfunctions seen during emergence with the various inhalational agents. In contrast, intravenous agents produce more stereotyped, but equally troublesome, sequelae during recovery from anesthesia: nausea and respiratory depression for narcotics, hallucinations and disorientation from the belladonna alkaloids and ketamine, and prolonged somnolence and loss of muscle tone after the administration of anesthetic doses of barbiturates and benzodiazepines.

Postoperative analgesia may be provided by the residual effects of systemic narcotics given intraoperatively, by agents given during or before emergence from anesthesia, or by peripheral nerve blocks or other forms of regional or infiltration anesthesia. Except for diagnostic procedures without painful sequelae, every anesthetic plan should include some provision for analgesia during anesthetic emergence and recovery.[55] The severity of postoperative pain is usually assessed by the anesthesiologist or by the recovery room nurse. They estimate the apparent level of autonomic stress as evidenced by hypertension, diaphoresis, or tachycardia, although verbal or nonverbal somatic expressions of pain, such as posturing, may be even more specific and therefore more useful.

There are other techniques of postoperative pain control, such as patient-controlled anesthesia (PCA), in which patients themselves may determine both the timing and the dose of their postoperative analgesic therapy.[56, 57] Physicians consistently underestimate the severity of pain experienced by their patients,[58] especially when therapy with parenteral narcotics is the only approach available.[59] PCA adds the psychologic element of control to the direct advantage of metered, continuous analgesia.

Incisional pain is the most obvious and common problem seen during the transition from anesthesia to full recovery of nervous system function. However, there are other considerations that contribute significantly to a smooth, aesthetic, and safe emergence. A good anesthetic plan includes provision for minimizing coughing and straining (responses that raise intra-abdominal, intraocular, intracranial, and venous pressures), disorientation, retching or vomiting, and uncontrolled shivering. Antiemetics can be used preoperatively or intraoperatively; modern, halogenated inhalational agents produce less intrinsic gastric irritation and postoperative vomiting than did diethyl ether, but all retain some general, perhaps nonspecific, emetic properties.[46] For patients viewed at particular risk of regurgitation and aspiration, a histamine-receptor blocking drug, an anticholinergic agent, or liquid antacids can minimize gastric volume or increase the pH of gastric contents.

PREMEDICATION

Historical Perspective

With the possible exception of Clover's preference for a "teaspoon full of brandy, without water, a few minutes beforehand, . . . ," techniques of preoperative medication were not commonly described until sometime after the turn of this century. Certainly they were not widely appreciated until 1920, when the term *premedication* came into general usage.[60] Premedication before general and regional anesthesia, however, has never been consistently practiced. Textbooks of anesthesia commonly present a table of the goals of premedication as if their use is, and always has been, based purely on holistic considerations of the patient's perioperative experience. In fact, premedication evolved as a necessary antidote to the undesirable side effects of the inhalational anesthetics then available for use.[61]

The high incidence of bradyarrhythmias after anesthetic induction with chloroform precipitated the widespread use of atropine premedication in the United Kingdom.[62] Scopolamine, because it afforded both amnesia and relief from intense salivary and bronchial secretions, was recognized to have the ideal adjunctive properties needed to minimize the psychic trauma associated with the slow, stormy induction of anesthesia with open-drop ether. The addition of morphine to anesthetic plans with use of either of these prototype inhalational agents provided sufficient additional analgesia to obviate the need to achieve the very deep, and dangerous, levels of general anesthesia otherwise once required for successful surgery.

Objectives

In contemporary use, premedication is most commonly employed to achieve a desired psychologic and pharmacologic state at the time of anesthetic induction. Therefore, premedication strategies are determined directly by the patient's physical and mental status, as well as by the anesthetist's overall plan for anesthetic management (Fig 1–8). The most obvious function of premedication in current clinical practice is anxiolysis, the alleviation of anxiety and emotional stress. While

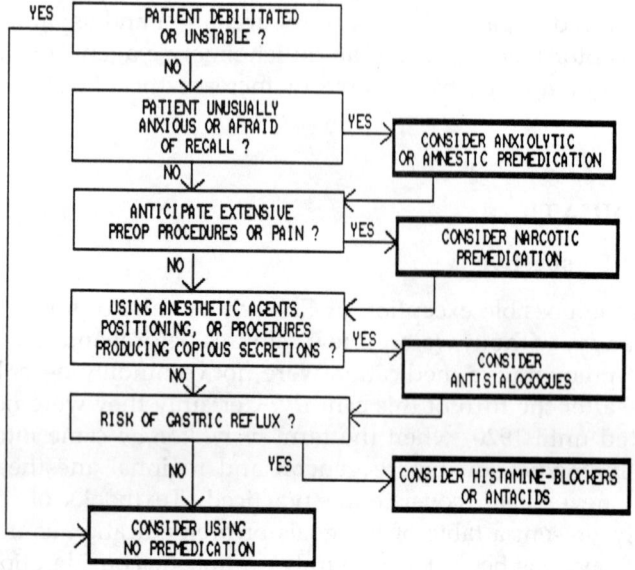

FIG 1—8.
Decision-making schematic for selecting premedication. Options are determined largely by specific objectives in minimizing the neuroendocrine response to stress and the risk of anesthetic side effects.

there is some evidence that an effective preoperative visit by the anesthesiologist may often achieve this goal through psychologic means alone,[63-65] the brevity of a typical preoperative consultation and the personality of either the anesthesiologist or the patient may make its routine achievement difficult. In addition, many of the fears and concerns disturbing patients facing surgery are not anesthesia related.[66]

Analgesia as an objective of premedication is clearly desirable in patients with pain related to their illness. A reasonable case can also be made for its provision if patients require invasive cardiovascular monitoring preoperatively, or if they will undergo multiple injections as part of a regional anesthetic technique. Although historically rooted in the observations of Claude Bernard that morphine reduced the anesthetic requirement, and the mortality, of experimental animals, the practice of routinely providing a preoperative analgesic "foundation" before general anesthesia is now mostly a matter of personal preference and anesthetic "style."

In contrast, preoperative use of an anticholinergic drug such as atropine may be pragmatic if the anesthetic to be used, such as ketamine, has specific sialagogue properties, where prolonged peroral en-

TABLE 1-4.

Commonly Stated Goals of Premedication

Anxiolysis
Amnesia
Vagolysis
Antacid/antihistaminic effects
Antisialagogue effects
Antiemetic effects
Reduced anesthetic requirement
Anticonvulsive effects (regional anesthesia)

doscopy is required, or if the patient will have surgery in the prone position, since the normal route of drainage for oral and tracheal secretions is reversed under these circumstances.

Patient preference appears to be for narcotic or narcotic-based premedication.[67] However, convincing arguments can be made for the need to accomplish any one of a long number of specific effects under certain circumstances (Table 1-4). The characteristics and side effects of the inhalational and intravenous agents currently used for general anesthesia are now sufficiently benign and controlled, however, to make premedication no longer mandatory. This approach is also realistic, since premedication is often impractical or limited to some form of intravenous supplementation immediately before anesthetic induction in the increasing fraction of patients having outpatient surgery.

SUMMARY

The patient's general state of health is directly related to perioperative morbidity and mortality and is a major determinant of the anesthetic plan. The preoperative assessment of organ system function and functional reserve required for assignment of an ASA physical status classification also permits rational selection of an anesthetic approach from among the various major categories of anesthetic drugs and techniques. Specific operative details, such as the site and duration of surgery, usually dictate the subsequent choices that must be made from within these categories for specific drugs or routes of administration.

Inhalational agents provide comprehensive but stereotyped anesthetic effects of predictable duration, even in patients with multiple organ system disease. Anesthetic techniques that require the use of multiple intravenous drugs offer individual control of the major components of the anesthetic state, but the resulting polypharmacy can be more difficult to manage intraoperatively. Because of their pharmacokinetic variability, the duration of the effects of intravenous anesthetic drugs may also be less consistent than that of the effects of inhalational agents. Regional anesthesia is a valuable option if not excluded by difficulties of access, controllability, or patient acceptance. Details of anesthetic premedication, induction, emergence, and postoperative analgesia should reflect the same priorities already established for the plan for anesthetic maintenance.

REFERENCES

1. Roizen MF: Routine preoperative evaluation, in Miller RD (ed): *Anesthesia,* ed 2. New York, Churchill-Livingstone, 1986, pp 225–253.
2. Carson JL, Eisenberg JM: The preoperative screening examination, in Goldmann DR, et al (eds): *Medical Care of the Surgical Patient.* Philadelphia, JB Lippincott, 1982, pp 16–30.
3. Hirsh RA: An approach to assessing perioperative risk, in Goldmann DR, et al (eds): *Medical Care of the Surgical Patient.* Philadelphia, JB Lippincott, 1982, pp 31–39.
4. American Society of Anesthesiologists, Inc.: New classification of physical status. *Anesthesiology* 1963; 24:111.
5. Saklad M: Grading of patients for surgical procedures. *Anesthesiology* 1941; 2:281–284.
6. Dripps RD, Lamont A, Eckenhoff JE: The role of anesthesia in surgical mortality. *JAMA* 1961; 178:261–266.
7. Owens WD, Felts JA, Spitznagel EL Jr: ASA physical status classifications: A study of consistency of ratings. *Anesthesiology* 1978; 49:239–243.
8. Keats AS: The ASA classification of physical status—a recapitulation. *Anesthesiology* 1978; 49:233–236.
9. Keats AS: What do we know about anesthetic mortality? *Anesthesiology* 1979; 50:387–392.
10. Del Guercio LR, Cohn JD: Monitoring operative risk in the elderly. *JAMA* 1980; 243:1350–1355.
11. Goldman L, Caldera DL, Nussbaum SR, et al: Multifactorial index of cardiac risk in noncardiac surgical procedures. *N Engl J Med* 1977; 297:845–850.
12. Marx GF, Mateo CV, Orkin LR: Computer analysis of postanesthesia deaths. *Anesthesiology* 1973; 39:54–58.
13. Lewin I, Lerner AG, Green SH, DelGuercio LRM, Siegel JH: Physical class and physiologic status in the prediction of operative mortality in the aged sick. *Ann Surg* 1972; 174:217–231.
14. Cooper JB, Newbower RS, Long CD, McPeek B: Preventable anesthesia mishaps: A study of human factors. *Anesthesiology* 1978; 49:399–406.
15. Lunn JN, Mushin WW: *Mortality Associated With Anaesthesia.* London, Nuffield Provincial Hospitals Trust, 1982.

16. Vacanti CF, VanHouten RJ, Hill RC: A statistical analysis of the relationship of physical status to postoperative mortality in 68,388 cases. *Anesth Analg* 1970; 49:564–566.
17. Hatton F, Tiret L, Vourch G, Desmonts JM, Otteni JC, Scherpereel P: Morbidity and mortality associated with anesthesia—French survey: Preliminary results, in Vickers MD, Lunn JN (eds): *Mortality in Anaesthesia.* Berlin, Springer-Verlag, 1983, pp 23–38.
18. Keys TE: *History of Surgical Anesthesia.* Mineola, N.Y., Dover, 1963, pp 1–193.
19. Wildsmith JAW, Scott DB: Local anesthetics: Actions and applications, in Stevens JA (ed): *Preparation for Anaesthesia.* Baltimore, University Park Press, 1980, pp 263–285.
20. Katz J: Intravenous regional anesthesia. *Semin Anesth* 1983; 2:50–57.
21. Holmdahl MH: A hundred years of local anesthesia. *Semin Anesth* 1986; 5:13–134.
22. Sise LF: Pontocain-glucose solution for spinal anesthesia. *Surg Clin North Am* 1935; 15:1501–1511.
23. Sheskey MC, Rocco AG, Bizzarri-Schmid M, Francis DM, Edstrom H, Covino BG: A dose-response study of bupivacaine for spinal anesthesia. *Anesth Analg* 1983; 62:931–935.
24. Bromage PR: Spread of analgesia solutions in the epidural space and their site of action: A statistical study. *Br J Anaesth* 1962; 34:161–178.
25. Erdemir HA, Soper LE, Sweet RB: Studies of factors affecting peridural anesthesia. *Anesth Analg* 1965; 44:400–405.
26. Greene N: Area of differential block in spinal anesthesia with hyperbaric tetracaine. *Anesthesiology* 1958; 19:45–50.
27. McCollum DE, Stephen CR: The use of graduated spinal anesthesia in the differential diagnosis of pain of the back and lower extremities. *South Med J* 1964; 57:410–416.
28. Ward RJ, Bonica JJ, Freund FG, Akamatsu T, Danziger F, Englesson S: Epidural and subarachnoid anesthesia. *JAMA* 1965; 191:275–278.
29. DeJong RH: Arterial carbon dioxide and oxygen tensions during spinal block. *JAMA* 1965; 191:698–702.
30. Kennedy F, Effron AS, Perry G: The grave spinal cord paralyses caused by spinal anesthesia. *Surg Gynecol Obstet* 1950; 91:385–398.
31. Dripps RD, Vandam LD: Long-term follow-up of patients who received 10,098 spinal anesthetics. *JAMA* 1954; 156:1486–1491.
32. Rubin AP: Spinal and epidural anesthesia, in Stevens AJ (ed): *Preparation for Anesthesia.* Baltimore, University Park Press, 1980, pp 286–308.
33. Thompson GE: Pharmacology, physiology, and use of spinal and epidural anesthesia. *Semin Anesth* 1983; 2:24–29.
34. Gold MI, Berkowitz S: Spinal anesthesia for surgery in patients with previous lumbar laminectomy. *Anesth Analg* 1980; 59:881–882.
35. Kane RE: Neurologic deficits following epidural or spinal anesthesia. *Anesth Analg* 1981; 60:150–161.
36. Armstrong-Davison MH: *Evolution of Anaesthesia.* Altrincham, England, John Sheratt, 1963, pp 1–236.

37. MacQuitty B: *The Battle for Oblivion: The Discovery of Anesthesia.* London, Harrap, 1969.
38. Rupreht J, van Lieburg MJ, Lee JA, Erdmann W (eds): *Anaesthesia: Essays on Its History.* Berlin, Springer-Verlag, 1985.
39. Hatton F, Tiret L, Maujol L: Study of the overall risk in anaesthesia: Methodology used, in Conseiller C, et al (eds): *Complications of Anaesthesia: Operative Risk.* New York, Elsevier, 1982, pp 199–209.
40. Sykes WS: *Essays on the First Hundred Years of Anesthesia,* vol 1. Huntington, N.Y., Krieger, 1972.
41. Attia RR, Grogono AW, Domer FR: Inhalation agents, in Attia RR, Grogono AW (eds): *Practical Anesthetic Pharmacology,* ed 2. East Norwalk, Conn., Appleton & Lange, 1978, pp 11–37.
42. Suckling CS: Halothane (fluothane)—the chemical approach to nonexplosive volatile anesthetic agents. *Anaesthesia* 1958; 13:194.
43. Sykes WS: *Essays on the First Hundred Years of Anesthesia,* vol 2. Huntington, N.Y., Krieger, 1972.
44. Dundee JW, Wyant GM: *Intravenous Anaesthesia.* Edinburgh, Churchill-Livingstone, 1974, p 341.
45. Dundee JW: Early problems in establishing intravenous anaesthesia, in Rupreht J, et al (eds): *Anaesthesia: Essays on Its History.* Berlin, Springer-Verlag, 1985, pp 88–91.
46. Eger EI II: *Isoflurane: A Compendium and Reference,* ed 2. Madison, Wis., Anaquest, 1985.
47. Smith WDA: *Under the Influence: A History of Nitrous Oxide and Oxygen Anesthesia.* London, Macmillan, 1982.
48. Eger EI II, Saidman LJ: Hazards of nitrous oxide anesthesia in bowel obstruction and pneumothorax. *Anesthesiology* 1965; 26:61–66.
49. Miller JD, Katz RL: General anesthetic agents, in Bevan JA, Thompson JH (eds): *Essentials of Pharmacology,* ed 3. Philadelphia, Harper & Row, 1983, pp 272–283.
50. Little DM Jr, Stephen CR: Modern balanced anesthesia: A concept. *Anesthesiology* 1954; 15:246–261.
51. Takeshima K, Noda K, Higaki M: Cardiovascular response to rapid anesthesia induction and endotracheal intubation. *Anesth Analg* 1964; 43:201–208.
52. Fusciardi J, Godet G, Bernard JM, Bertrand M, Kieffer E, Viars P: Roles of fentanyl and nitroglycerin in prevention of myocardial ischemia. *Anesth Analg* 1986; 65:617–624.
53. Yakaitis RW, Blitt CD, Anguilo JP: End-tidal halothane concentration for endotracheal intubation. *Anesthesiology* 1977; 47:386–388.
54. Rosenberg H, Clofine R, Bialik O: Neurologic changes during awakening from anesthesia. *Anesthesiology* 1981; 54:125–130.
55. Dodson ME: *The Management of Postoperative Pain.* London, Edward Arnold, 1985.
56. Church JJ: Continuous narcotic infusion for relief of postoperative pain. *Br Med J* 1979; 1:977–979.

57. White PF: Postoperative pain management with patient controlled analgesia. *Semin Anesth* 1986; 2:116–122.
58. Marks RM, Sachar EJ: Undertreatment of medical inpatients with narcotic analgesic. *Ann Intern Med* 1973; 78:173–181.
59. Donovan M, Dillon P, McGuire L: Incidence and characteristics of pain in a sample of medical-surgical inpatients. *Pain* 1987; 30:69–78.
60. Shearer WM: The evolution of premedication. *Br J Anaesth* 1960; 32:554–562; 1961; 33:219–225.
61. Baker AB: Preoperative medication, in Stevens AJ (ed): *Preparation for Anaesthesia*. Baltimore, University Park Press, 1980, pp 83–100.
62. Mirakhur RK, Clarke RSJ, Dundee JW, McDonald JR: Anticholinergic drugs in anaesthesia. *Anaesthesia* 1978; 33:133–138.
63. Egbert LD, Battit GE, Turndorf H, Beecher HK: The value of the preoperative visit by an anesthetist. *JAMA* 1963; 185:553–555.
64. Leigh JM, Walker J, Janaganathan P: Effect of preoperative anaesthetic visit on anxiety. *Br Med J* 1977; 2:987–989.
65. Schlesinger HJ, Mumford E, Glass GV: Effects of psychological intervention on recovery from surgery, in Guerra F, Aldrete JA (eds): *Emotional and Psychological Responses to Surgery*. Orlando, Fla., Grune & Stratton, 1980, pp 9–18.
66. Norris W, Baird WLM: Preoperative anxiety: A study of the incidence and aetiology. *Br J Anaesth* 1967; 39:503–509.
67. Wilson SL, Vaughan RW, Stephen CR: Subjective patient evaluations of commonly used preanesthetic medications. *Anesthesiology Rev* 1979; 6:35–41.
68. Fineberg HV, Pearlman LA, Gabel RA: The case for abandonment of explosive anesthetic agents. *N Engl J Med* 1980; 303:613–617.

2

Defining and Measuring the Anesthetic State

Despite the universal euphemism for anesthesia suggesting that patients are "put to sleep" for surgery, very little is known about the anesthetic state *except* that it has virtually nothing in common with physiologic sleep. Nor is anesthesia, as the term implies, a state of absent perception. General anesthesia, classically called "narcosis," encompasses a variety of reversible, drug-induced coma states characterized by three clinically evident phenomena: loss of consciousness ("hypnosis"), which is usually assumed to provide, but does not guarantee, absence of recall (amnesia) and loss of perception of painful stimulation (analgesia); the elimination or blunting of somatomotor, cardiovascular, respiratory, and neuroendocrine reflexes; and, to varying degrees, loss of spontaneous movement and reduction of resting skeletal muscle tone.

Elimination of apprehension (anxiolysis) may be produced in the conscious, sedated patient with use of drugs having tranquilizing or analgesic properties, but, like analgesia, it is also assumed to accompany hypnosis. Both regional and local anesthesia provide analgesia in a less ambiguous form: they eliminate perception of pain without alteration or loss of consciousness and without modifying affect or memory (Fig 2–1).

General anesthesia and hypnosis, in particular, are terms that are difficult to define and to measure for fundamental reasons: "the prob-

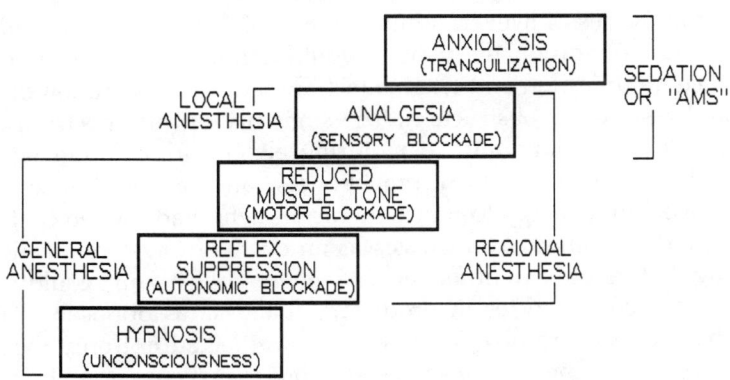

FIG 2–1.
Fundamental characteristics of various forms of anesthesia. *Analgesia, amnesia,* and *anxiolysis* are implied components of the depressed consciousness, or hypnosis, which characterizes general anesthesia. *Regional anesthesia* is major neural blockade produced at or around the segmental spinal cord level, or at large peripheral nerves proximal to the site of surgery, and includes "field block" techniques. *Local anesthesia* refers to nonspecific neural blockade produced by direct infiltration of skin and subcutaneous tissues at the surgical site. "*AMS*" signifies monitoring and sedation by anesthesia personnel, and is sometimes indicated as "MAC" (monitored anesthesia care).

lem of narcosis is intimately connected with the question of what the physiological correlate of consciousness will be."[1] Nevertheless, detailed clinical observations of induction into and emergence from general anesthesia have been made for more than a century, and they provide considerable empirical data regarding the sequence and the characteristics of these processes. That information and pertinent observations from experimental studies will be summarized in this chapter.

THEORIES OF NARCOSIS AND "ANESTHESIA"

The goal of surgical analgesia seems simple enough: the elimination of conscious perception of acute pain. From the first days of surgical anesthesia, however, it was clear that analgesia is at once both distinct from, and inextricably linked to, the far more complex drug-induced state we now call anesthesia. The practical use of nitrous oxide for relief of surgical pain arose directly from the chance observation of Horace Wells that this substance provided sufficient analgesia that a mobile, communicative young man was nevertheless oblivious to what would otherwise have been a painful abrasion. The same agent was also known to be capable of producing bizarre, uninhibited voluntary and reflex motor activity, events that amused audiences during demonstrations yet for which the subject himself appeared amnesic.

In most cases, however, administration of nitrous oxide would produce a state of stupor: the patient would demonstrate no response to verbal communication and was, in fact, in danger of aspiration of vomitus and respiratory obstruction. The similarity of this spectrum of responses to that commonly seen during alcohol intoxication was not overlooked by contemporary practitioners, and James Simpson used this convenient analogy to refute detractors who had argued that chloroform-induced unconsciousness was an event so mysterious and forbidding that its utilization for relief of "mere bodily pain" could not be justified.[2] Inconsistencies in producing analgesia as opposed to other anesthetic effects are now known to have reflected not only the complex neurophysiology of consciousness, but also the nonspecific nature of the physical chemistry of traditional anesthetic agents.

Lipid Solubility

The nervous system is composed predominantly of lipid. Anesthetic agents, despite the fact that their molecular structures are heterogeneous in almost every other respect, are found in high concentrations in virtually every part of this complex organ system specifically because of their lipid solubility. In 1901 both Meyer and Overton suggested (simultaneously but independently) that there was a fundamental correlation between anesthetic potency and lipid solubility.[3] This relationship was subsequently invoked repeatedly by proponents of various "theories of narcosis" seeking to describe a unitary mechanism, although anesthesia is now thought more likely to be an assortment of similar but complex clinical phenomena than to reflect a single, discrete neuropharmacologic event.

Contemporary data do, however, provide some support for the classic "lipid theories." Lipid bilayers can be configured in vitro in a manner roughly analogous to simple cell membranes, and they have been found to be reversibly disrupted or "disordered" by volatile anesthetic agents, steroids, amines, and barbiturates, all of which also possess anesthetic properties.[4] Observations of "pressure reversal" or antagonism of general anesthesia by high ambient atmospheric pressures (50 to 100 atm)[5] suggest that disruption of normal neuronal membrane structures or increases in lipid membrane volumes (by interposition of small molecules highly soluble in lipid) are mechanisms capable of producing anesthetic effects. However, neither hyperthermia nor several other means of membrane "disordering" produce narcosis, and serious discrepancies have been demonstrated between the membrane volume effects and the potency of intravenous anesthetics.[6]

Anesthetic-induced changes at the level of the neuronal membrane, therefore, may not be a unique and unitary mechanism by which these molecules produce loss of consciousness. In fact, cell membranes are not the only hydrophobic areas containing anesthetic molecules in high concentration. One recent hypothesis suggests that anesthetics may inhibit the electron mobility essential for the normal changes in protein conformation that occur in excitable membranes.[7] Thus while lipid solubility is a consistent characteristic of molecules with anesthetic effects, there still is considerable doubt that lipid solubility per se is the essential quality that confers to these substances their ability to produce anesthesia.[8]

Other Physicochemical Theories

Other physicochemical theories of narcosis and anesthesia suggest that anesthetics produce a gross disruption of cellular function by impairing oxidative metabolism, and in this way produce drug-induced unconsciousness.[4, 8] A few investigators have speculated that anesthetics produce an increase, rather than a decrease, in the ordering of water and other intracellular constituents, or that they reversibly alter the structure of intracellular components. Most recent studies, however, have concentrated their attention on neuronal electrophysiology (Table 2–1).

Altered Electrophysiology

The essential macromolecular functional unit of the nervous system is the synapse, an electrically excitable system of membranes that exhibit cycled, phasic increases in ionic conduction in response to chemical transmitter molecules. Some recently proposed mechanisms for general anesthesia suggest that anesthetic molecules change end-plate depolarization thresholds,[9] produce selective occlusion of membrane ion channels or "pores,"[4] or change the protein conformation of the "gatekeeper" molecules that modulate synaptic function.[10]

A prototype for ion channel mechanisms does, in fact, exist: local anesthetics produce their characteristic neural blockade in this manner, interfering with the influx of sodium required for dendritic depolarization and subsequent propagation of nerve action potentials. All local anesthetic molecules are closely related in configuration by a common terminal tertiary amine, however. In contrast, there is a much more diverse spectrum of structural variety for substances with general anesthetic effects.

If general anesthesia were an agent-specific phenomenon without a unitary mechanism, one would expect to find multiple sites of anes-

TABLE 2–1.
Major Proposed Theories and Mechanisms of General Anesthetic Action

Physicochemical
  Semicoagulation of intracellular proteins
  Disordering of membrane lipid fine structure
  Physical obstruction of membrane ion channels
  Formation of intracellular microcrystalline hydrates
  Depressed neuronal oxidative metabolism
  Inhibited protein conformability
Neurophysiologic
  Decreased influx of metabolic substrate
  Generalized depression of neuronal oxidation
  Impaired neuronal electrical conduction
  Presynaptic inhibition of neurotransmitter release
  Depressed postsynaptic excitatory transmission
  Enhanced postsynaptic inhibitory transmission
  Hyperpolarization due to altered ion conductance

thetic action on the cell membrane.[11] Alternatively, one ubiquitous, nonspecific receptor that controlled transmembrane ionic conduction might be activated by any of the molecular variations represented in the anesthetic armamentarium.[12] The anesthetic state produced by a nonspecific receptor should be qualitatively the same, regardless of the agent used. The vast numbers of neuronal pathways involved in wakefulness and pain perception might make unconsciousness a "statistical phenomenon" that occurs when some critical fraction of electrically conducting pathways, rather than a specific site, is blocked sufficiently to depress nervous system function on a clinical level.[13] Specific receptors at multiple sites would, however, more easily explain the somewhat different characteristics of anesthesia produced by different anesthetic agents.

Neuronal Effects

Most recent investigations have concluded that the neurophysiologic actions of various anesthetics are selective, highly specific, and not necessarily depressant. Isolated neurons exposed to typical clinical concentrations of halothane, diethyl ether, enflurane, and isoflurane exhibit a distinct and unique pattern of electrical activity in response to each agent.[14] These discharge patterns include both suppression of electrical discharge and bursts of electrical excitation.

In fact, global hyperexcitation and electroencephalographic (EEG) activation are characteristic of anesthesia induced with diethyl ether, enflurane, and ketamine; gross electrical evidence of convulsive activity can be seen with an overdosage of any of these agents. In contrast, halothane and the barbiturates produce progressive, dose-related depression of electrical discharge, findings suggesting that the clinical state of anesthesia can be produced by either depression or stimulation of various determinants of nervous system electrical activity.[15]

It has become increasingly difficult, therefore, to reconcile these findings with any unitary cellular mechanism of general anesthesia. There appears to be growing consensus that the fundamental mechanism by which general anesthetics produce unconsciousness is not their effect on electrical activity at the subcellular level, but rather their ability to disrupt, by diverse mechanisms, communication between neurons. As predicted almost 40 years ago,[16] all anesthetic agents are now known to be selectively disruptive of the normal patterns of chemically mediated synaptic transmission.[17] Halothane and thiopental appear to potentiate inhibitory neurotransmission mediated by synapses secreting γ-aminobutyric acid (GABA)[18]; depression of excitatory synaptic transmission in most areas of the nervous system is also well documented.[13, 19] Various combinations of reduced excitatory activity coincident with increases in transmission along inhibitory pathways could easily produce the global state of "depressed" overall neuronal excitability that is characteristic of general anesthesia.[20]

Theories of anesthesia invoking multiple sites of action are also far easier to accommodate on a polycellular, neuronal level than on a molecular basis. From this perspective, "hypnosis" or anesthesia is the result of either coincident, multiple mechanisms or is produced by agents having similar actions at diverse sites within the nervous system. Because of the richness of its synaptic network, the reticular formation would be particularly vulnerable to disruption; in fact, generalized depression of consciousness is the sine qua non of agents that produce general anesthesia. With either multiple sites or unique mechanisms of action, however, the precise pattern and quality of anesthesia would, as is observed, vary somewhat with the agent employed.

HYPNOSIS AND ANESTHESIA

The sequence of transient confusion, excitement, and obtundation produced by general anesthetics during the complex process of loss of consciousness was first described by Plomley in 1847, only 6 months after the introduction of chloroform into general use in England. His initial description of the anesthetic action of chloroform underwent additional elaboration by John Snow in 1858. Based on observations of the administration of diethyl ether, which had a more prolonged period of induction (and therefore provided greater opportunity for observation), virtually the same sequence of events was formally itemized by Guedel in 1920.[21] During slow induction of general anesthesia, there was progressive loss of orientation, then diffuse motor and reflex excitement, and, subsequently, loss of consciousness with decreased muscle tone and absence of spontaneous movement. Increasing the time of exposure to the agent or using greater inhaled concentrations of either of these agents progressively reduced movement in response to surgical stimulation of increasing intensity.

In modern practice, this sequence of overt neurologic dysfunction can still be easily observed during slow inhalational induction of anesthesia with any of the contemporary potent agents. The consistency with which this chemically diverse group of vapors produces the same sequence and pattern of neurologic dysfunction suggests that the process reflects the organization of the nervous system itself, rather than the specific chemical characteristics of the anesthetic molecules employed.[22] At any given concentration, each of these agents appears to exert effects on some areas of the nervous system but not on others; the substructures of the brain therefore exhibit a "differential sensitivity" to general anesthetics.

Stages of Anesthesia

During slow induction of general anesthesia and the production of "hypnosis" by anesthetics with depressant properties, the functions provided by the hierarchical layers of neurologic development disappear in reverse order of their ontogenic appearance. First, subtle and diffuse depression of cortical areas produces loss of social awareness, self-control, and orientation. Dysfunction then progresses rapidly to a grossly evident state of unconsciousness characterized by loss of response to verbal command and loss of reflexive eye blinking in response to the stroking of the eyelash ("stage I," "intoxication," or, unique to diethyl ether, "stage of anesthesia").

With continuing anesthetic uptake, transient release of the tonic inhibition of cortical and subcortical areas then produces hyperreflexia, diffuse, random motor activity, and an irregular respiratory pattern ("stage II," "excitement," or "unconsciousness with exaggerated reflex activity"). Unmodulated, exaggerated orotracheal reflex activity appears and then disappears rapidly (Fig 2–2).

Finally, more profound depth of anesthesia results in neurologic dysfunction sufficiently complete that the patient is motionless except for rhythmic, shallow respiration. Surgical stimuli fail to produce reflex motor withdrawal and they generate progressively smaller cardiovascular, respiratory, and neuroendocrine responses ("stage III," "surgical anesthesia," or "unconsciousness with reflex depression").

These phases or "stages" describe comprehensively the general transition from the awake to the fully anesthetized state.[23–25] At the most profound levels of anesthesia produced by high concentrations of potent inhalational anesthetics, the patient may exhibit apnea (even in the absence of neuromuscular blockade) and, subsequently, cardiovascular collapse ("stage IV," "respiratory paralysis," or "stage of anesthetic overdosage"). These last signs of nervous system depression, however, reflect more the toxic side effects of high concentrations of anesthetic agents than a natural progression of the neurologic manifestations of "hypnosis."

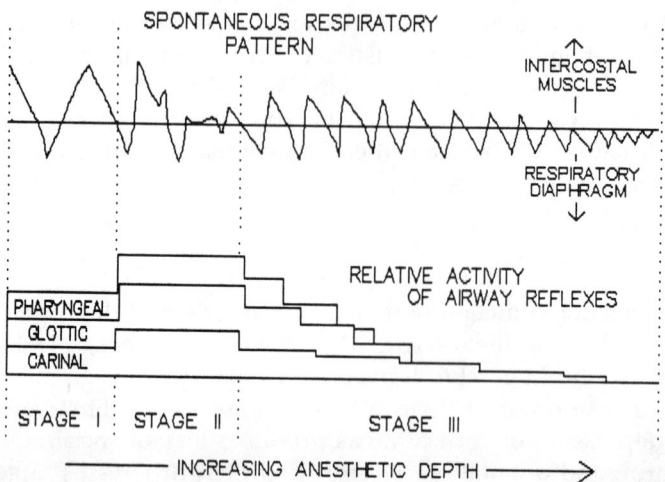

FIG 2-2.
Changes in spontaneous respiratory pattern and the sensitivity of airway reflexes at various levels of inhalational anesthesia. *Stage II* (excitement) has an irregular respiratory pattern with transient apnea ("breath holding") and disinhibited tracheobronchial reflex activity that may trigger laryngospasm. Deeper levels of *stage III* anesthesia produce progressive depression of the intercostal muscle contribution to spontaneous ventilation and imply a greater dependence on diaphragmatic movement alone. (Adapted from Gillespie NA: *Anesth Analg* 1943; 27:275–281.)

Awareness During Surgery

Given the complexity of this sequence and our inability to identify either the site or the mechanism of anesthetic action, hypnosis is used simply as a synonym for unconsciousness, or the antithesis of awareness. Where in the continuum of transitory events that constitute an anesthetic induction awareness is lost, or amnesia or analgesia begins, is extraordinarily difficult to establish. The absence of recall is generally assumed to accompany hypnosis at a "surgical" level of anesthesia, but the use of neuromuscular blockade and tracheal intubation in contemporary anesthetic practice makes even the determination of level of anesthesia problematic, since inadequate anesthesia may be masked because the patient is unable to speak or to move in response to surgical stimulation.[26] Nor may changes in vital signs be helpful, since autonomic responses are also frequently blunted or abolished by the widespread use of cardiovascular and antihypertensive medication.

"Awareness" refers to the capacity to integrate sensory input into an emotional context and to store it as memory.[27] By definition, then, intraoperative awareness and the perception of surgically induced pain constitute inadequate depth of anesthesia. In the absence of purposeful responses to pain, awareness can be verified only by the demonstration of postoperative recall for intraoperative events. Definitive evidence of inadequate anesthesia is available only retrospectively, when it is too late to remedy. Awareness can be present either at a conscious level, determined by conversation with the patient, or by means of hypnotic interview of suggestible patients. Postoperative reports of perceptions and emotional responses that do not appear to correlate with known intraoperative events are usually relegated to the category of hallucinations or dreams.

Data regarding the incidence of recall during general anesthesia administered according to modern standards are limited. Many anesthesiologists are reluctant to disclose the existence of episodes that they, patients, and surgeons will consider evidence of their failure to provide an expected and essential service. Extensive postoperative interviews are required, and there is always some lack of certainty in distinguishing between true recall as opposed to dreamlike, delusional, and hallucinatory phenomena.[28] Subconscious recall may, in addition, be evident only in the form of subtle behavioral patterns not apparent even to the patient himself: more than 20% of patients who undergo surgery and general anesthesia have persistent disturbance of sleep patterns or undergo changes in mood postoperatively.[29-31]

Fortunately, few anesthetized patients have a true "traumatic neurosis," a syndrome producing anxiety, phobias, and a general feeling of loss of control and mistrust.[32] Even 1 month after a deep ether anesthetic, however, 40% of a small series of hypnotically suggestible patients were found to have had subconscious recall of specific audible intraoperative events.[33] After minimal anesthesia for severe trauma, the incidence of conscious and specific recall may be as high as 43%.[34]

Nevertheless, although some investigators insist that recall is effectively nonexistent during well-conducted, elective general anesthesia,[35-37] true awareness of intraoperative events may occur in about 2% of elective anesthetics.[38, 39] Neither the type of anesthetic selected nor the patient's prior anesthetic experiences appear to influence the incidence. Nor does the addition of low inspired concentrations of potent inhalational anesthetic agents to narcotic-based anesthetics guarantee absence of recall.[40] Therefore, in the absence of the clear demonstration of a relationship between the anesthetic technique selected and the incidence of awareness, it has been suggested that "sacrificing the advantages of light surgical anesthesia merely to obviate awareness, hallucinations, or dreaming would be a retrogressive step in anesthetic care."[28] However, many anesthesiologists incorporate scopolamine, benzodiazepines, or other anesthetic drugs into their anesthetic routine in an attempt to reduce the possibility of awareness.

SUPPRESSION OF REFLEXES AND LOSS OF MUSCLE TONE

Derived from clinical observations, the classic indices of anesthetic depth are purely descriptive. Subsequent attempts to improve these signs have assessed the anesthetic state *in relation to* the intensity of surgical stimulation.[24, 41] These measures of reflex responsiveness acknowledge, appropriately, that the depth of anesthesia is a relative, not an absolute, state of drug-induced dysfunction. In contemporary practice, therefore, reflex responsiveness, or its absence, is almost continually evaluated, and this form of assessment has become the most reliable and useful clinical index of the adequacy of depth of anesthesia.

Anesthesiologists evaluate responsiveness to surgical pain in one of two ways: as somatomotor reflexes, the patient moving away from the site of stimulation, or as a change in continuously monitored respiratory pattern or variation in cardiovascular signs. More elaborate, but less utilitarian, estimates of responsiveness attempt to quantitate the neuroendocrine response to pain by analysis of plasma catecholamines, especially norepinephrine,[42] or they monitor the cerebral cortical electrical responses to various stimuli with raw or processed EEG data[15, 22, 43, 44] or specialized evoked potential (EP) apparatus.[45] Both resting and evoked esophageal motility have also been used to assess the adequacy of anesthetic depth.[46]

Minimum Alveolar Concentration

Movement in response to surgical incision is the simplest and oldest form of assessment of reflex responsiveness. John Snow observed that "Ether contributes other benefits besides preventing . . . pain. It keeps patients still, who otherwise would not be."[17] In the second stage of anesthesia, withdrawal in response to incision represents a segmental or suprasegmental reflex response; at the third or "surgical" level, this response is abolished. Movement, therefore, is still the "gold standard" by which the potencies of inhalational anesthetic agents are compared. Minimum alveolar concentration (MAC) is the inhalational equivalent of a median effective anesthetic dose (ED_{50} or AD_{50}). It is determined by noting movement in response to pain under conditions of pharmacokinetic equilibrium in which end-tidal anesthetic concentrations are assumed to be similar or identical to alveolar concentrations.[47, 48]

MAC does not distinguish explicitly between purposeful and reflex withdrawal movements, but values for a given anesthetic agent are remarkably similar in both human and laboratory animal species. In addition, MAC values appear to be virtually independent of patient gender or the duration of exposure to the anesthetic, of variations in acid-base status, or of other moderate changes in the physiologic environment, including carbon dioxide and oxygen tensions or blood pressure.[17] Physiologic factors that do alter MAC significantly include pregnancy[49] and the processes of physical maturation and aging: across the adult years of life, MAC values for all inhalational agents studied[50-53] fall at virtually identical rates, declining about 25% between the ages of 20 and 80 years (Fig 2-3).

Pharmacodynamics

Alternative measures such as concentration of unconsciousness (CUNC)[22] and other "scientific" indices have failed to achieve general and sustained acceptance in studies of anesthetic dose-and-effect relationships, the discipline of pharmacodynamics. In contrast, MAC has become the established pharmacodynamic standard for both clinical and research efforts, although it defines only the midpoint of the relationship between anesthetic dose and its effect, and is therefore useful primarily for comparisons of relative anesthetic potency.

Additional measurements at higher and lower end-tidal concentrations establish the variability of responsiveness and provide reliable estimates of end-points closer to the clinically relevant dosages of anesthetic agents, concentrations needed to achieve 95% of maximal efficacy.[54] Some of these issues have, in fact, been addressed in work that has investigated AD_{95}[55] and MAC Awake[56] for inhalational anesthetics, thus broadening the range of available data to permit comparisons of potency at constant anesthetic end-points (Table 2-2).

Questions remain, however, regarding the additivity of MAC fractions. Additivity is a valid assumption only if the slopes of the dose-effect relationships for the various inhalational anesthetic agents are parallel to each other.[57] Although there appears to be a general state of parallelism between halothane and enflurane (Fig 2-4), these are the only agents that have been studied extensively, and even minor errors in statistical methodology could confound interpretation of these data.[58] MAC additivity both for inhalational anesthetics and

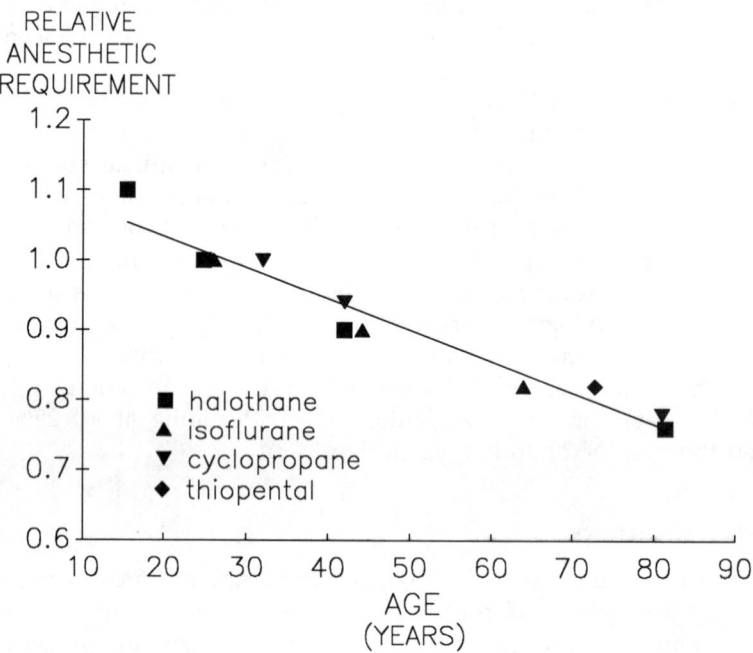

RELATIVE
ANESTHETIC
REQUIREMENT

- ■ halothane
- ▲ isoflurane
- ▼ cyclopropane
- ◆ thiopental

AGE
(YEARS)

FIG 2–3.
Relative anesthetic requirement as a function of the average age of different subject groups studied. Relative MAC (inhalational agents) or ED_{50} (thiopental) was calculated as the ratio of the measured value for a given patient group when compared with the "standard" AD_{50} value derived from studies of anesthetic requirements in healthy adults in the third decade of life. Data are from studies of unpremedicated subjects.[50, 52, 81] By linear regression analysis, the relationship suggests that anesthetic requirement, expressed as a percentage of the "standard" value, is approximately 115 less one half of the subject's age.

for narcotics and other central nervous system depressants appears to be a clinically relevant phenomenon, however, and this assumption is utilized frequently to estimate median effective anesthetic dosages when, for example, nitrous oxide is used as an anesthetic carrier gas.

Unlike measurements of inhalational anesthetic concentrations, which can be obtained easily under conditions of relative dynamic equilibrium, concentrations of intravenous agents in plasma change rapidly. Uncertainty as to the temporal relationship between injected dose, subsequent plasma concentration, and end-point of anesthetic effect has hampered studies of the pharmacodynamics of intravenous agents. A newer standard for anesthetic potency in which the plasma drug concentration is related to one half of a maximal drug-induced re-

TABLE 2–2.

Alveolar Concentrations Associated With Various Anesthetic End-Points*

Agent	MAC/AD$_{50}$	AD$_{95}$	MAC BAR$_{50}$	MAC BAR$_{95}$	MAC Awake
Cyclopropane	9.2%	10.1%	—	—	5.3%(est.)
Diethyl ether	1.92%	2.22%	—	—	1.41%
Enflurane	1.69%	1.88%	2.70%	4.34%	—
Halothane	0.74%	0.90%	1.07%	1.55%	0.41%
Isoflurane	1.16%	1.63%	—	—	—
Methoxyflurane	0.16%	0.22%	—	—	0.08%
Nitrous oxide	101%	N/A	—	—	59% (est.)
Sevoflurane	1.71%	2.07%	—	—	—

*All values as percent atmosphere at sea level; determined in, or adjusted for, unpremedicated young subjects. MAC/AD$_{50}$ = minimum alveolar anesthetic concentration or its pharmacodynamic equivalent, median anesthetic dose, delivered in oxygen; AD$_{95}$ = anesthetic dose or concentration effective in 95% of population; MAC BAR$_{50}$ = estimated median effective anesthetic concentration for blocking neuroendocrine response to skin incision, assuming MAC additivity; MAC BAR$_{95}$ = estimated anesthetic concentration effective in blocking neuroendocrine response to skin incision in 95% of population studied; MAC Awake = equilibrium alveolar anesthetic concentration midway between values permits and prevents simple response to verbal command; — = not measured.

duction in electroencephalographic spectral edge is known as median inhibiting concentration (IC$_{50}$).[59] This concept is one step closer to the site of anesthetic action than the design of studies utilizing only measurements of injected dosage, and it eliminates distortions of the traditional dose-effect relationship produced by unsuspected variations in the plasma drug concentrations. However, the addition of theoretical "effect compartments" to modify the traditional pharmacologic model is required to reconcile discrepancies between the time at which peak plasma drug concentrations are achieved and the time to subsequent maximal anesthetic effect. In fact, there is also little empirical evidence that concentration-effect relationships are more precise than the more traditional dose-effect curves.[58, 60]

Ventilatory Responsiveness

Ventilatory responses to surgical stimulation, once widely used to determine the adequacy of anesthetic depth, are of little practical value in contemporary practice because of the widespread use of neuromuscular blockade and controlled ventilation. Classic observation of the changes in spontaneous respiratory pattern and altered laryngotracheal and bronchial reflex responses after manipulation or surgical stimulation were first clearly outlined more than 50 years ago.[23, 61]

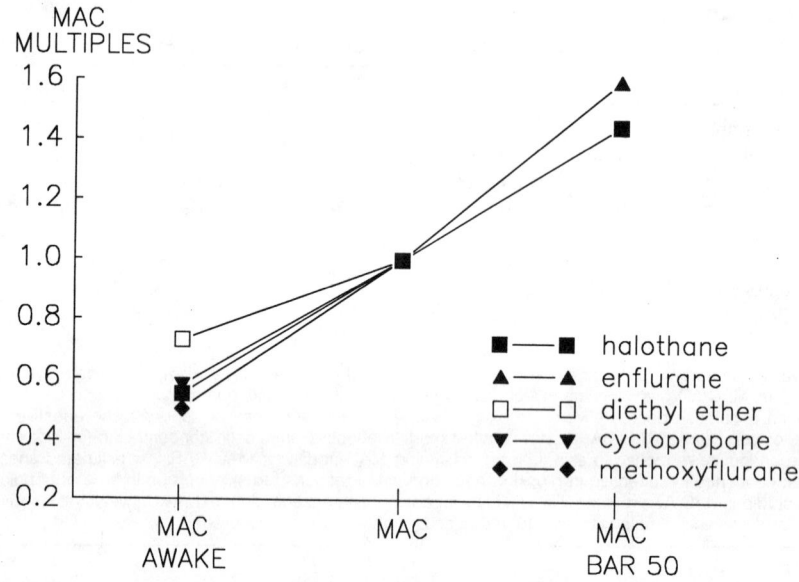

FIG 2–4.
MAC multiples required for *MAC*,[47, 48, 50] *MAC Awake*,[56] and *MAC BAR$_{50}$*.[42] General parallelism for a diverse group of chemical structures across this range of anesthetic endpoints supports the concept that these drugs have the same, or similar, sites or mechanisms of anesthetic action.

Although minor differences in the respiratory patterns are observed during progressively deeper levels of anesthesia with various inhalational agents because of their specific chemistry or side effects, a general, stereotyped pattern can be evoked reliably in the clinical setting when spontaneous respiration is maintained and neuromuscular blocking drugs are avoided. With increasing inspired concentrations of potent inhalational anesthetics, there is a progressive, dose-related increase in respiratory rate. Reciprocal reduction in tidal volume reflects the reduced contributions of intercostal muscles to ventilatory effort. Ultimately, depression of responsiveness to carbon dioxide and cessation of diaphragmatic action produce apnea.

After a brief period of exaggerated responsiveness, tracheobronchial reflex activity fades progressively, in a cephalad-to-caudad direction: the laryngeal reflexes, then the tracheal reflexes, and, last of all, the carinal cough reflex are suppressed, and then abolished. These ventilatory and reflex functions return in reverse order with spontaneous breathing during emergence from anesthesia.[61]

Cardiovascular Responsiveness

Pupillary signs do not provide reliable estimates of the depth of anesthesia with any of the anesthetic drugs currently employed.[62] Similarly, the cardiovascular properties of modern anesthetics are sufficiently unique that observation of vital signs alone is unreliable for determining the depth of anesthesia, at least over the usual range of anesthetic concentrations required for surgery. In a comparative study of the median effective inhalational anesthetic concentrations required for blocking neuroendocrine responses to skin incision, MAC BAR$_{50}$, the heart rate response to surgical incision was abolished by alveolar concentrations of halothane close to MAC, but no clinically appropriate inspired concentration of enflurane effectively accomplished the same result.[42]

Some aspects of cardiac function are, however, similarly affected: all inhalational agents exert a common, almost generic form of myocardial and vasomotor depression, discussed in more detail in Chapter 6. Therefore, although arterial hypotension is almost invariably the final common sign of anesthetic overdosage with inhalational anesthetics, it is neither a predictable nor a reliable indicator of depth of anesthesia at surgical levels.

Muscle Tone

Purposeful withdrawal of the patient in response to painful stimulation during surgery is clearly undesirable, since it indicates that anesthetic depth is inadequate for surgery. The origins of a complaint by the surgeon that a patient is "tight," however, may be obscure, and thus the solution can be less obvious. Even in the adequately anesthetized patient, persistent skeletal muscle tone or unexpected reflex motor phenomena can compromise abdominal, orthopedic, or microscopic surgical procedures.

With loss of consciousness, purposeful movements quickly evolve into diffuse hypertonic activity, reflecting the greater sensitivity of inhibitory, as opposed to facilitatory, motor neuron functions. After this transient period of muscle rigidity and hyperreflexia, however, increasing depth of inhalational anesthesia is accompanied by a rapid and marked decline in skeletal muscle tone, which eventually gives way to simple resistance to passive movement. Finally, although spontaneous ventilation is maintained, there is a progressive loss of intercostal and abdominal wall muscle tone and a persistent, shallow pattern of diaphragmatic breathing.

With more profound neuromuscular depression there may be tracheal "tug," a caudad movement of the larynx and trachea during inspiration. This phenomenon reflects the fact that diaphragmatic motion is no longer effectively opposed by the pharyngeal and cervical skeletal muscle tone that normally anchors the tracheobronchial tree. At this level, surgical or "stage III" anesthesia, segmental somatomotor responses can be evoked only with stimuli of great intensity because both afferent and efferent limbs of the reflex arc are depressed by the action of general anesthetics. Electromyographic recordings from the abdominal wall suggest that acute increases in the depth of anesthesia per se, as would be produced by a bolus injection of thiopental, for example, can produce transient total suppression of spontaneous skeletal muscle electrical activity.[63]

Enflurane has been described as stimulating some forms of cerebrocortical electrical activity[64] and, under some circumstances, may produce the corresponding clinical manifestations of clonic motor disturbances.[65] Like other inhalational anesthetics, however, it appears, in general, to reduce resting muscle tone and may also suppress evoked neuromuscular responses directly. Some intravenous anesthetic agents also selectively stimulate central components of the nervous system, increasing resting muscle tone and producing random or reflex somatomotor phenomena. Ketamine produces electrocortical activation, ocular nystagmus, increased skeletal muscle tone, and exaggerated reflex activity. Similarly, chest wall rigidity produced by rapid injection of intravenous narcotics probably represents a central phenomenon, since it occurs in tourniquet-isolated extremities,[66] and, like ketamine-induced movement, it appears to resolve with either neuromuscular blockade or additional depression of the central nervous system produced by adjuvant anesthetic drugs.

At inspired concentrations adequate for clinical purposes, all potent inhalational anesthetics not only reduce resting muscle tone because of generalized nervous system effects but also potentiate blockade of evoked neuromuscular responses by relaxant drugs such as curare and pancuronium.[67] In addition, the halogenated ethers isoflurane and enflurane, true to the legacy established by their nonhalogenated prototypes, have significant intrinsic neuromuscular blocking properties (Chapter 5).[68]

Traditionally, neuromuscular blockade has been monitored by evaluating neurally evoked muscle responses. The stimulation patterns test specifically for the mobilization, release, and reception of acetylcholine, which are functions of the neuromuscular junction. However, absolute force of mechanical response is not routinely evaluated after the antagonism of neuromuscular blockade, nor is it common to do any form of direct comparison of muscle strength before and after general anesthesia. Depression of calcium-mediated contractile mechanisms, a ubiquitous quality of potent inhalational anesthetic agents probably responsible for their familiar capacity to depress cardiac contractility,[69] may also exert a similar, but more limited, direct effect on the contraction of skeletal muscle. Although there appears to be a general correlation between neurally evoked responses and clinical evidence of strength, some instances of inadequate or marginal muscle strength after exposure to inhalational agents may be due not to blockade of the neuromuscular junction but to residual direct depression of the skeletal muscle contractile apparatus.

ANALGESIA

Pain is extremely complex, for it encompasses physiologic, psychologic, social, and cultural components. *Analgesia* is the elimination or modification of this "constellation of unpleasant perceptual and emotional experiences,"[70] and it can be provided by any of a variety of anesthetic techniques. In the unconscious patient, analgesia is achieved as a component of hypnosis. The patient apparently does not perceive or experience anxiety, displeasure, or any other cerebrocortical response to painful stimuli.

It is less clear, however, whether inability to discriminate the location, intensity, and quality of a painful stimulus abolishes pain per se, or merely interferes with its perception. Does pain exist if it is not experienced on a cortical level? The persistence of a variety of consistent and predictable autonomic reflex responses to stimulation or tissue-damaging injury in the unconscious patient supports the concept that pain is a physiologic as well as a psychologic phenomenon. Analgesia in this context, however, is the elimination not of pain but of its perception. Pain, in the absence of its perception, appears to exist as a major component of what is generally described as the "stress response," a complex sequence of physiologic disruption, autonomic responses, and metabolic changes that may actually be a major determinant of perioperative morbidity.[71]

Pain Pathways

At segmental reflex levels, surgical pain in both awake and unconscious patients can produce skeletal and smooth muscle contractions, with withdrawal or spasticity of the injured extremity, abdominal or chest wall rigidity, or arterial hypertension. A segmental reflex response to tissue trauma may also release norepinephrine from sympathetic nerve endings. If low spinal anesthesia is used to produce afferent blockade, it suppresses this polysegmental reflex in proportion to the level of blockade.[72] At higher, suprasegmental levels, surgically induced tissue trauma evokes tachycardia, hyperventilation, and an increase in plasma concentrations of epinephrine, cortisol, glucagon, and growth hormone. These clinical responses to tissue injury may be suppressed by extensive neural blockade of the efferent limbs of the appropriate reflex arc in an "all-or-none" fashion, or they can be partially or completely suppressed by progressively deeper levels of anesthesia, since they require participation of higher centers.[30]

Somatic Pain

Considerable progress has been made in defining both the pathways and the modulating and integrative centers for pain transmission (Fig 2–5). Somatic pain, classically described as "epicritic" or "discriminative" because of the precision with which its quality and location can be described, travels along lateralized spinothalamic pathways. In the substantia gelatinosa of the spinal cord, however, it is subject to significant amplification or demodulation by corticospinal, thalamic, or other influences. This integrative area of the spinal cord may provide the anatomic locus of the "gate theory" of pain transmission.[73]

Somatic pain, after modulation at a segmental level, proceeds cephalad with some input to the brain stem (suprasegmental reflex responses), to the midbrain (arousal), and then to the primary subcortical pain-processing area, the thalamus. After modification here, afferent input from the spinothalamic tracts is directed to the cerebral cortex where it is transformed from diffuse to discrete pain by the assignment of positional, qualitative (postcentral gyrus), and emotional (frontal lobes) characterization.[74]

Visceral Pain

In contrast, visceral pain is nondiscriminative or "protopathic." Visceral pain retains this nonspecific quality even after it has gained access to the cardiovascular and respiratory centers of the brain stem, and to higher centers. Visceral pain also has a dominant influence, especially in anesthetized or cortically depressed individuals, on state of arousal, as determined by activity within the midbrain reticular formation. Eventually it gains access to the cerebral cortex via two routes: in-

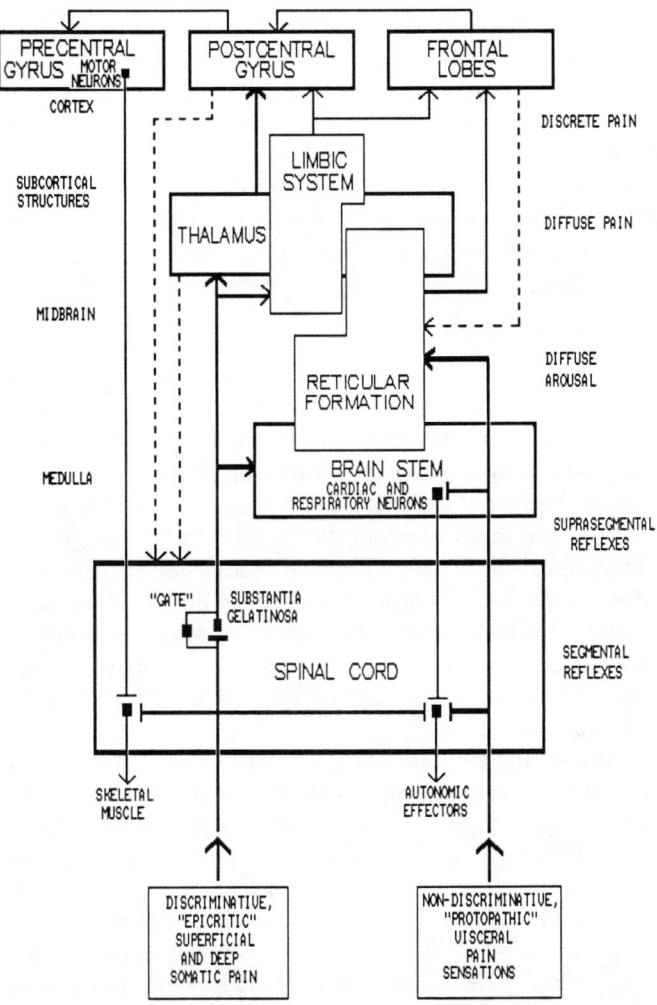

FIG 2–5.
Schematic representation of pain pathways organized according to both anatomic and functional hierarchy. *Solid lines* indicate major conducting pathways; *dashed lines* represent inhibitory "feedback" systems that modulate pain transmission at the level of the spinal cord "gate" and at the midbrain. Both visceral and somatic pain can provide the afferent component of segmental reflex arcs with skeletal muscle motor and autonomic efferents. The thalamus is probably the major processing area for somatic pain at higher levels. The reticular formation appears ultimately to mediate the ability of pain of any type to alter arousal state.

directly, through the thalamus, or by a more direct path, to the associational areas of the frontal lobes.

This latter mechanism provides the emotional component of the experience of diffuse visceral pain in surgical patients. For both somatic and visceral pain, segmental and suprasegmental reflex responses are stereotyped and predictable during general anesthesia. In the conscious patient, however, pain of any type is an idiosyncratic interaction of personality, psychology, and neurophysiology.[75]

Therapy for Acute Pain

Pain pathways are complex and lengthy, providing numerous points at which they can be interrupted. Virtually all are utilized by some form of analgesic therapy.[76] Traditional opiates and opioids provide receptor-mediated interruption of transmission of painful stimuli at the level of the spinal cord, the brain stem, or the thalamus. Analgesics with anti-inflammatory properties inhibit the release of bradykinin, prostaglandins, or other neurohumoral mediators of pain. Regional anesthesia interrupts the afferent and efferent limbs of segmental or suprasegmental pain reflex arcs. "Hypnotic" general anesthetics, such as the barbiturates, eliminate the conscious perception of painful stimuli, or may have additional depressant effects at lower centers that modulate pain transmission.

Less traditional forms of analgesia have still other mechanisms of action. The term *neuroleptanalgesia* describes a robotlike state of emotional indifference to pain.[77] Classically, neuroleptanalgesia is established with a butyrophenone, such as haloperidol or droperidol, and a short-acting narcotic. The effect of the narcotic is to produce traditional analgesia. The butyrophenone adds a unique psychologic element of apparent apathy, described best as drug-induced parkinsonism, a term that conveys the expressionless facies and lack of spontaneous movement characteristic of these patients.

This analogy is also pharmacologically consistent with the dopaminergic blocking properties of butyrophenone drugs. Similar qualities and states of apparent indifference to pain have also been described for drug combinations using phenothiazines. Because of the inability of neuroleptic agents to reliably make the patient amnestic or to provide anxiolysis, current application is largely as anesthetic adjuvants and induction agents, or, in some cases, for short-term sedation or anesthesia for diagnostic procedures.[78]

An alternative approach to analgesia is the use of a cataleptic phencyclidine derivative, ketamine. Once called "dissociative anesthesia," a ketamine-induced state of coma is a unique combination of potent analgesia and amnesia not associated with depression of respiration or loss of skeletal muscle tone.[79] The mechanism of action of ketamine-induced anesthesia is similarly novel: it interrupts neuronal communication between the thalamus and the cerebral cortex, producing a "dissociation" between cortical and midbrain electrical activity, thus eliminating any arousal effect on the reticular formation. The resultant clinical state of depressed consciousness is paradoxical relative to the coincident phenomenon of cerebral cortical hyperexcitation, which may produce hallucinations, arterial hypertension, and hyperreflexia.

Specific binding of ketamine to opiate receptors has also been demonstrated; it may explain the obvious intensity and specificity of the analgesia produced by this drug.[80] Ketamine is particularly useful for providing intense, short-term analgesia for diagnostic or surgical procedures, especially where unassisted spontaneous ventilation is desired. Rapid parenteral uptake and short duration of action suggest a primary clinical application as an anesthetic adjuvant or induction agent.

SUMMARY

Anesthesia and hypnosis appear to be far better defined on a clinical and functional level than on a mechanistic neurochemical or physicochemical basis. Many attempts to provide a unitary hypothesis for anesthesia have been advanced, but current research suggests that general anesthesia and its components of hypnosis, amnesia, anxiolysis, analgesia, loss of muscle tone, and reflex suppression, most likely reflect impaired synaptic transmission, probably produced at multiple sites by a variety of cellular or subcellular mechanisms. Effects on the reticular formation appear to explain the universal quality of depressed consciousness that virtually defines general anesthesia. Segmental effects on pain and motor pathways and some cortical disinhibition may contribute to the overall characteristics of anesthesia produced by any specific agent.

The clinical characteristics of intentional, drug-induced coma have been observed and organized into systems to permit determination of "adequate" levels of anesthesia. Quantification of anesthetic effects relies largely on measurements of depressed somatomotor and cardiorespiratory responsiveness to surgical pain. Relative anesthetic potency, as quantified by MAC, is a consistent and apparently additive phenomenon when multiple agents are used as part of the anesthetic plan.

Awareness of pain and subsequent recall of intraoperative events on a conscious or subconscious level are rare but demonstrable even when anesthetic depth is maintained at "surgical" levels. Suppression of the neuroendocrine response to pain and to tissue injury can be accomplished to a graded or a relatively complete extent, but the effectiveness with which even deep levels of inhalational anesthesia protect, rather than jeopardize, the patient remains uncertain and controversial.

REFERENCES

1. Schaefer H: Remarks on the theory of narcosis. *Int Anesthesiol Clin* 1963; 1:977–979.
2. Hyman AI: Chloroform and controversy. *Semin Anesth* 1986; 5:255–257.
3. DeBon FL, Muehlbaecher C: Integration of the theories of anesthesia. *Int Anesthesiol Clin* 1963; 1:927–935.
4. Firestone LL, Kitz RJ: Anesthetics and lipids: Some molecular perspectives. *Semin Anesth* 1986; 5:286–300.
5. Lever MJ, Miller KW, Paton WDM, Smith ED: Pressure reversal of anaesthesia. *Nature* 1971; 231:368.
6. Halsey MJ, Wardley-Smith B, Green CJ: Pressure-reversal of general anaesthesia — a multi-site expansion hypothesis. *Br J Anaesth* 1979; 50:1091–1097.
7. Hameroff SR, Watt RC: Do anesthetics act by altering electron mobility? *Anesth Analg* 1983; 62:936–940.
8. Koblin DD, Eger EI II: Theories of narcosis. *N Engl J Med* 1979; 301:1222–1224.
9. Nicoll RA, Madison DV: General anesthetics hyperpolarize neurons in the vertebrate central nervous system. *Science* 1982; 217:1055–1056.
10. LaBella FS: Is there a general anesthesia receptor? *Can J Physiol Pharmacol* 1981; 59:432–442.
11. Trevor AJ, Miller RD: General anesthetics, in Katzung BG (ed): *Basic and Clinical Pharmacology*, ed 2. East Norwalk, Conn., Appleton & Lange, 1984, pp 283–292.
12. Norman J: Mechanisms of anaesthesia (editorial). *Br J Anaesth* 1983; 55:189–190.
13. Richards CD: Actions of general anesthetics on synaptic transmission in the CNS. *Br J Anaesth* 1983; 55:201–207.
14. Weston GA, Roth SH: Differential actions of volatile anaesthetic agents on a single isolated neurone. *Br J Anaesth* 1986; 58:1390–1396.
15. Winters WD: Neurophysiologic correlates of the anesthetic state, in Brechner VL (ed): *Pathological and Pharmacological Considerations in Anesthesiology.* Springfield, Ill., Charles C Thomas, 1973, pp 48–60.
16. Larabee MG, Posternak JM: Selective action of anesthetics on synapses and axons in mammalian sympathetic ganglia. *J Neurophysiol* 1952; 15:91–114.

17. Eger EI II: *Anesthetic Uptake and Action*. Baltimore, Williams & Wilkins, 1974.
18. Fontenot HJ: The GABA system: New evidence of neurotransmitter involvement in the mechanism of anesthesia. *Anesthesiology* 1984; 61:A327.
19. Judge SE: Effect of general anesthetics on synaptic ion channels. *Br J Anaesth* 1983; 55:191–200.
20. Rosner BS, Clark DL: Neurophysiologic effect of general anesthetics. II. Sequential regional actions in the brain. *Anesthesiology* 1973; 39:59–81.
21. Guedel AE: Third stage ether anesthesia: A subclassification regarding the significance of the position and movements of the eyeball. *Am J Surg* 1920; 34:53–57.
22. Clark DL, Rosner BS: Neurophysiologic effects of general anesthetics. I. The electroencephalogram and sensory evoked response in man. *Anesthesiology* 1973; 38:564–582.
23. Gillespie NA: The signs of anesthesia. *Anesth Analg* 1943; 27:275–281.
24. Laycock JD: Signs and stages of anaesthesia; a restatement. *Anaesthesia* 1953; 8:15–20.
25. Dornette WL: The anatomic basis of the signs of anesthesia. *Anesth Analg* 1964; 43:71–81.
26. Anonymous: Consciousness during surgical operations (editorial). *Br Med J* 1959; 2:810–811.
27. Guerra F: Awareness and recall. *Int Anesthesiol Clin* 1986; 24:75–99.
28. Wilson SL, Vaughan EW, Stephen CR: Awareness, dreams, and hallucinations associated with general anesthesia. *Anesth Analg* 1975; 54:609–616.
29. Bennett HL, Davis HS, Giannini JA: Non-verbal response to intraoperative conversation. *Br J Anaesth* 1985; 57:174–179.
30. Phillips GD, Cousins MJ: Neurological mechanisms of pain and the relationship of pain, anxiety, and in sleep, in Cousins MJ, Phillips GD (eds): *Acute Pain Management*. New York, Churchill-Livingstone, 1986, pp 21–48.
31. Guerra F: Awareness under general anesthesia, in Guerra F, Aldrete JA (eds): *Emotional and Psychological Responses to Anesthesia and Surgery*. New York, Grune & Stratton, 1980, pp 1–8.
32. Blacher RS: On awakening paralyzed during surgery: A syndrome of traumatic neurosis. *JAMA* 1985; 234:67–68.
33. Levinson BW: States of awareness during general anesthesia. *Br J Anaesth* 1986; 37:544–546.
34. Bogetz MS, Katz JA: Recall of surgery for major trauma. *Anesthesiology* 1984; 61:6–9.
35. Terrell RK, Sweet WO, Gladfelter JH, Stephen CR: Study of recall during anesthesia. *Anesth Analg* 1969; 48:86–90.
36. Eich E, Reeves JL, Katz RL: Anesthesia, amnesia, and the memory/awareness distinction. *Anesth Analg* 1985; 64:1143–1148.
37. Wilson J, Lewis SA, Jenkinson JL: Electroencephalographic investigation of awareness during anaesthesia. *Br J Anaesth* 1970; 42:804–805.
38. Hutchinson R: Awareness during surgery: A study of its incidence. *Br J Anaesth* 1960; 33:463–469.

39. Utting JE: Awareness in anesthesia. *Anaesth Intensive Care* 1975; 3:334–340.
40. Saucier N, Walts LF, Moreland JR: Patient awareness during nitrous oxide, oxygen and halothane anesthesia. *Anesth Analg* 1983; 62:239–240.
41. Woodbridge PD: Changing concepts concerning depth of anesthesia. *Anesthesiology* 1958; 18:536–550.
42. Roizen MF, Horrigan RW, Frazer BM: Anesthetic doses blocking adrenergic (stress) and cardiovascular responses to incision-MAC BAR. *Anesthesiology* 1981; 54:390–398.
43. Levy WJ, Shapiro HM, Maruchak G, Meathe E: Automated EEG processing for intraoperative monitoring. *Anesthesiology* 1980; 53:223–236.
44. Maynard DE, Jenkinson JL: The cerebral function analysing monitor. *Anaesthesia* 1984; 39:678–690.
45. Grundy BL: Intraoperative monitoring of sensory evoked potentials. *Anesthesiology* 1983; 58:72–87.
46. Evans JM, Davies WL, Wise CC: Lower esophageal contractility: A new monitor of anaesthesia. *Lancet* 1984; 2:1151–1154.
47. Eger EI II, Saidman LJ, Brandstater B: Minimum alveolar anesthetic concentration: A standard of anesthetic potency. *Anesthesiology* 1965; 26:756–763.
48. Saidman LJ, Eger EI II, Munson ES, Babad AA, Muallem M: Minimum alveolar concentrations of methoxyflurane, halothane, ether and cyclopropane in man: Correlation with theories of anesthesia. *Anesthesiology* 1967; 28:994–1002.
49. De Rosayro AM, Vogel M, Knight PR: Halothane MAC and pregnancy: Endorphins, progesterone, or "?". *Anesthesiology* 1984; 61:A336.
50. Gregory GA, Eger EI II, Munson ES: The relationship between age and halothane requirement in man. *Anesthesiology* 1969; 30:488–491.
51. Nicodemus HF, Nassiri-Rahimi C, Bachman L, Smith TC: Median effective doses (ED50) of halothane in adults and children. *Anesthesiology* 1969; 31:344–348.
52. Munson ES, Hoffman JC, Eger EI II: Use of cyclopropane to test the generality of anesthetic requirement in the elderly. *Anesth Analg* 1984; 63:998–1000.
53. Stevens WC, Dolan WM, Gibbons RT: Minimum alveolar concentrations (MAC) of isoflurane with and without nitrous oxide in patients of various ages. *Anesthesiology* 1985; 42:197–200.
54. Waud BE, Waud DR: On dose-response curves and anesthetics (editorial). *Anesthesiology* 1970; 33:1–4.
55. DeJong RH, Eger EI II: MAC expanded: AD50 and AD95 values of common inhalation anesthetics in man. *Anesthesiology* 1975; 42:384–389.
56. Stoelting RK, Longnecker DE, Eger EI II: Minimum alveolar concentrations in man on awakening from methoxyflurane, halothane, ether, and fluroxene anesthesia: MAC Awake. *Anesthesiology* 1970; 33:5–9.
57. Teplick R: MAC additivity: Reality or analytic error? *Anesthesiology* 1984; 61:A335.

58. Teplick R: Methodological errors in the estimation of MAC. *Anesthesiology* 1984; 61:A334.
59. Scott JC, Ponganis KV, Stanski DR: EEG quantitation of narcotic effect: The comparative pharmacodynamics of fentanyl and alfentanil. *Anesthesiology* 1985; 62:234–241.
60. Waud BE, Waud DR: Dose-response curves and pharmacokinetics (editorial). *Anesthesiology* 1986; 65:355–358.
61. Miller AH: Ascending respiratory paralysis under general anesthesia. *JAMA* 1925; 84:201.
62. Cullen DJ, Eger EI II, Stevens WC, et al: Clinical signs of anesthesia. *Anesthesiology* 1972; 36:21–36.
63. Fink BR: A method of monitoring muscular relaxation by the integrated abdominal electromyogram. *Anesthesiology* 1960; 21:178–185.
64. Rosenberg H, Clofine R, Bialik O: Neurologic changes during awakening from anesthesia. *Anesthesiology* 1981; 54:125–130.
65. Flemming DC, Fitzpatrick J, Fariello RG, Duff T, Hellman D, Hoff BH: Diagnostic activation of epileptogenic foci by enflurane. *Anesthesiology* 1980; 52:431–433.
66. Freund FG, Martin WE, Wong KC, Hornbein TF: Abdominal rigidity induced by morphine and nitrous oxide. *Anesthesiology* 1973; 38:358–362.
67. Fogdall RP, Miller RD: Neuromuscular effects of enflurane, alone and combined with *d*-tubocurarine, pancuronium, and succinylcholine in man. *Anesthesiology* 1975; 42:173–178.
68. Miller RD, Eger EI II, Way WL, Stevens WC, Dolan WM: Comparative neuromuscular effects of Forane and halothane alone and in combination with *d*-tubocurarine in man. *Anesthesiology* 1971; 35:38–42.
69. Merin RG: Inhalation anesthetics and myocardial metabolism. *Anesthesiology* 1973; 39:216–255.
70. Bonica JJ: Past and current status of pain research and therapy. *Semin Anesth* 1986; 5:82–99.
71. Kehlet H: Pain relief and modification of the stress response, in Cousins MJ, Phillips GD (eds): *Acute Pain Management*. New York, Churchill-Livingstone, 1986, pp 49–75.
72. Pflug AE, Halter JB: Effect of spinal anesthesia on adrenergic tone and the neuroendocrine response to surgical stress in humans. *Anesthesiology* 1981; 55:120–126.
73. Melzack R, Wall PD: Pain mechanisms: A new theory. *Science* 1965; 150:971–979.
74. Mehta M: *Intractable Pain*. London, WB Saunders, 1973, p 287.
75. Melzack R, Dennis SG: Neurophysiological foundations of pain, in Sternbach RA (ed): *The Psychology of Pain*. New York, Raven Press, 1978, pp 1–26.
76. Cannon JT, Liebeskind JC, Frenk H: Neural and neurochemical mechanisms of pain inhibition, in Sternbach RA (ed): *The Psychology of Pain*. New York, Raven Press, 1978, pp 27–47.

77. Foldes FF: Neuroleptanesthesia for general surgery. *Int Anesthesiol Clin* 1973; 11:1–35.
78. Morrison JD: Neuroleptic techniques, in Dundee JW, Wyant GM, (eds): *Intravenous Anaesthesia*. Edinburgh, Churchill-Livingstone, 1974; pp 217–218.
79. White PF, Way WL, Trevor AJ: Ketamine—its pharmacology and therapeutic uses. *Anesthesiology* 1982; 56:119–136.
80. Finck AD, Ngai SH: Opiate receptor mediation of ketamine analgesia. *Anesthesiology* 1982; 56:291–297.
81. Muravchick S: Effect of age and premedication on thiopental sleep dose. *Anesthesiology* 1984; 61:333–336.

3

Central Nervous System Function During and After Anesthesia

Only a few generations ago, the brain was thought to be a homogenous lipid tissue mass with an inert circulation. Brain blood flow was assumed to be determined passively by the difference between systemic arterial and venous pressures; maintained at constant levels by the homeostatic reflexes of the autonomic nervous system, these parameters seemed well matched to what were thought to be the constant metabolic requirements of brain tissue. By 1940, however, published observations of spontaneous fluctuation of cerebrovascular diameters viewed through pial "windows" suggested that the cerebral circulation had spontaneous, active adjustments of vascular diameter in response to changes in blood pressure.[1] Speculation was subsequently replaced by quantitative, scientific measurements of cerebral blood flow and metabolism in the intact human subject,[2] work that reopened what was to become one of the most productive and important areas of modern circulatory physiology.

Subsequent improvements in methodology have revealed the intricacy of cerebral circulatory control. Since anesthetic drugs, by design, produce temporary disruption of nervous system function in the form of neural blockade, autonomic disruption, and drug-induced coma, recent developments in brain neurochemistry and transmitter systems are of special interest to those who anesthetize patients. To anticipate and limit the effects of these drugs and to make their actions compatible with preexisting patient disease states, it is also necessary to be familiar with the integrated physiology of nervous system functioning, summarized in the sections that follow.

INTRINSIC CONTROL OF CEREBRAL BLOOD FLOW

Authors of early studies measuring cerebral blood flow (CBF) could determine only "global" values reflecting overall hemispheric perfusion. It appeared to be symmetric and relatively constant at 45 to 55 mL per 100 g tissue per minute, independent of a wide range of physical and mental activities, suggesting a constant requirement for 600 to 800 mL of blood flow per minute.[3] However, improved methodology subsequently provided the precision necessary to measure regional cerebral blood flow (rCBF) in as many as 40 areas of the cerebral cortex and basal ganglia simultaneously, revealing a sixfold variation in regional brain perfusion rates.[4]

Coupling

Spatial (place-to-place) or temporal (moment-to-moment) differences in metabolic and electrical activity produce rCBF values that range from about 20 mL/100 g/min in white matter to almost 140 mL/100 g/min in active gray matter.[5] These variations in rCBF are directly and proportionally related, or *"coupled,"* to short-term, regional variations in the rate of cerebral metabolic consumption of oxygen ($CMRO_2$).[6] Level of consciousness, sensory stimulation, rapid eye movement (REM) sleep, seizure activity, motor function, body temperature, and the presence of anesthetic agents (or other drugs that depress or stimulate nervous system function) all influence nervous system activity. Therefore, they also alter both regional $CMRO_2$ ($rCMRO_2$) and rCBF, although perhaps not by the same mechanism.[7]

The physiologic mechanism that provides coupling appears to be a localized, regional adjustment of cerebral arteriolar smooth muscle tone. Adenosine, a potent vasodilator substance, is also a by-product of oxidative phosphorylation; it appears in rapidly increasing concentrations in the extracellular fluid of metabolically active nervous system tissues.[8] Adenosine may be a key component of the metabolic link between increased neuronal activity and reduced regional cerebrovascular resistance (rCVR). Alternative possibilities include the local vasomotor effects of hydrogen, potassium, or calcium ions. The mechanism of cerebral vasomotion in any one area may, in fact, be multifactorial, but it is almost certain to be metabolically mediated.[7] Observations of *increased* regional oxygen tensions in cortical areas having epileptiform activity suggest that the development of local tissue hypoxia does not explain the coupling of rCBF and $rCMRO_2$.[9]

Autoregulation

For full effectiveness, coupling requires the simultaneous functioning, on a hemispheric scale, of CBF *autoregulation*. This term describes the direct and proportional relationship between cerebral perfusion pressure (CPP) and hemispheric cerebrovascular resistance (Fig 3–1). Autoregulation is an organ-level, relatively coarse mechanism that provides a platform of constant hemispheric CBF upon which regionally controlled coupling mechanisms can maintain a precise balance between cerebral metabolic supply and demand at tissue and cellular levels. Autoregulation, in effect, buffers the cerebral circulation from transient disruptions of arterial blood pressure homeostasis over a substantial range of systemic arterial pressures.[6]

Pathologic or age-related increases in overall level of sympathetic tone may influence the set-point of autoregulation.[7] Sparse, but apparently functional, sympathetic innervation of the cerebral circulation arises from the cervical sympathetic chain. It may provide a neurally integrated component of CVR, at least in some brain areas.[10] A neu-

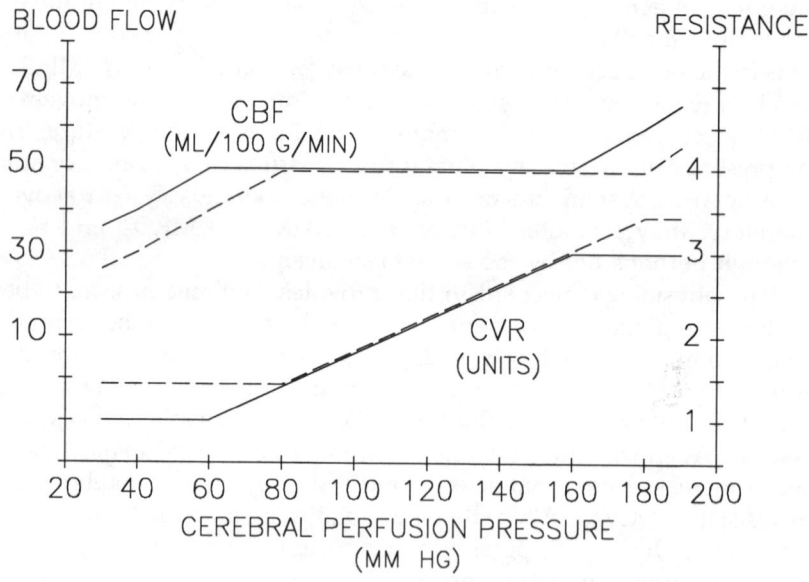

FIG 3–1.
Cerebral blood flow *(CBF)* autoregulation, defined as spontaneous adjustment of cerebrovascular resistance *(CVR)* in response to changes in cerebral perfusion pressure (mean arterial minus cerebral venous or CSF pressures). Patients with chronic arterial hypertension *(dashed lines)* demonstrate a rightward *CBF* "shift" and an upward and rightward *CVR* shift.

rovascular, rather than an ionic,[11] mechanism may also mediate hemorrhage-induced cerebral vasospasm,[12] but it probably does not play an important role in the moment-to-moment functioning of autoregulation.

The classic "myogenic" hypothesis of Bayliss, proposed more than 80 years ago, maintains that the intrinsic active muscular and passive elastic properties of cerebrovascular smooth muscle can provide rapid, virtually automatic adjustment of CVR in response to changes of CPP. Evidence that, in fact, blood pressure–mediated vascular distention (or collapse) produces direct myogenic autoregulation exists in the form of observations of spontaneous, active changes in cerebral vascular diameter: even in isolated middle cerebral arteries, vascular responses to arterial pressure changes are comparable to those that occur within the intact cerebral circulation.[13] Although a metabolic mechanism cannot be excluded, the rapidity of autoregulatory responses is generally such that they appear to occur before sufficient time has elapsed for hypoperfusion to generate any form of metabolic disruption.

Whatever their exact mechanisms, both autoregulation and coupling work together to provide both *consistency* and *constancy* of cerebral perfusion in a manner that appears to be both qualitatively and quantitatively unique to this organ system. This interaction of global and regional control systems may be essential, since the tissues of the nervous system have a high, and absolute, requirement for continuous delivery of oxygen at a rate of 40 to 50 mL/min, or about 3.5 mL O_2/100 g tissue/min. About 60% of the oxygen is required for the metabolism needed to synthesize neurotransmitters, and the balance is largely to sustain ionic transport and cellular integrity.

Unlike muscle or blood, brain tissues lack iron-containing pigments and are therefore unable to store oxygen. Cerebral blood volume occupies only about 5% of total intracranial contents, and consequently does not represent a source of significant oxygen reserve. Although 20% of cardiac output is distributed to this organ, which represents less than 2% of total body mass, the brain cannot be considered a vascular organ in the anatomic sense. It is more precisely described as a metabolically active organ system that requires a high relative rate of overall perfusion; CBF is then regionally distributed in proportion to local metabolic requirements.

Blood-Brain Barrier

Water-soluble dyes injected into the systemic circulation do not stain central nervous system (CNS) tissues. The anatomic basis for this phenomenon has been the subject of speculation for decades. Currently the blood-brain barrier (BBB) is defined largely in functional terms. It is a complex of both anatomic and physiologic constraints that permit free movement of water and small molecules between the vasculature and the brain tissue, yet prevent the parallel movement of molecules that are polar, large, or not highly lipid soluble.[14] Continuous tight junctions between adjacent capillary endothelial cells of the cerebral circulation provide passive restrictions to the movement of molecules larger than 0.5 nm. This excludes molecules not having the specific active or carrier-mediated transport systems that provide larger molecules their access to the CNS.[15]

These characteristics maintain the fragile, extremely critical biochemical environment that permits normal function of nervous system tissues. The BBB, in effect, provides "ground rules" for the movement of water and molecular species. It has no apparent direct relationship to the hemodynamic, myogenic, or metabolic mechanisms believed to be involved in autoregulation or coupling of CBF. Uncomplicated general anesthesia per se does not appear to disrupt the BBB; one study, however, suggests that deep levels of halothane anesthesia may produce brain concentrations high enough to have a toxic effect on the endothelial cells that maintain normal barrier function.[16] The process of aging itself also does not appear to disrupt the BBB in man. In the absence of neurologic or cerebrovascular disease, trauma, or intracranial hemorrhage, therefore, it can be assumed to be functionally intact in all healthy patients during and after general anesthesia.

INTRACRANIAL CONTENTS

Volume

Unique among major organs, the brain is enclosed in a rigid container. The skull dictates absolute constraints on the total volume of its contents. The three normal components of intracranial volume (ICV) are brain tissue itself, the vascular structures of the cerebral circulation and cerebral blood volume (CBV), and cerebrospinal fluid (CSF), an extension of brain interstitial fluid.

Brain tissue accounts for just over 80% of ICV; CBV represents 5% to 8% of the intracranial contents, and CSF occupies the remaining 7% to 10%. A pathologic fourth component consisting of brain tumor, hematoma, or foreign body may appear as part of a clinical syndrome. Brain tissue and CSF are both essentially liquid, and therefore not internally compressible, but both can expand acutely or chronically by processes of osmotic edema or failure of CSF reabsorption.[17]

Pressure

CSF is constantly produced by both active secretion and passive filtration at the choroid plexus at a rate of 20 to 25 mL/hour. CSF is reabsorbed at the arachnoid granulations at a rate directly proportional to CSF or ICP. Rates of CSF production and reabsorption are at equilibrium at ICP levels of 15 mm Hg or less, and therefore intracranial CSF volume remains constant at this pressure.[18] Abrupt reduction of intracranial CSF volume occurs after surgical drainage of CSF by cisternal or lumbar puncture, or after gross displacement of CSF from the intracranial to the lumbar subarachnoid compartments when there are sudden increases in the volumes of brain tissue or dilation of the cerebral vasculature. Slower changes in CSF volume reflect altered rates of CSF production or reabsorption, subacute changes in cerebrovascular or brain tissue volume, or accommodation for a slowly developing tumor or hematoma.

By virtue of its connection to the systemic circulation and the distensible or "floppy" nature of the cerebral veins, the cerebral vasculature and its blood volume function as a capacitor for intracranial volume change. This anatomy minimizes acute fluctuations in mean intracranial pressure. At equilibrium intracranial pressures, ICP is directly related to central venous pressure. In fact, continuous measurements of CSF pressure reveal phasic components that are produced by low-pressure cardiac pulsations transmitted retrograde along venous pathways. Gravitationally induced reductions in intravascular pressures are imposed on both the arterial and the venous sides of the cerebral circulation as, for example, during the negative "G forces" typical of aerospace activity. Loss of consciousness rarely reflects inadequacy of CPP under these circumstances, therefore, but rather is due to a fall in cardiac output resulting from pooling of blood in extracranial tissues.[19]

Cerebral venous pressure (CVP) is normally fractionally greater than ICP, and CPP therefore is defined as the hydrostatic gradient between mean arterial and cerebral venous pressures. Under these conditions, CPP is simply the driving pressure across the cerebral microcirculation. However, the definition of CPP changes to mean arterial minus CSF pressure when ICP exceeds CVP. The cerebral veins function as a network of "Starling resistors": pathologic elevations in ICP limit CBF by collapsing those intracranial venous segments not protected by the dura or by the cranium itself from external compression. Luminal collapse of these venous segments increases CVR and reduces CPP, thus compromising CBF even when mean arterial pressure remains unchanged.[20]

Compliance

The intracranial compliance curve describes the nonlinear, nearly exponential relationship between ICP and increases in the volumes of intracranial tissues. Increases in the volume of one or more intracranial components may occur without significant elevation of ICP if they are offset by enhanced rates of CSF reabsorption or by the bulk displacement of intracranial CSF to the vertebral subarachnoid compartment. When edematous brain tissue or dilated cerebral blood volume can no longer be easily accommodated by CSF displacement, however, the pressure/volume relationship undergoes abrupt transition from a compliant to a noncompliant state (Fig 3–2).

In a noncompliant state, intracranial contents may be subject to large increases in ICP that develop rapidly even when the volumetric increases in brain or vascular volume are very small. Intravenous fluid therapy that elevates central venous, and therefore cerebral venous,

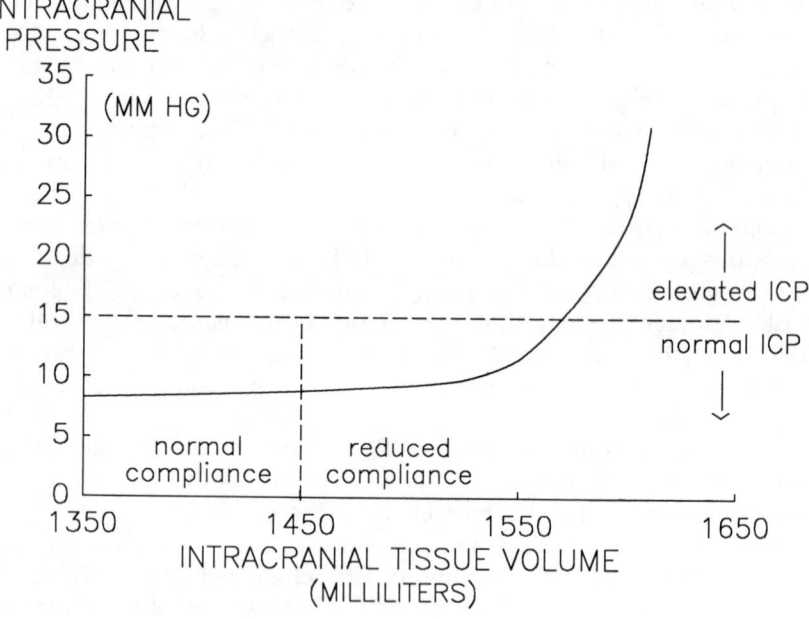

FIG 3–2.

Idealized representation of the relationship between intracranial pressure *(ICP)* and volume, generally referred to as the "intracranial compliance curve."[116] Brain tissue volumes are generalized for illustrative purposes; the "critical loading volume" required for transition to a state of reduced compliance varies with the site of its introduction into the cranial and vertebral compartments.[117]

pressures can further aggravate elevated ICP in patients with reduced compliance.[21] The diagnosis of reduced intracranial compliance is presumptive in any patient with a mass lesion exceeding 2 cm in diameter, or in whom there is evidence of reduced CSF volume, regardless of ICP. The principles of anesthetic management for patients with reduced compliance are essentially the same as those for patients with overt intracranial hypertension.

DISRUPTION OF CEREBRAL BLOOD FLOW HOMEOSTASIS

Autoregulation is effective over a range of CPP spanning approximately 100 mm Hg; with normal ICP, the cerebral circulation is maximally dilated at a mean arterial pressure of 50 or 60 mm Hg (see Fig 3–1). Once CVR is at its minimum value, CBF becomes a passive function of CPP, although it may still meet cerebral metabolic requirements. Even further reduction of CPP and CBF may be tolerated if the oxygenation of cerebral capillary blood is maximal and if cerebral metabolism is depressed. Autoregulation also occurs in other parts of the nervous system: adequate perfusion of the spinal cord is reportedly well maintained down to mean pressures of 50 mm Hg or less.[22]

Arterial Hypertension

Chronic arterial hypertension displaces the CBF autoregulation curve. CVR rises in direct proportion to CPP, but the relationship begins at the same relative lower limit of mean arterial blood pressures, about 60% of resting values.[23] The rightward shift of the autoregulation curve suggests that there is some CBF autoregulation even at systolic pressure values as high as 180 mm Hg. Intrinsic myogenic responses may be reinforced under these circumstances by an increase in sympathetic nervous system activity, since autoregulation during hypertension can be ablated by the administration of α-adrenergic blocking agents, or simulated in normal individuals by direct electrical stimulation of the cervical sympathetic ganglia.[24]

Nevertheless, an autoregulation "breakthrough" phenomenon with rising CBF is seen in acutely hypertensive individuals when mean arterial blood pressures exceed 150 mm Hg. Inability to further increase CVR under these circumstances may reflect either failure of myogenic control within the cerebral circulation or direct damage to the endothelial cells of the cerebral capillary bed, with subsequent release of substances capable of acting as arteriolar vasodilators or attacking the integrity of the tight junctions forming the anatomic basis of the BBB. This loss of barrier function produces vasogenic brain edema; consequent increases in brain tissue volume reduce intracranial compliance. Poorly controlled hypertensive patients, in fact, do experience a higher incidence of postoperative neurologic deficits than do well-controlled hypertensive patients.[25] Since effective CBF autoregulation returns with adequate antihypertensive therapy, preoperative evaluation and therapy may improve surgical outcome under these circumstances.[26]

Aging

Autoregulation of CBF is well maintained in the elderly individual, even in the presence of hypothermia and nonpulsatile flow.[27] Despite significant neuronal attrition and loss of brain mass, the tight functional coupling between regional brain metabolism and its blood flow also appears to be intact in healthy individuals across the entire range of human life span. Nor does age itself appear to disrupt tissue or vascular responsiveness to the cerebral metabolic environment.[28] By age 80 years, however, specific hemispheric CBF falls 20% to 30% to values of about 35 to 40 mL/100 g of tissue/min, however, because of reduced neuron density and age-related declines in perfusion needed for the lessened metabolic demands associated with the synthesis of fewer neurotransmitter molecules.[29, 30]

Intravenous Anesthesia

There is no evidence that anesthesia or other processes that simply alter levels of consciousness disrupt either CBF autoregulation or regional coupling significantly. During general anesthesia, there are localized increases in brain perfusion in those areas of the cerebral cortex that have increased electrical and metabolic activity. Acute afferent stimulation of the cortex by pain, laryngoscopy, or activation of skeletal muscle spindle pathways during succinylcholine fasciculation, for example, still produces increases in rCBF large enough to alter ICP.[31-33]

Intravenous anesthetic agents themselves generally produce reductions of hemispheric and regional CBF that are proportional to the depression of $CMRO_2$ characteristic of narcosis, loss of spontaneous skeletal muscle activity, and drug-induced coma (Fig 3–3). Narcotics, etomidate, barbiturates, benzodiazepines, and steroidal agents such as Althesin all depress rCBF as a secondary consequence of their primary

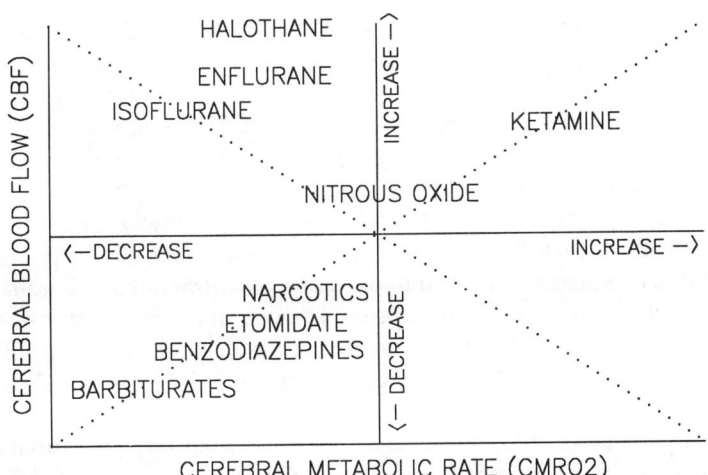

FIG 3–3.
General effects of anesthetic agents and adjuvants on cerebral blood flow *(CBF)* and metabolic rate *(CMRO₂)* in normotensive subjects. Distance from the intersection of the axes is proportional to the magnitude of the changes observed. Unlike intravenous anesthetics, inhalational agents uncouple the normal proportioning of *CBF* and *CMRO₂*, increasing CBF by decreasing CVR despite the fact that nervous system depression reduces perfusion requirements.

effect, the reduction of cortical electrical activity and cerebral metabolic rate.[34–38]

Brain concentrations sufficient to totally suppress electroencephalographic activity provide the maximal depression of CBF obtainable with the use of barbiturates.[39] The use of barbiturates to control $CMRO_2$, CBF, and, therefore, ICP, is therapeutically important for patients with head injuries. In contrast, anesthetic doses of ketamine induce cortical electrical and metabolic hyperactivity,[40, 41] and this agent, in fact, generates a significant increase in CBF and ICP.

Inhalational Anesthesia

The halogenated inhalational anesthetics, in contrast to the intravenous agents, uncouple CBF from its normal relationship to cerebral activity and $CMRO_2$.[36] Although halothane, enflurane, and isoflurane depress $CMRO_2$, they simultaneously decrease CVR and produce *increases* in CBV, perhaps by interfering with the calcium flux required for active contraction of vascular smooth muscle. Nitrous oxide does not appear to have any direct cerebral vasodilator properties.

The potent inhalational anesthetics do not, therefore, increase CBF directly. CBF increases only when CPP is maintained, or when it declines less than does CVR. Thus the *net* effect of an inhalational anesthetic on both intracranial and systemic hemodynamics ultimately determines whether it will produce increased CBF. When blood pressure and cardiac output are well maintained, halogenated inhalational agents produce mild to moderate increases in CBF (Fig 3–3). These changes are greatest initially, and then return slowly toward control values over a period of several hours. Because of the expansion of CBV, there is a corresponding decrease in intracranial compliance.[42] Presumably because it superimposes hypocapnic cerebral vasoconstriction mediated by a different mechanism, increases in both CBF and CBV produced by inhalational agents appear to be minimized by prior hyperventilation.[43]

The direct vasodilator effects of the potent halogenated inhalational anesthetics abolish intrinsic autoregulation of CBF at inspired concentrations at or above 0.5 to 1.0 minimum alveolar concentration (MAC).[44] This side effect may therefore produce a certain element of cerebral protection by establishing a state of "luxury" perfusion, since increases in CBF at normal mean arterial pressure significantly exceed the minimum perfusion requirements associated with the reduced $CMRO_2$ of a depressed functional state. Clinical studies of patients undergoing carotid endarterectomy do, in fact, suggest that adequate cerebral perfusion is maintained at lower carotid stump pressure during inhalational anesthesia than is required by unanesthetized patients, or by those receiving a narcotic-based, nitrous oxide–relaxant anesthetic.[45]

Cerebrospinal Fluid Dynamics

The direct effect of anesthetic agents on cerebrospinal fluid (CSF) dynamics has only recently been investigated. Enflurane appears to be unique among the inhalational anesthetics, increasing the rate of CSF formation while simultaneously increasing the resistance to its reabsorption. Steady increase of CSF volume and a consequent reduction of intracranial compliance become clinically significant after a period of several hours.[46] Halothane produces a smaller increase in the resistance to reabsorption of CSF and does not stimulate CSF production.[43] Similarly, isoflurane does not increase the rate of CSF formation, and may actually accelerate its reabsorption.[47]

Narcotic-based nitrous oxide anesthesia may also facilitate CSF reabsorption, increasing intracranial compliance significantly. Barbiturates, benzodiazepines, and etomidate have inconsistent effects on CSF dynamics, but probably depress CSF production to some degree, at least in high dosages.[48] For patients with reduced intracranial compliance, the interdependence between CSF dynamics and intracranial blood flow and blood volume is sufficiently important that the net effect of a given anesthetic approach on ICP reflects simultaneous changes both in actual CSF dynamics and in the total metabolic environment experienced by brain tissues perioperatively. The neuroendocrine response to stress itself may reduce CSF production by causing constriction of the choroid plexus.[49]

Carbon Dioxide

The systemic cardiovascular and respiratory control systems that maintain oxygenation and excretion of carbon dioxide are extraordinarily effective in maintaining these parameters within normal limits. Consequently, there is rarely a conflict between the adjustments of cerebral vasomotor tone initiated by CBF autoregulatory mechanism and those that would occur as a consequence of gross abnormalities of respiratory gases. However, cerebral vasomotion in direct response to arterial carbon dioxide levels is particularly relevant to anesthetic management because it has become common practice to control pulmonary ventilation, and therefore modify arterial blood gases, during general anesthesia.

Carbon dioxide can be a potent, direct modulator of CBF, in a manner that is independent of its other metabolic or autonomic effects. The relationship between CVR and partial pressure of CO_2 in arterial blood (Pa_{CO_2}) is inverse and nearly linear: CBF increases 2%, or about 1 mL/100 g/min, for every 1 mm Hg increase in carbon dioxide tension over a range of arterial values from 20 to 60 mm Hg.[50] Seen in physiologic perspective, however, carbon dioxide probably plays a relatively small role in the minute-to-minute maintenance of regional and hemispheric CBF. Arterial carbon dioxide tensions are kept tightly controlled within a very narrow range of normal values by sensitive central mechanisms of carbon dioxide ventilatory responsiveness (Chapter 7). Therefore, adjustments of CVR in response to altered arterial Pa_{CO_2} appear to represent an "override" function of greatest importance in anesthetized patients who are subject to controlled ventilation, blood gas abnormalities, altered CO_2 responsiveness, or perioperative respiratory insufficiency.

Cerebral Hypoxia

Superimposed hypocapnia or hypercapnia frequently produces graded, even dramatic changes in perioperative CBF. Hypoxemia, however, is rarely encountered by the cerebral circulation under normal circumstances. The profound and powerful cerebral hypoxic vasodilator response is essentially an all-or-none, pathophysiologic mechanism triggered at oxygen partial pressures of 40 mm Hg or less, when saturation falls below 60%. It is probably unrelated to the phenomena of coupling and autoregulation that operate in normal intact brain.

Both autoregulation and coupling of CBF are fragile mechanisms. They are disrupted by virtually any form of acute intracranial pathology or generalized systemic disruption, as well as by exposure to anesthetic agents and adjuvants with direct vasodilator properties. Diffuse cerebral vasodilation may accompany head trauma, profound arterial or intracranial hypertension, and all forms of circulatory collapse or gross systemic hypoxemia, hypercapnia, or acidosis. Intracranial hemorrhage, in contrast, can produce localized areas of vasospasm[51] that further extend the initial ischemic injury.[52]

When hemispheric CBF is compromised by inadequate cardiac output or by profound arterial hypotension to levels below those required for adequate CBF, cerebral tissue ischemia produces a sequence of symptoms described as the "ischemic penumbra."[53] Progressively severe cerebral dysfunction is suggested by electroencephalographic (EEG) abnormalities when CBF falls to 30 mL/100 g/min; loss of consciousness and gross EEG suppression occur as CBF approaches 20 mL/100 g/min; and neurally evoked electrical potentials disappear at 15 mL/100 g/min. Membrane-based ionic transport fails at CBF values of 10 mL/100 g/min or less, with irreversible nervous tissue injury if the perfusion deficit is not quickly repaid.[54]

BRAIN PROTECTION

Despite the frequency of very marked changes in arterial blood pressure, nonhypoxemic intraoperative cerebral injury is rare, 1 per 5,000 anesthetics or less, at least in patients having procedures other than carotid, cardiac, or intracranial surgery. The abolition of CBF autoregulation by halogenated inhalational anesthetics therefore probably does not in itself endanger the metabolic environment of the brain if adequate levels of perfusion and oxygenation are maintained. There appear to be no residual psychologic, intellectual, or behavioral consequences of a well-conducted, uncomplicated inhalational anesthetic.[55]

Brain protection by adjuvant drugs or techniques becomes an issue only when hemispheric CBF or rCBF is compromised, or when the patients are subject to profound hypotension, cardiac arrest, embolic events, or sustained systemic hypoxemia. The vulnerability of the brain to injury, and therefore the emphasis on its protection, reflects the inability of neural tissue to generate its energy requirements through mechanisms other than oxidative phosphorylation, as well as the catastrophic, irreversible consequences of hypoxic brain injury.

The complex interrelationships between mechanical, vascular, and metabolic elements within the skull and their associated pathologic conditions (Fig 3–4) determine the clinical strategies useful for management of specific patients. The primary step in brain protection,

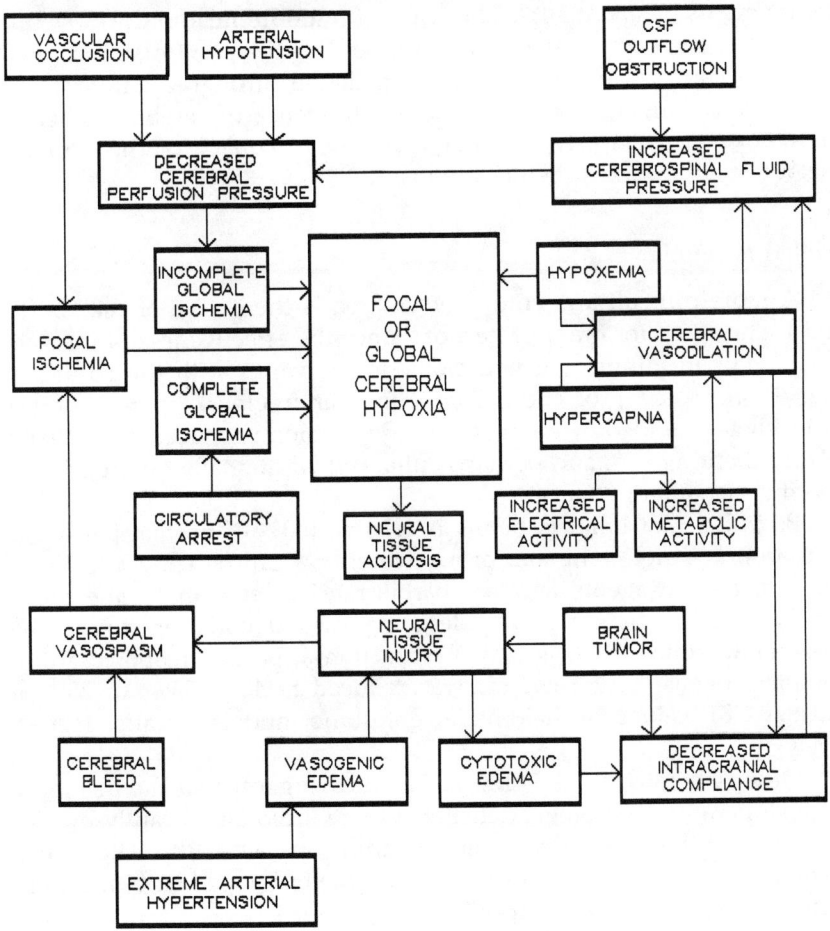

FIG 3–4.
Schematic representation of the complex interrelationships between the various pathophysiologic and mechanical phenomena associated with cerebral injury. Virtually all abnormalities ultimately produce neurologic injuries by leading directly, or indirectly, to focal or global cerebral tissue hypoxia.

however, is always maintenance of a benign cerebral metabolic environment. Adequacy of oxygen delivery is implicit in every rational anesthetic plan; maintenance of cardiac output, systemic arterial blood pressure, and full arterial oxygenation are always fundamental goals.

A favorable balance between oxygen supply and demand in neural tissues may be further enhanced by the depressed functional state of the nervous system during anesthesia, or by the incidental hypothermia common in the operating room. Every degree centigrade of reduction of the core body temperature further depresses most tissue oxygen requirements by about 10%. The effect of hypothermia on $CMRO_2$, unlike that of the barbiturates, continues beyond the point of cortical isoelectricity, and is therefore probably mediated through a different cellular mechanism. In general, however, tolerance of cerebral ischemia or hypoxemia is largely dependent on the adequacy of the cerebral metabolic environment before the insult.[56]

Global Ischemia

A more difficult and controversial area is the choice of the "best" anesthetic agent for brain protection, since the effectiveness of the various agents in minimizing neurologic injury varies with the nature of the lesion. Some protection from injury after global brain ischemia probably is provided by the metabolic depression produced by virtually all anesthetic agents, and perhaps enhanced additionally by drugs with specific vasodilator effects.

Provided that brain ischemia is relative (60% of normal perfusion or more), and not complete, protective effects can be shown for both the inhalational agents and the barbiturates at customary anesthetic dosage levels.[57] In patients undergoing carotid endarterectomy, the CBF below which EEG signs of dysfunction appear in response to incomplete hemispheric ischemia was reduced to 40%, 35%, or 25% of normal CBF values by halothane, enflurane, and isoflurane, respectively.[45]

Other laboratory[57] and clinical[58] studies suggest that the incidence of postoperative neurologic deficit can be reduced significantly by barbiturates if they are given before reductions of CPP. After head trauma, however, there is no evidence of the efficacy of barbiturates as a treatment for cerebral injury.[59]

Focal Ischemia

Focal brain ischemia due to local mechanical or obstructive phenomena produces a different pattern of neural injury than that seen after generalized reduction of hemispheric CBF. Since increased hemispheric CBF obviously cannot compensate for localized interruption of regional CBF, anesthetic plans for patients at risk must utilize metabolic depression rather than generalized cerebral vasodilation; brain tissue distal to the obstructed circulation is, in effect, isolated from the hemispheric cerebral dilator effects of these drugs. Isoflurane has been shown to provide a significant degree of protection from focal ischemic injury, but measurements of cerebral energy state in animal models suggest that barbiturates and benzodiazepines may be superior.[60] Intentional hypothermia has additional $CMRO_2$-suppressing qualities, but is rarely employed in current practice because of its cardiovascular side effects and technical complexity.

An anesthetic plan for perioperative brain protection includes, therefore, a threefold approach: (1) ensuring an optimal metabolic environment through the fundamental safeguards of adequate systemic hemodynamics and full arterial oxygenation; (2) pharmacologic and/or thermal suppression of functional, and therefore metabolic, brain activity to prolong the "safe" ischemia time; and (3) use of inhalational agents to minimize cerebral vascular resistance, allowing maximal CBF for any given level of CPP. Metabolic suppression with barbiturates may be an additional strategy for patients likely to experience focal insults.

For patients at high risk of global ischemia or sustained arterial hypotension, a combination of cerebral vasodilator and metabolic depressant drugs should be considered. Hyperglycemia accelerates the accumulation of lactic acid, producing vasomotor paralysis and "cerebral steal," intensifying cellular injury after an ischemic or hypoxic insult.[61, 62] Diabetic patients at high risk for neurologic injury must therefore be very tightly controlled,[63] and other patients at risk should have appropriate modification of intravenous fluid therapy to eliminate the possibility of iatrogenic hyperglycemia.[64]

Therapy

There is, for all practical purposes, no metabolic or therapeutic treatment for cerebral injuries due to profound ischemia or hypoxemia. The rapid depletion of neuronal adenosine triphosphate (ATP) and the subsequent efflux of intracellular potassium and ingress of calcium produce rapidly deteriorating conditions in a matter of minutes. Although ATP is rapidly regenerated and electrical activity may resume in many areas after reperfusion,[54] many of these apparently recovered tissues subsequently die during the course of "delayed neuronal necrosis." Destruction of cell and organelle membranes by free radicals or other mechanisms may, in fact, be accelerated by rapid imposition of an oxygen-rich environment.[65]

NEUROTRANSMITTERS AND ANESTHETIC REQUIREMENT

The brain is not a homogenous organ composed of repetitive subunits, but is instead a collection of neuronal subpopulations characterized by differing capacities for chemical synthesis and a variety of electrical responses to neurohumoral transmitter molecules. Neurotransmitters and associated neurotrophic hormones are the features unique to the CNS that make it possible for this organ, unlike others, to change, adapt, and adjust to external influences by altering communication patterns between its component tissues and cells.

A relationship between brain neurotransmitters and anesthetic requirement is also generally accepted, although the mechanism remains poorly understood. Measurements of anesthetic requirement for inhalational anesthesia suggest that MAC values may decline as much as 30% as a consequence of the depletion of brain catecholamines by antihypertensive drug therapy with α-methyldopa or reserpine[66]; amphetamine intoxication, in contrast, increases brain catecholamines and can double anesthetic requirement.[67]

Aging produces generalized reductions in excitatory neurotransmitters such as dopamine, norepinephrine, tyrosine, and serotonin; simultaneously, there is an associated, linear decline in relative anesthetic requirement (Chapter 2). Additional mechanisms through which aging may alter anesthetic requirement include the consequences of increased concentrations of the catabolic brain enzymes used to destroy neurotransmitters, the reduced affinity of specific brain receptors for neurotransmitters, or a generalized loss of fluidity in the membrane systems in which these receptors reside.[68]

INTRAOPERATIVE MONITORING OF NEUROLOGIC FUNCTION

Raw Electroencephalogram

Detection and recording of spontaneous electroencephalographic (EEG) activity at the scalp during general anesthesia were used almost 40 years ago in an attempt to establish quantitative, objective, and unambiguous assessment of the functional state of the nervous system during various levels of general anesthesia. It has not, however, yet fulfilled that objective. EEG does not provide reliable assessment of depth of anesthesia because of the relative subtlety of the continuum of EEG patterns associated with increasing depth of anesthesia. Interpretation is further complicated by the variability seen with the use of different anesthetic agents, and by inability to distinguish between drug-specific and event-specific forms of spontaneous electrical discharge, such as those seen with surgical stimulation or acute hypercarbia.[69]

Classically, seven levels of progressive EEG depression were observed for ether anesthesia.[70] Currently, depression of EEG is generally accepted to mean a progressive reduction in frequency from the normal range of 4 to 30 Hz toward an ultimate state of isoelectricity, with absence of perceptible wave-form activity. Halothane, isoflurane, barbiturates, and the benzodiazepines all produce transient initial increases in frequency and voltage, followed by sustained, progressive decreases in frequency and increases in voltage as anesthesia proceeds from the lightest to the deepest stages.[71]

Except for the brief periods of excitation, these EEG phenomena are not easily subdivided into discrete stages. However, some anesthetics have idiosyncratic effects: epileptiform spikes appear abruptly during light surgical levels of enflurane anesthesia, but are then rapidly suppressed at deeper levels.[72] In the absence of surgical stimulation virtually all anesthetic agents produce EEG isoelectricity at profoundly deep levels of anesthesia; this event is neither clinically relevant nor a practical routine measure of anesthetic depth.

Processed Electroencephalogram

Traditional intraoperative EEG analysis relies on subjective interpretation of raw EEG wave-forms derived from multiple channels. While sensitive and unlikely to give erroneous information, this form of monitoring requires considerable expertise and experience, and is therefore impractical for large-scale or routine "on-line" monitoring of anesthetized patients. Computerized signal processing and interest in quantitative assessment of the relationship between drug concentrations and effects have generated techniques of automated EEG processing, such as compressed spectral array (CSA) and density spectral array (DSA).[73] By portraying frequency, voltage, and time on a three-dimensional display generated by the sampling of electrical activity during discrete time intervals known as "epochs," these techniques preserve the sensitivity and richness of the raw EEG, yet facilitate analysis by a process of pattern recognition.

The cerebral function monitor (CFM), in contrast, reduces the complexity of the information contained in the raw EEG to a single numerical parameter. Although this eliminates the need for subjective interpretation, it sacrifices sensitivity, and may be useful only as an indicator of gross anesthetic overdosage or generalized, profound metabolic disruption.[69]

In either its raw or processed form, the EEG is a reliable indicator of mass electrical activity near the cortical surfaces of the brain; as such, it is appropriately utilized when the integrity of hemispheric brain metabolism is at significant risk.[74] During carotid endarterectomy, for example, decreases in EEG amplitude and frequency that last more than 10 minutes may predict postoperative neurologic sequelae[75]; both EEG changes and postoperative clinical findings are directly related to the duration of arterial occlusion.[76] When EEG signs of ischemia are noted, therefore, the insertion of a carotid shunt may reduce the incidence or severity of neurologic deficit under these circumstances. The value and practicality of EEG monitoring for patients having other procedures, such as cardiopulmonary bypass or controlled arterial hypotension, remain controversial, however.

Evoked Potentials

Monitoring of evoked potentials (EPs) provides access to cortical, subcortical, and spinal cord electrical signals that are generated in response to sensory stimuli.[77] Unlike the passive recording of continuous mass electrical activity used to obtain the EEG, this approach to neurologic monitoring excludes random activity by assessing specific, localized somatosensory (SSEP), auditory (AEP), or visual (VEP) evoked potential events.

Equipment requirements for EP are greater than for EEG, since stimulation intensity and timing must be precisely controlled. Measurements of the time lag between stimulus and response, or "latency," and of the amplitude of the EP can also be more difficult in anesthetized than in conscious patients. Inhalational anesthetics themselves have neuronal and synaptic effects that increase latency and decrease electrical amplitude of EP in proportion to their inspired concentrations,[78] although light to moderate levels of halothane, enflurane, or isoflurane do not preclude the use of the EP.

EP appears to have no compelling advantage over EEG when used for determination of depth of anesthesia. The primary application of EP at the present time remains the evaluation of electrical transmission along specific pathways during surgery in which there is a high probability of neurologic deficit. A practical example of EPs, in their simplest form, is the "wake-up test," which requires that anesthetic levels be reduced to the point where the patient responds physically to a spoken command to move his lower extremities at intervals during spinal fusion surgery for scoliosis or similar operations.[79]

Electrode-generated EP in anesthetized patients also appears to be a reliable indicator of spinal cord insult. Similarly, SSEP may be of value in identifying spinal cord ischemia during general anesthesia for thoracoabdominal aortic surgery. Brain stem auditory evoked potentials (BAEP) have had unique value for monitoring the integrity of the auditory nerve and its connections within the brain stem during neurosurgical procedures.

POSTANESTHETIC NEUROLOGIC DYSFUNCTION

Emergence From Anesthesia

If the metabolic requirements of the nervous system have been continuously met intraoperatively, normal neurologic function should return quickly and completely. Although most patients exhibit purposeful movements and are able to follow a command within minutes of the discontinuation of nitrous oxide, about 50% exhibit transient, and perhaps 5% exhibit sustained excitement or delirium, especially if the anesthetic routine includes the use of scopolamine or barbiturates.[80] Generally the transition from surgical levels of anesthesia to the fully awake state, like the induction of anesthesia, is characterized by a predominance of excitatory over inhibitory functions producing unmodulated shivering (Chapter 4), skeletal muscle hypertonicity, and transient deep hyperreflexia. These and other components of an abnormal neurologic examination, in fact, usually persist in varying degrees for up to 40 minutes after the inhalational anesthetic has been discontinued.[81]

Postanesthetic Phenomena

Persistent drowsiness, a sense of heaviness, headache, nausea and vomiting, anorexia, and malaise are nonspecific postanesthetic phenomena.[82] More common in women than in men, these symptoms are usually seen after general anesthetics of more than 20 minutes' duration despite meticulous attention to the pharmacologic details of the anesthetic technique,[83] although they occur with decreasing frequency and severity in adults of increasing age. While certain pharmacologic combinations may either exaggerate or suppress their incidence, these side effects are reflections of the general process of gross disruption of nervous system function, and commonly persist for up to 48 hours.[55]

Persistent somnolence after halothane anesthesia, however, may be drug specific. The degree and duration of residual neurologic depression after the use of this agent have been correlated with the total dosage of drug and exposure to its metabolic by-product, inorganic bromide.[84, 85] An additional element, direct metabolic toxicity, may occur after exposure to sustained concentrations of halothane that exceed 3 MAC: depleted brain high-energy stores, falling $CMRO_2$, and rising tissue lactate levels have been measured in animal studies. Under these circumstances, this agent may actually disrupt aerobic metabolism and poison the metabolic machinery of neural tissues.[86] Although the clinical relevance of these studies has yet to be established,[87] these data suggest that although all inhalational agents produce cerebral vasodilation and maximize CBF, depression of $CMRO_2$ per se may not guarantee an optimum cerebral metabolic environment.

The hallmark of direct neurotoxicity produced by general anesthetics is irritability, presenting clinically as convulsions or other signs of uninhibited electrocortical discharge.[88] For inhalational anesthetic molecules, a direct relationship between the degree of molecular halogenation, anesthetic potency, and epileptogenicity is well established.[89] Convulsions are also generally regarded as presumptive clinical evidence of gross nervous system toxicity when they follow the administration of narcotics, etomidate, Althesin, propranidid, and ketamine.[90-92] Ketamine may also produce sustained psychotic effects, hallucinations, and general cortical excitation.[93, 94]

Persistent Perioperative Dysfunction

Diffuse central nervous system depression or other persistent sequelae after emergence from anesthesia are, until proved otherwise, the manifestations of residual drug effects. Overt neurologic toxicity, a rare complication of anesthesia if it is administered with clinically approved agents, generally implies massive inadvertent overdosage or grossly inappropriate application. More commonly, acute perioperative brain syndromes are produced by underlying metabolic abnormalities, such as hyponatremia from water intoxication, or hypoglycemia or hyperglycemia in patients with diabetes or in those receiving drugs that cause disruption of normal carbohydrate metabolism. Other causes of acute brain syndrome immediately after surgery include hypothermia, hyperthermia, hypoxia, hypercarbia, or a combination of these mechanisms.[95]

Prompt identification of the source of prolonged CNS dysfunction after anesthesia is exceptionally important because cerebrovascular or metabolic insults, especially hypoxia, can be catastrophic and irreversible. They are distinguished from less-ominous residual drug effects by the greater severity or "denseness" of their symptoms and by their focal nature, especially if they reflect a cerebrovascular event. Also conspicuous is the absence of marked improvement in the first few hours after discontinuation of the anesthetic.

Persistent and severe neurologic deficits after anesthesia are usually caused by a metabolically destructive cerebral environment due to protracted arterial hypotension, cerebral embolism, cerebrovascular accident, or hypoxemia. The overall incidence of ultimately fatal or catastrophic perioperative cerebrovascular accident is only about 0.5%, a rate surprisingly low considering the high prevalence of cerebrovascular disease in the typical surgical population.[96]

Intermediate-Term Effects

In healthy young volunteers, the maximum postemergence alteration of mental function after 4 hours or more of routine, uncomplicated general anesthesia occurs the second day postoperatively. Presenting signs appear as weakness, lethargy, headache, and other somatic symptoms that rapidly become less severe and usually disappear by the end of the first week. In one out of every ten patients, more diffuse changes in nervous system function, such as altered affect, sleep disturbances, and loss of appetite, may persist, however, even after the first postoperative week.[82]

The cause of these intermediate-term patterns of nervous system dysfunction, 1 to 4 weeks after anesthesia and surgery, remains unknown. Comparison of psychologic functioning after general and regional anesthesia suggests that the process of general anesthesia itself is not responsible for residual neurologic dysfunction in this period.[97] The intermediate-term patterns may be due to exposure to specific anesthetic agents such as nitrous oxide, which has extremely subtle, subclinical effects on nervous system enzymatic function.[98]

More likely, however, these phenomena represent a functional reaction to tissue injury and the neuroendocrine stress response associated with surgery and illness. Most of the available data suggest that environmental factors are sufficiently important that they actually influence recovery from anesthesia. In general, favorable outcome seems to be determined primarily by mental status before surgery, the success and appropriateness of the surgical procedure involved, and the general level of emotional and material support available to the patients in the first 2 weeks postoperatively.[99] Prompt, continuous, and effective treatment of postoperative pain must be included as a support function: it minimizes stress and allows for sufficient rest, alleviating the deleterious effects of sleep deprivation and generalized fatigue associated with surgery and hospitalization in the shortest possible time.

NEUROLOGIC DYSFUNCTION AND REGIONAL ANESTHESIA

Acute Toxicity

In clinical practice, acute anesthetic toxicity is seen clinically in almost 2% of all patients receiving regional anesthesia; the primary manifestation is CNS irritability.[100] Inadvertent intravascular injection or unexpectedly high rates of local absorption of anesthetic solutions produces a spectrum of cortical disinhibition progressing from paresthesias to light-headedness, generalized tingling, trembling, and twitching. If severe, symptoms may proceed to convulsions and coma with respiratory arrest.

Cardiac arrest is almost always a late event, resulting from systemic hypoxemia, although in rare cases it may be a direct consequence of CNS effects.[101] Local anesthetics exhibit nervous system toxicity in direct proportion to their potency,[102] and they pass the blood-brain barrier easily and quickly.[103] Principles of therapy for CNS toxicity due to local anesthetics, therefore, include prompt ventilatory and circulatory support and pharmacologic suppression of persistent seizure activity to minimize the generation of areas of focal cerebral ischemia.[100]

Residual Effects and Sequelae

Although more limited in extent, the residual disruption of nervous system function that follows regional anesthesia may be as profound and, in many cases, more prolonged than that after general anesthesia. A protracted but qualitatively normal recovery period is not an adverse effect of regional anesthesia, but usually a manifestation of variability in individual pharmacokinetics of local anesthetic agents. Headache after lumbar puncture for spinal anesthesia is common and predictable with use of large-gauge needles and in patients who ambulate soon after surgery. Treatment of lumbar puncture headache with epidural blood patch, while usually successful, itself introduces the risk of infection and new neurologic injury.[104]

Other less frequent consequences of the mechanics of lumbar puncture include paresis of cranial nerves[105] and transient hearing loss.[106] Decreased hearing acuity may also occur, without headache, after lumbar puncture.[107] Postoperative backache occurs in 10% to 20% of all patients, regardless of choice of general or regional anesthetic technique, and is related largely to the duration of surgery, especially in procedures exceeding 2 hours' duration.[108]

Persistent adverse effects and neurologic deficit after regional anesthesia may reflect traumatic, ischemic, or toxic insults to the peripheral nervous system. The incidence of protracted neurologic sequelae or even permanent injury despite technically "correct" administration of regional anesthesia appears to be very low. Fear of permanent paralysis, once sufficiently promoted to almost eliminate the practice of spinal anesthesia,[109] has been largely discounted by objective, long-term studies of outcome.[110] However, the available data do suggest that significant long-term neurologic dysfunction after spinal, epidural, or plexus block anesthesia is a rare, but not unknown, phenomenon.[111] Two to four patients in every thousand who have received regional anesthesia of some type subsequently experience transient paresis, persistent numbness, or residual muscle weakness well after a period of time more than ample to dissipate the intended effects of local anesthetics.[112, 113]

Intraneural injection and other forms of trauma to peripheral nerves produced by the needles used to accomplish regional anesthesia appear to be the major source of residual nerve injury after conduction anesthesia.[114] Modifications of technique to eliminate the use of paresthesias for location of peripheral nerves and the choice of less-traumatic short-beveled needles may further reduce the incidence of traumatic injury.[111]

Residual dysfunction due to ischemia may also be reduced by the use of long-acting local anesthetics, instead of the more common current practice of adding vasoconstrictor drugs to short-acting local anesthetics to extend the duration of their effect. Finally, although virtually all attempted studies of neural toxicity have been done in the laboratory rather than under clinical circumstances, the results of these investigations are consistent: in high concentrations, and especially when prepared in solutions of high pH, local anesthetics appear to be capable of producing irreversible nerve injury and permanent neural blockade.[115] Consequently, the epidemiologic consequence of alkalinization of local anesthetics to accelerate the onset of nerve block remains to be established, since this is a relatively recent practice.

SUMMARY

The requirement of nervous system tissues for a continuous, consistent supply of oxygen and carbohydrate is met on an organ system level by myogenic autoregulation of cerebral blood flow, and at regional tissue sites by the active coupling of tissue metabolism and blood flow. Cerebral vasodilation by hypercapnia and hypoxia are superimposed on the underlying mechanisms that distribute CBF in proportion to local electrical activity in metabolic requirements. The relationship between the volume of intracranial contents and intracranial pressure is complex. However, even small increases in cerebral blood volume, such as those produced by halogenated inhalational anesthetics, can compromise CBF in patients with reduced intracranial compliance.

Since the anesthetic state itself does not appear to impair, and may actually improve, the balance between cerebral oxygen supply and demand, the fundamental principle of brain protection is the maintenance of cardiovascular and respiratory homeostasis. However, for patients at high risk of vascular occlusion, hypotension, or hypoxemia, various pharmacologic strategies utilizing metabolic depression or cerebral vasodilation have been advocated. Raw and processed EEG and evoked potentials have been used both to monitor depth of anesthesia and to identify intraoperative neurologic injury.

The "emergence phenomena" commonly seen after general anesthesia usually represent hyperreflexia due to transient disinhibition and persistent cortical depression. More subtle forms of dysfunction may persist for days, or, in rare cases, weeks, but these appear to be nonspecific responses to the stress of the perioperative environment. True drug-induced nervous system toxicity generally manifests itself as seizures or other forms of nervous system irritability. Persistent dysfunction after regional anesthesia is due most often to traumatic techniques of peripheral nerve identification, but may reflect, to some extent, the direct, drug-specific actions of local anesthetic agents.

REFERENCES

1. Fog M: Cerebral circulation. The reaction of the pial arteries to a fall in blood pressure. *Arch Neurol* 1937; 37:351–364.

2. Kety SS, Schmidt CF: The determination of cerebral blood flow in man by the use of nitrous oxide in low concentrations. *Am J Physiol* 1945; 143:53.
3. Kety SS: Circulation and metabolism in the human brain in health and disease. *Am J Med* 1950; 9:205–217.
4. Ingvar DH, Lassen NA: Regional blood flow of the cerebral cortex determined by Krypton-85. *Acta Physiol Scand* 1962; 54:325–338.
5. Landau WM, Freygang WH, Rowland LP, Sokoloff L, Kety SS: The local circulation of the living brain; values in the unanesthetized and anesthetized cat. *Trans Am Neurol Assoc* 1955; 80:125–129.
6. Lassen NA, Christensen MS: Physiology of cerebral blood flow. *Br J Anaesth* 1976; 45:719–734.
7. Kuschinsky W, Wahl M: Local chemical and neurogenic regulation of cerebral vascular resistance. *Physiol Rev* 1978; 58:656–689.
8. Winn HR, Rubio GR, Berne RM: The role of adenosine in the regulation of cerebral blood flow (editorial). *J Cereb Blood Flow Metab* 1981; 1:239–244.
9. Purves MJ: Control of cerebral blood vessels: Present state of the art. *Ann Neurol* 1978; 3:377–383.
10. Sercombe R, Aubineau P, Edvinsson L, et al: Neurogenic influence on local cerebral blood flow. *Neurology* 1975; 25:954–963.
11. Harder DR, Dernbach P, Waters A: Possible cellular mechanism for cerebral vasospasm after experimental subarachnoid hemorrhage in the dog. *J Clin Invest* 1989; 80:875–880.
12. James JM, Millar RA, Purves MJ: Observation on the extrinsic neural control of cerebral blood flow in the baboon. *Circ Res* 1969; 25:77–93.
13. Yoshida K, Meyer JS, Sakamoto K, Handa J: Autoregulation of cerebral blood flow. *Circ Res* 1966; 19:726–738.
14. Davson H: The blood brain barrier. *J Physiol (Lond)* 1976; 255:1–28.
15. Pollay M, Roberts PA: Blood brain barrier: A definition of normal and altered function. *Neurosurgery* 1980; 6:675–685.
16. Anderson RE, Michenfelder JD, Sundt TM Jr: Brain intracellular pH, blood flow, and blood brain barrier differences with barbiturate and halothane anesthesia in the cat. *Anesthesiology* 1980; 52:201–206.
17. Fishman RA: Brain edema. *N Engl J Med* 1975; 293:706–711.
18. Wood JH: Physiology, pharmacology, and dynamics of cerebrospinal fluid. In Wood JH (ed): *Neurobiology of Cerebrospinal Fluid.* New York, Plenum Press, 1980, pp 1–16.
19. Henry JP, Gauer OH, Kety SS, Kramer K: Factors maintaining cerebral circulation during gravitational stress. *J Clin Invest* 1951; 30:292–300.
20. Kety SS, Shenkin HA, Schmidt CF: The effects of increased intracranial pressure on cerebral circulatory functions in man. *J Clin Invest* 1948; 27:493–499.
21. Shenkin HA, Bezier HS, Bouzarth WF: Restricted fluid intake: Rational management of the neurosurgical patient. *J Neurosurg* 1976; 45:432–436.
22. Spargo PM, Tait AR, Knight PR, Kling TF: Effect of nitroglycerin-

induced hypotension on canine spinal cord blood flows. *Br J Anaesth* 1987; 59:640–647.

23. Kety SS, Hafkenschiel JH, Jeffers WA, Leopold JH, Shenken HA: The blood flow, vascular resistance and oxygen consumption of the brain in essential hypertension. *J Clin Invest* 1948; 27:511–514.
24. Rosenblum WI: Neurogenic control of cerebral circulation. *Stroke* 1971; 2:429–439.
25. Assidao CB, Donegan JH, Whitesell RC, Kalbfleisch JH: Factors associated with perioperative complications during carotid endarterectomy. *Anesth Analg* 1982; 61:631–637.
26. Strandgaard S: Autoregulation of cerebral blood flow in hypertensive patients. *Circulation* 1976; 53:720–727.
27. Brusino FG, Reves JG, Prough DS, Stump DA: The effect of age on cerebral blood flow autoregulation during hypothermic cardiopulmonary bypass. *Anesthesiology* 1987; 67:A10.
28. Schieve JF, Wilson WP: The influence of age, anesthesia and cerebral arteriosclerosis on cerebral vascular activity to CO_2. *Am J Med* 1953; 11:171–174.
29. Melamed E, Lavy S, Bentin S, Cooper G, Rinot X: Reduction in blood flow during normal aging in man. *Stroke* 1980; 11:31–35.
30. McGeer EG, McGeer PL: Age changes in the human for some enzymes associated with metabolism of catecholamine, GABA, and acetylcholine. *Adv Behav Biol* 1975; 16:287–305.
31. Burney R, Winn R: Increased cerebrospinal fluid pressure during laryngoscopy and intubation for induction of anesthesia. *Anesth Analg* 1975; 54:687–690.
32. Lanier WL, Milde JH, Michenfelder JD: Cerebral stimulation following succinylcholine in dogs. *Anesthesiology* 1986; 64:551–559.
33. Stirt JA, Grosslight KR, Bedford RF, Vollmer D: "Defasciculation" with metocurine prevents succinylcholine-induced increases in intracranial pressure. *Anesthesiology* 1987; 67:50–53.
34. Michenfelder JD, Theye RA: Effects of fentanyl, droperidol, and Innovar on canine cerebral metabolism and blood flow. *Br J Anaesth* 1971; 43:630–635.
35. Renou AM, Vernhiet J, Macrez P, et al: Cerebral blood flow and metabolism during etomidate anaesthesia in man. *Br J Anaesth* 1978; 50:1047–1051.
36. Smith AL, Wollman H: Cerebral blood flow and metabolism: Effects of anesthetic drugs and techniques. *Anesthesiology* 1972; 36:378–400.
37. Fitch W, McGeorge AP, MacKenzie ET: Anaesthesia for studies of the cerebral circulation: A comparison of phencyclidine and Althesin in the baboon. *Br J Anaesth* 1978; 50:985–991.
38. Rockoff MA, Naughton KVH, Shapiro HM, et al: Cerebral circulatory and metabolic response to intravenously administered lorazepam. *Anesthesiology* 1980; 53:215–218.
39. Steen PA, Newberg LA, Milde JH, Michenfelder JD: Hypothermia and

barbiturates: Individual and combined effect on canine cerebral oxygen consumption. *Anesthesiology* 1983; 58:527–532.

40. Dawson B, Michenfelder JD, Theye RA: Effects of ketamine on canine cerebral blood flow and metabolism. *Anesth Analg* 1971; 50:443–447.

41. Nelson SR, Howard RB, Cross RC, Samson F: Ketamine-induced changes in regional glucose utilization in the rat brain. *Anesthesiology* 1980; 52:330–334.

42. Schettini A, Moreshead G: Effects of halothane and sodium thiopentone on surface brain pressure and brain electrical impedance in dogs with normal intracranial tension. *Br J Anaesth* 1978; 50:1003–1012.

43. Artru AA: Relationship between cerebral blood volume and CSF pressure during anesthesia with halothane or enflurane in dogs. *Anesthesiology* 1983; 58:533–539.

44. Smith AL, Neigh JL, Hoffman JC: Effects of general anesthesia on autoregulation of cerebral blood flow in man. *J Appl Physiol* 1970; 29:665–669.

45. Michenfelder JD, Sundt TM, Fode N, Sharbrough FW: Isoflurane when compared to enflurane and halothane decreases the frequency of cerebral ischemia during carotid endarterectomy. *Anesthesiology* 1987; 67:336–340.

46. Artru AA, Nugent M, Michenfelder JD: Enflurane causes a prolonged and reversible increase in the rate of CSF production in the dog. *Anesthesiology* 1982; 57:255–260.

47. Artru AA: Isoflurane does not increase the rate of CSF production in dogs. *Anesthesiology* 1984; 60:193–197.

48. Artru AA: Dose-related changes in the rate of cerebrospinal fluid formation and resistance to reabsorption of cerebrospinal fluid following administration of thiopental, midazolam, and etomidate in dogs. *Anesthesiology* 1988; 69:541–546.

49. Faraci FM, Mayhan WG, Farrell WJ, Heistad DD: Humoral regulation of blood flow to choroid plexus: Role of arginine vasopressin. *Circ Res* 1988; 63:373–379.

50. Kety SS, Schmidt CF: The effects of altered tensions of carbon dioxide and oxygen on cerebral blood flow and cerebral oxygen consumption of normal young men. *J Clin Invest* 1948; 27:487–492.

51. Harder DR, Dernbach P, Waters A: Possible cellular mechanism for cerebral vasospasm after experimental subarachnoid hemorrhage in the dog. *J Clin Invest* 1987; 80:875–880.

52. Steen PA, Newberg LA, Milde JH, Michenfelder JD: Cerebral blood flow and neurologic outcome when nimodipine is given after complete cerebral ischemia in the dog. *J Cereb Blood Flow Metab* 1984; 4:82–87.

53. Astrup J, Siesjo B, Symon L: Thresholds in cerebral ischemia—the ischemic penumbra (editorial). *Stroke* 1981; 12:723–725.

54. Nilsson B, Norberg K, Siesjo BK: Biochemical events in cerebral ischaemia. *Br J Anaesth* 1975; 47:751–760.

55. Storms LH, Stark AH, Calverley RK, Smith NT: Psychological functioning after halothane or enflurane anesthesia. *Anesth Analg* 1980; 59:245–249.

56. Siesjo B: Cerebral circulation and metabolism. *J Neurosurg* 1984; 60:883–903.
57. Newberg LA, Michenfelder JD: Cerebral protection by isoflurane during hypoxemia or ischemia. *Anesthesiology* 1983; 59:29–35.
58. Nussmeier NA, Arlend C, Slogoff S: Neuropsychiatric complications after cardiopulmonary bypass: Cerebral protection by a barbiturate. *Anesthesiology* 1986; 64:165–170.
59. Ward JD, Becker DP, Miller JD: Failure of prophylactic barbiturate coma in the treatment of severe head injury. *Neurosurgery* 1985; 62:383–388.
60. Nugent M, Artru AA, Michenfelder JD: Cerebral metabolic, vascular and protective effects of midazolam maleate. *Anesthesiology* 1982; 56:172–176.
61. Siemkowicz E: The effect of glucose on restitution after transient cerebral ischemia: A summary. *Acta Neurol Scand* 1985; 71:417–427.
62. Lanier W, Stanland KJ, Scheithauer BW, Milde JH, Michenfelder JD: The effects of dextrose infusion and head position on neurologic outcome after complete cerebral ischemia in primates: Examination of a model. *Anesthesiology* 1987; 66:39–48.
63. D'Alecy LG, Lundy EF, Barton KJ, Zelenock GB: Dextrose-containing intravenous fluid impairs outcome and increases death after eight minutes of cardiac arrest and resuscitation in dogs. *Surgery* 1986; 100:505–511.
64. Longstreth WT, Inui T: High blood glucose level on hospital admission and poor neurological recovery after cardiac arrest. *Ann Neurol* 1984; 15:59–63.
65. Kirino T: Delayed neuronal death in the gerbil hippocampus following ischemia. *Brain Res* 1982; 239:57–69.
66. Miller RD, Way WL, Eger EI II: The effects of alpha-methyldopa, reserpine, guanethidine, and iproniazid on minimum alveolar requirement (MAC). *Anesthesiology* 1968; 29:1094–1098.
67. Johnston RR, Way WL, Miller RD: Alterations of anesthetic requirement by amphetamine. *Anesthesiology* 1972; 36:357–363.
68. Muravchick S: Immediate and long-term nervous system effects of anesthesia in elderly patients. *Clin Anesthesiol* 1986; 4:1035–1045.
69. Levy WJ, Shapiro HM, Maruchak G, Meathe E: Automated EEG processing for intraoperative monitoring. *Anesthesiology* 1980; 53:223–236.
70. Courtin RF, Bickford RG, Faulconer A: The classification and significance of electroencephalographic patterns. *Proc Mayo Clin* 1950; 25:197–206.
71. Eger EI II, Stevens WC, Cromwell TH: The electroencephalogram in man anesthetized with Forane. *Anesthesiology* 1971; 35:504–508.
72. DeJongh RH, Heavner JE: Correlation of the Ethrane electroencephalogram with motor activity in cats. *Anesthesiology* 1971; 35:474–481.
73. Sebel PS, Bovill JG, Wauguier A, Rog P: Effects of high-dose fentanyl anesthesia on the electroencephalogram. *Anesthesiology* 1981; 55:203–211.
74. Anderson EM, Carney AL, Page L: Carotid and vertebral artery surgery, EEG monitoring, and the operating room. *Adv Neurol* 1981; 30:361–377.

75. Rampil IJ, Holzer JA, Quest DO, Rosenbaum SH, Correll JW: Prognostic value of computerized EEG analysis during carotid endarterectomy. *Anesth Analg* 1983; 62:186–192.

76. Collice M, Arena D, Fontana RA, Mola M, Galbiati N: Role of EEG monitoring and cross-clamping duration in carotid endarterectomy. *J Neurosurg* 1986; 65:815–819.

77. Grundy BL: Monitoring of sensory evoked potentials during neurosurgical operations: Methods and applications. *Neurosurgery* 1982; 11:556–575.

78. Pathak KS, Ammadio M, Kalamchi A, Scoles PV, Shaffer JW, Mackay W: Effects of halothane, enflurane, and isoflurane on somatosensory evoked potentials during nitrous oxide anesthesia. *Anesthesiology* 1987; 66:753–757.

79. Vauzelle C, Stagnara P, Jouvinroux P: Functional monitoring of spinal cord activity during spinal cord surgery. *Clin Orthop* 1973; 93:173–178.

80. Eckenhoff JE, Kneale DH, Dripps RD: The incidence and etiology of post-anesthetic excitement; a clinical survey. *Anesthesiology* 1961; 22:667–673.

81. Rosenberg H, Clofine R, Bialik O: Neurologic changes during awakening from anesthesia. *Anesthesiology* 1981; 54:125–130.

82. Davison LA, Steinhelber JC, Eger EI II, Sevens WC: Psychological effects of halothane and isoflurane. *Anesthesiology* 1975; 43:313–324.

83. Fahy A, Marshall M: Post-anesthetic morbidity in outpatients. *Br J Anaesth* 1969; 41:433–438.

84. Tinker JH, Gandolfi AJ, VanDyke RA: Elevation of plasma bromide levels in patients following halothane anesthesia: Time correlation with total halothane dosage. *Anesthesiology* 1976; 44:194–196.

85. Meldgaard OT, Cold GE: Serum bromide after general anaesthesia with halothane. *Acta Anaesthesiol Scand* 1979; 23:513–518.

86. Michenfelder JD, Theye RA: *In vivo* toxic effects of halothane on canine cerebral metabolic pathways. *Am J Physiol* 1975; 299:1050–1055.

87. Kofke WA, Hawkins RA, Davis DW, Biebuyck JF: Comparison of the effects of volatile anesthetics on brain glucose metabolism in rats. *Anesthesiology* 1987; 66:810–813.

88. Steen PA, Michenfelder JD: Neurotoxicity of anesthetics. *Anesthesiology* 1979; 50:437–453.

89. Rudo FG, Krantz JC Jr: Anaesthetic molecules. *Br J Anaesth* 1974; 46:181–189.

90. Clarke RSJ, Dundee JW, Garrett RT: Adverse reactions to intravenous anesthetics. A survey of 100 reports. *Br J Anaesth* 1975; 47:575–585.

91. Thompson GE: Ketamine-induced convulsions. *Anesthesiology* 1972; 37:662–663.

92. Barron DW: Propranidid in epilepsy. *Anaesthesia* 1974; 29:445–447.

93. Johnson BD: Psychosis and ketamine. *Br Med J* 1971; 4:428–429.

94. Meyers EF, Charles P: Prolonged adverse reactions to ketamine in children. *Anesthesiology* 1978; 49:39–40.

95. Haugen FP: The failure to regain consciousness after general anesthesia. *Anesthesiology* 1961; 22:657–666.
96. Djokovic JL, Hedley-Whyte J: Prediction of outcome of surgery and anesthesia in patients over 80. *JAMA* 1974; 242:2301–2306.
97. Ghonheim MM, Hinrichs JV, O'Hara MW, et al: Comparison of psychologic and cognitive functions after general or regional anesthesia. *Anesthesiology* 1988; 69:507–515.
98. Deacon R, Lumb M, Perry J, et al: Inactivation of methionine synthase by nitrous oxide. *Eur J Biochem* 1980; 104:419–423.
99. Weissberg MP: Suicide and surgery, Guerra F, Aldrete JA (eds): in *Psychological Responses to Anesthesia and Surgery*, Orlando, Fla., Grune & Stratton, 1980, pp 27–35.
100. Moore DC, Bridenbaugh LD: Oxygen: The antidote for systemic toxic reactions from local anesthetic drugs. *JAMA* 1960; 174:842–847.
101. Blumhart LD, Smith PEM, Owen L: Electrocardiographic accompaniments of temporal lobe epileptic seizures. *Lancet* 1986; 1:1051–1056.
102. Reynolds F: Adverse effects of local anesthetics. *Br J Anaesth* 1987; 59:78–95.
103. Usubiaga JE, Moya F, Wikinski JA, et al: Relationship between the passage of local anesthetics across the blood brain barrier and their effects on the central nervous system. *Br J Anaesth* 1967; 39:943–947.
104. Cornwall RD, Dolan WM: Radicular back pain following lumbar epidural blood patch. *Anesthesiology* 1975; 43:692–693.
105. Lee JJ, Roberts RB: Paresis of the fifth cranial nerve following spinal anesthesia. *Anesthesiology* 1978; 49:217–218.
106. Vandam LD, Dripps RD: Long-term follow-up of patients who received 10,098 spinal anesthetics. Part II: Incidence and analysis of minor sensory neurologic defects. *Surgery* 1955; 38:463–469.
107. Wang LP, Fog J, Bove M: Transient hearing loss following spinal anesthesia. *Anaesthesia* 1987; 42:1258–1263.
108. Middleton MJ, Bell CR: Postoperative backache: Attempts to reduce incidence. *Anesth Analg* 1965; 44:446–448.
109. Kennedy F, Effron AS, Perry G: The grave spinal cord paralyses caused by spinal anesthesia. *Surg Gynecol Obstet* 1950; 91:385–398.
110. Dripps RD, VanDam LD: Long-term follow-up of patients who received 10,098 spinal anesthetics: Failure to discover major neurological sequelae. *JAMA* 1954; 156:1486–1491.
111. Selander D, Edshage S, Wolff T: Paresthesiae or no paresthesiae? *Acta Anaesthiol Scand* 1979; 23:27–33.
112. Thorsen G: Neurological complications after spinal anaesthesia. *Acta Chir Scand* 1947; 95(suppl 121):1–272.
113. Kane RE: Neurologic deficits following epidural or spinal anesthesia. *Anesth Analg* 1981; 60:150–160.
114. Wooley EJ, VanDam L: Neurological sequelae of brachial plexus nerve block. *Ann Surg* 1959; 149:53–60.
115. Truant AP, Takman B: Differential physico-chemical and neuropharma-

cologic properties of local anesthetic agents. *Anesth Analg* 1959; 38:478–484.

116. Miller JD, Garibi J, Pickard JD: Induced changes of cerebrospinal fluid volume. *Arch Neurol* 1973; 28:265–269.

117. Sullivan HG, Miller JD, Griffith RL III, Becker DP: CSF pressure transients in response to epidural and ventricular volume loading. *Am J Physiol* 1978; 234:R167–R171.

4

Autonomic Homeostasis During Anesthesia

The autonomic nervous system monitors and controls the general maintenance of vital body functions. Implied in the term *autonomic* is the automatic self-regulation of metabolic functions. Physiologic variables are maintained within normal limits despite inevitable variations of activity and environment.

Although it is relatively easy to examine and measure the activity of isolated tissues and organs, studies of discrete organ systems do not explain or describe the integrated, moment-to-moment determination of cardiac output, arterial oxygenation, renal plasma flow, and other essential clinical indices of bodily function in the awake or in the anesthetized state. The integrated, overall metabolic activity of the human body is, in effect, more than the simple sum of the organs and tissues of which it is composed. In the absence of disease, the capacities of end-organs themselves do not determine physiologic status. Rather, end-organs are components within a complex system; they function at various levels of activity, modulated by the interplay of local receptor feedback activity and central neuronal and circulating hormonal and chemical elements.

General and regional anesthetics have important, and in some cases even predominant, effects on specific end-organs, but the extent to which anesthetic agents disrupt metabolic homeostasis almost always reflects the degree to which they impair the functioning of autonomic control systems. No meaningful discussion of the role of the autonomic nervous system is possible without appreciation of some basic concepts of control system theory. The chapter that follows also discusses the physiology and pathophysiology of the autonomic nervous system as it functions in the anesthetized individual during and after exposure to specific anesthetic agents.

AUTONOMIC "ENGINEERING"

A system is a collection of interconnected components.[1] An "open-loop" system directs incoming (afferent) information to an effector end-organ, which then produces outgoing (efferent) activity (Fig 4–1). The efferent signal from this system will reflect both the intensity of the input and the degree of "gain" or amplification applied to this input before it is sent to the effector. The functional capacity of the effector itself defines the range of possible output levels from minimum to maximal. Whatever the intensity of the input signal or the degree of its amplification, the functional level of the system, as measured by output, cannot exceed the maximal capacity of the effector that generates the output. In systems with multiple effectors, if the output from one effector then provides the input for the next, maximal output of this system is limited by the maximal capacity of the least capable effector.

"Closed-loop" systems, by definition, have some form of interconnection between efferent and afferent signals. They "feed back" effer-

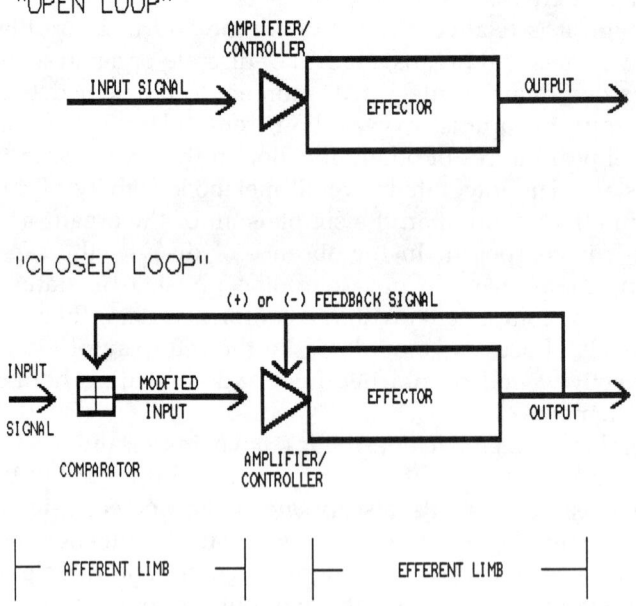

FIG 4–1.
Schematic diagram of open- and closed-loop circuit models for reflex arcs. In autonomic control systems, the amplifier/controller components are thought to be within the hypothalamus, but they may have no specific or discrete anatomic location. Comparators may exist at both spinal cord and higher levels.

ent information to the input side of the system, either directly or indirectly. Output is therefore related not only to the amount of input but also to the current functional level of the system. Feedback systems provide the basis for a self-regulating or "servo" capacity not possible in open-loop systems. The signal that is fed back to the input side of the system may be added to, or subtracted from, the original input signal before it is directed to the effector. Thus the feedback itself can be "negative," limiting further output as output increases, or it can be "positive," enhancing output at an accelerating rate as the activity of the system increases. In either case, the level of effector function becomes self-regulating.

The interaction between a driver, the engine in his automobile, and the speed of his vehicle provides a simple and familiar analogy for a closed-loop system. Just as organ system capacity itself is rarely a determinant of moment-to-moment functional level for physiologic parameters, the peak horsepower of an automobile does not control its speed in daily use. The engine is the effector for the system, controlled by a throttle. Functioning as an open loop, the engine would either idle at minimum throttle, or when the driver pressed the accelerator, the engine would produce power (output), which then translates mechanically into vehicle velocity. The vehicle would lurch forward, its speed a function only of the ability of its engine to produce horsepower and overcome aerodynamic and frictional resistance. In a closed-loop mode, however, the driver functions as the "comparator," sending input of variable magnitude through the throttle to adjust speed upward or downward. Speed is maintained at a constant or a desired level as the driver continually uses information regarding vehicle speed to modulate throttle position. The power developed by the engine is therefore a consequence, rather than a determinant, of the set-point for vehicle speed.

In a closed-loop system, maximal effector function will determine the output level of the system only when the set-point requires that the effector function at its maximum capacity. However, a seriously damaged power plant or a diseased organ system may be unable to provide adequate output even for modest demands. This situation represents a breakdown of one of the components of the system, not a characteristic of the normal functioning of a closed-loop system.

Perhaps the most well-described biologic closed-loop feedback system is that which provides control of arterial blood pressure by specialized baroreceptors. This feedback system, however, like virtually all such control loops, is part of yet a larger group of related feedback mechanisms for hemodynamic and metabolic function that are arranged in a hierarchical fashion (Fig 4–2). Individual set-points modulate output from each control loop, but to ensure functional levels compatible with the greater needs of the entire organism, there is a provision for communication between the various loops in this multilevel arrangement.

The driver of an automobile may consider increasing vehicle speed to minimize the time required to arrive at home, but he must also modulate this set-point in accordance with his awareness of local speed limits. Similarly, multilevel biologic systems control functional levels in an integrated fashion that provides conditions optimal for the entire organism. While none of the set-points can be mutually exclusive or grossly contradictory, all have a relative priority in the overall hierarchy that is based on the importance of their contribution to general metabolic balance. In the intact organism, no physiologic function occurs in isolation.

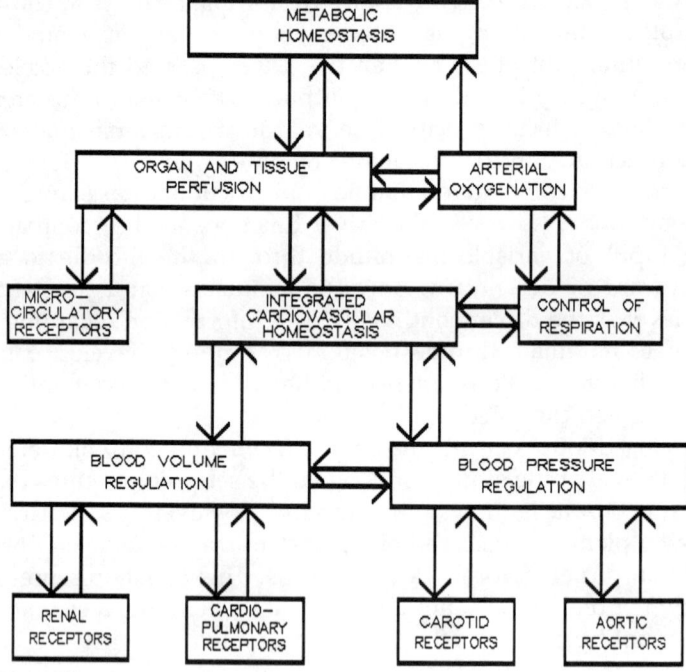

FIG 4–2.
Autonomic control systems exist within a hierarchy of interactive control systems. The extensive interrelationships make it unlikely that a single, rigid "set-point" exists for each function, and none are truly independent of overall metabolic status.

The primary role of the autonomic nervous system is to integrate this extraordinarily complex network of control loops in order to maintain a balanced flow of effector functions compatible with overall metabolic stability. Much remains to be known about the exceedingly complicated mechanisms that support Claude Bernard's deceptively simple concept of the milieu intérieur.[2]

BARORECEPTOR FUNCTION AND MAINTENANCE OF BLOOD PRESSURE

Baroreflexes

Baroreflex control of heart rate is the most completely studied biologic feedback control system relevant to anesthetic management.[3] The relationship between heart rate and blood pressure is also of special interest to anesthesiologists because these variables are the two most intensively and consistently monitored physiologic signs in clinical practice. They are valuable indices of the adequacy of anesthetic depth and provide a noninvasive means to assess the status of circulating blood volume. Assumptions and conclusions regarding overall intraoperative physiologic homeostasis are often based entirely on comparison of these vital signs with their usual or "normal" range.

The baroreflex system is a virtual prototype for biologic closed-loop feedback control systems: blood pressure is the input and heart rate the output of this system. Gain (amplification, or "responsiveness") is quantified by the slope of the curve that defines the relationship between systolic blood pressure and heart rate, frequently expressed as the R-R interval of the electrocardiogram on a beat-by-beat basis. Both the slope and the positioning of the curve relative to the axes are important characteristics of the relationship. The curve may be shifted relative to the axes independent of any changes in slope if the gain of the relationship between these two variables is maintained over a range of blood pressure or heart rate different from that encountered in the awake, unanesthetized state. Although linear across most of its range, like most biologic interactions this relationship is fundamentally sigmoid in nature, demonstrating a "threshold" or minimum value for input below which no change is seen in output. In addition, there is a plateau at the upper limits of the system that represents a rapid fall-off in responsiveness when its maximal capacity to effect further change is approached. Also, the gain or responsiveness of the system is modulated by influences from higher nervous system centers.

Carotid Sinus Mechanisms

Typically, tests of baroreflex responsiveness require acute distention of the baroreceptor elements of the carotid sinus, usually accomplished by elevating arterial pressure with peripherally acting pressor drugs, or by the application of negative pressure to the carotid sinus itself.[4] The responsiveness of the baroreflex system to acute reduction of arterial pressure achieved through gravitational tilt or acute arterial occlusion has also been studied, but less extensively.

In normal man, the rate at which the R-R interval increases in response to rising systolic arterial pressure averages about 20 to 30 msec/mm Hg, with considerable individual variation.[3] Heart rate slows because distortion of the tissues of the carotid sinus increases electrical activity in the carotid sinus nerves, stimulating the vagal nucleus and providing inhibitory (negative) feedback to the vasomotor and cardiac control centers of the brain stem. Although the exact medullary interconnections remain to be described, it is generally assumed that this negative feedback is actively processed by interconnecting neurons; stimulation of vagal efferent activity may be associated with reciprocal inhibition of the cell bodies for sympathetic efferent neurons, or may occur independently.[4, 5]

There is evidence that increased vagal tone is the predominant response to arterial hypertension in awake, unsedated individuals; in contrast, decreased sympathetic outflow may be the major consequence of carotid sinus stimulation in anesthetized subjects.[6] The carotid baroreflex system also appears to have greater sensitivity to falling than to rising arterial pressure.[7, 8] The slope or responsiveness of the carotid baroreflex response mechanism is reduced progressively by increasing age, and is impaired by the presence of chronic hypertension, with or without arteriosclerosis.[9] It may also be modified by hypercarbia or hypocarbia, although it appears to be independent of arterial oxygenation over a wide range of values.[10]

The primary function of the baroreflex system is the maintenance of arterial blood pressure homeostasis. The normal set-point for systolic blood pressure is more than adequate to provide a mean arterial pressure that permits perfusion of all bodily tissues. Cardiac output itself is not directly controlled by the baroreflex system, but is determined indirectly as a consequence of the changes in vascular resistance within each organ system, which serve to fine-tune local blood flow according to specific regional needs.

Blood Pressure Homeostasis During Anesthesia

Arterial hypotension is the most common hemodynamic complication that occurs during general or regional anesthesia. The anesthetic state itself, therefore, or the agents with which it is produced, must disrupt the effective functioning of this baroreflex mechanism. Patterns of change for blood pressure, heart rate, and autonomic activity during anesthesia are well established,[11] but the precise mechanism by which anesthetic agents disrupt homeostasis of blood pressure has been far more difficult to establish.[12]

Every potent inhalational anesthetic, including diethyl ether and cyclopropane, has direct depressant effects on both cardiac and vascular muscle. Ether and cyclopropane produce central sympathomimetic effects, however, and the release of catecholamines by this mechanism compensates for direct effector depression.[13] Blood pressure and heart rate are therefore maintained at or near the usual autonomic set-points when anesthesia is accomplished with these agents. Nevertheless, it is now also clear that even with normal blood pressure and heart rate, autonomic reactivity as measured by baroreflex responsiveness is significantly altered by virtually all anesthetic agents.

During general anesthesia, the self-regulation of vital functions, the essence of autonomic control, is disrupted, functioning at only 20% to 50% of its normal degree of effectiveness. The flattening of the slope of the baroreflex response curve may, in addition, be associated with an upward or downward shift, depending on the net effect of the anesthetic agent on heart rate and blood pressure (Fig 4–3). Baroreflex responsiveness is impaired by halothane in a dose-related manner, in contrast to the similarly potent, but dose-independent, effects of enflurane.[14] Isoflurane has lesser effects on baroreflex responsiveness, which become clinically significant as end-tidal concentrations approach 2 MAC.[15] The effects are rapidly reversible: both the slope and the set-point for baroreflex responsiveness return to normal within 10 to 20 minutes of discontinuation of either barbiturate or halothane anesthesia.[16]

Mechanism of Action

Analysis of anesthetic-induced changes in baroreflex responsiveness can be accomplished even without precise knowledge of normal anatomic or neurochemical mechanisms. Direct recording from the afferent limbs of this autonomic reflex arc suggests that, peripherally,

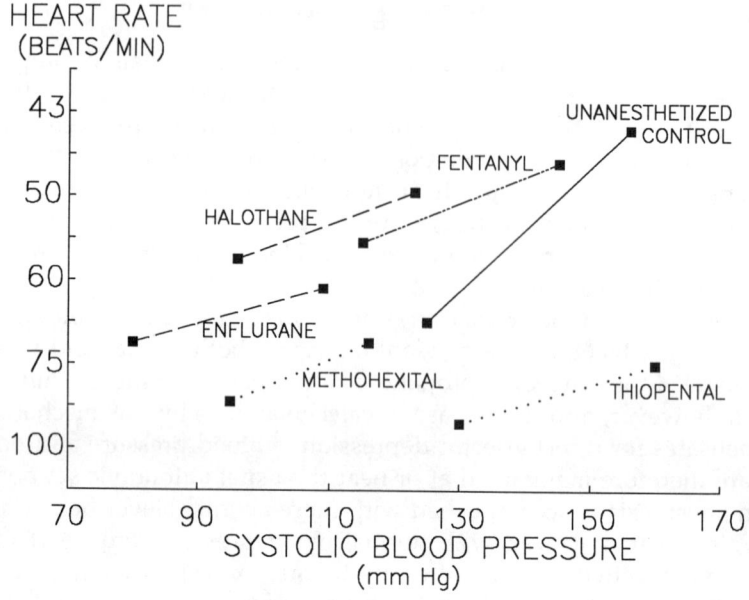

FIG 4–3.
Relationships between heart rate and systolic arterial blood pressure in the unanesthetized control state, and during general anesthesia produced by inhalational agents
(dashed lines), barbiturates *(dotted lines)*, and narcotics *(dashed-dotted lines)*. The lower
limit of the relationship represents the heart rate and blood pressure "set-point" at which
homeostasis is maintained during anesthesia; slope represents baroreceptor responsiveness after an acute hypertensive challenge.[20, 25, 26] General anesthesia with any agent
consistently reduces baroreflex responsiveness, but blood pressure and heart rate set-
points are agent specific.

these anesthetics actually sensitize the cells of the carotid sinus. Loss of
baroreflex responsiveness, therefore, probably reflects potent depressant effects at either central or efferent sites, or both.[17]

The consistent, dose-related decline in blood pressure set-point
seen during halothane anesthesia also suggests that there is some depression of the central, or integrative, components of this reflex arc.
Halothane has, in fact, been shown to depress the cardiac pressor
zones of the posterior hypothalamus, areas that produce tachycardia
when stimulated by isoflurane, enflurane, and other ethers.[12] The mild
sympathoadrenal-stimulating properties of nitrous oxide appear to reflect actions at levels above the pons.[18] Nevertheless, the role of these
central effects in anesthetic-induced baroreceptor depression is still
controversial.[17, 19, 20]

In fact, the major site of action for inhalational anesthetics appears to be the sympathetic ganglia.[21] Loss of blood pressure homeostasis may be further potentiated during anesthesia by those agents that have depressant effects on catecholamine release by the adrenal glands[19, 22, 23] or affect cardiovascular end-organs such as vascular or cardiac muscle. Blood pressure homeostasis is better maintained when anesthesia is produced by agents that cause significant stimulation of hypothalamic or medullary pressor areas, or by drugs that produce a generalized release of catecholamines.[24]

Thus, the summed pharmacologic actions of anesthetic agents on both central and peripheral structures ultimately determine whether these drugs reduce baroreflex responsiveness with, or without, a shift in the set-point and threshold.[25, 26] The state of general anesthesia itself does not appear to have a profound or consistent depressor effect on baroreflex responsiveness. Disruption of blood pressure homeostasis under these circumstances is a drug-specific, rather than a process-specific, phenomenon: other forms of altered consciousness such as sleep have been shown to produce enhanced, rather than depressed, baroreflex sensitivity.[7]

INTEGRATED CONTROL OF CARDIOVASCULAR HOMEOSTASIS

Because it is the most accessible, and thus the most well studied, autonomic reflex loop, the carotid sinus system is the prototype baroreflex, but it is only one of many discrete, integrated reflex arcs involved in moment-to-moment regulation of blood pressure. Although the precise hierarchy of these pathways is not yet known, it appears that the concept of an autonomous "vasomotor center" within the medulla subject to inhibition by input from the baroreceptor cells of the carotid sinus is overly simplistic. Current concepts[27] maintain that cardiovascular homeostasis reflects the continuing interaction of a far more diffuse network of pathways: ". . . all the major cardiorespiratory inputs connect at least to some degree with every autonomic effector. Autonomic activity is normally governed by the entire input profile, rather than by a single point."[28]

Supramedullary influences from the cerebral cortex and hypothalamus are also important, modulating and filtering nonautonomic visceral and somatic afferent input.[3] They directly modify the sensitivity of the medullary reticular formation that probably serves as the primary integrative zone. Chemoreceptor activity and ventilatory patterns, in particular the extent of lung inflation, can be additional forms of noncardiovascular input transmitted directly to medullary centers.[4] In effect, every type of neural input contributes to the determination of the autonomic set-point for cardiovascular homeostasis.

Carotid Baroreceptors

The anatomic location and the electrophysiology of the carotid sinus baroreceptors, both ideal to detect and correct acute arterial hypotension, appear to function in a way that maintains cerebral perfusion pressure as a primary objective.[3] In awake subjects, a fall in arterial pressure, especially if rapid, produces reflexly mediated increases of sympathoadrenal activity that elevate peripheral vascular resistance and increase cardiac output by increasing heart rate, thus restoring blood pressure toward its autonomic set-point. Classic concepts emphasize the importance of reflex withdrawal of chronic vagal influences on heart rate, and a simultaneous but lesser phenomenon of reciprocal stimulation of sympathoadrenal pathways. Gross changes in vagal activity, however, may be a primary effector pathway only as part of the control loop for acute arterial hypotension, or after direct mechanical distortion of the baroreceptors themselves, as occurs during carotid sinus massage. The carotid sinus baroreflex system certainly provides some antihypertensive function, but this role is probably secondary.[8]

Aortic Baroreceptors

In fact, strong negative feedback to the medullary cardiovascular areas during extremes of arterial hypertension occurs after the mechanical stretch or distention of mechanoreceptors in the aortic arch.[29] They initiate abrupt stimulation of the vagal nucleus, which reduces heart rate and, consequently, cardiac output, thus preventing increases in blood pressure resulting from augmented cardiac activity or cardiovascular stimulation. The carotid sinus baroreceptors correct arterial hypotension largely by increasing arteriolar resistance; aortic arch baroreceptors, in contrast, limit cardiac output by suppressing heart rate.

The aortic arch mechanism is sufficiently potent to override the carotid baroreflex if stimulation is intense: sustained arterial hypotension is occasionally produced by the clamping and cannulation of the aortic arch before initiation of cardiopulmonary bypass. In normal day-to-day functioning, however, the aortic arch baroreflex mechanism appears to be largely subordinate to the carotid baroreflex mechanism.

Cardiac Receptors

Other important cardiodepressor mechanisms that involve noncarotid mechanoreceptors include the cardiopulmonary receptors located in the septa between the cardiac chambers, and those at the junctions between cardiac chambers and great vessels. Receptors are also distributed, to a lesser extent, in the epicardium and other areas of the heart. Many of these receptors discharge continuously at frequencies that vary throughout the cardiac cycle. This electrical activity is conducted through the afferent components of the vagus nerve to the spinal cord, and then on to the medulla for integration into the network of baroreceptor and mechanoreceptor input, which ultimately determines the cardiovascular set-point for blood pressure homeostasis.

Other receptor arcs in the cardiovascular system remain silent at normal ventricular volumes, but are activated at extremes of cardiac size. Acute left ventricular distention produces vagal stimulation and withdrawal of sympathetic tone, thereby reducing cardiac output and lowering vascular resistance, especially in the renal circulation. Venous capacitance is also increased.[29] In contrast, distention of the right atrium, and perhaps the right ventricle, will initiate an enhancement of sympathoadrenal activity characterized by tachycardia and the release of adrenal epinephrine. These observations suggest that intrathoracic cardiopulmonary mechanoreceptor reflexes play an important role in the continuous regulation of central blood volume[8] and complement the activity of the carotid sinus mechanism, helping to avoid arterial hypotension.

Aortic arch and left ventricular reflex arcs therefore function synergistically to provide an effective antihypertensive control system. The primary interaction of these diverse sympathetic and parasympathetic reflex mechanisms occurs centrally at medullary and higher levels. There is evidence suggesting some degree of both local synergism and antagonism at the level of myocardial and neuronal receptors, however. Acetylcholine shortens the action potential of cardiac muscle and depresses adenylate cyclase activity, but it also facilitates the release of norepinephrine from myocardial depots[9] and enhances cardiac contractility. Halothane, and perhaps other inhalational anesthetics, may actually alter postsynaptic responsiveness to acetylcholine directly.[30]

Chemoreceptors and Hormones

The hierarchy of autonomic control systems for arterial blood pressure also includes input from the chemoreceptors of the carotid body, and it is probable that they play some role in the moment-to-moment control of cardiovascular homeostasis.[31] Similarly, there is growing evidence that receptors that respond to myocardial and to circulating bradykinins and prostaglandins have afferent connections to the same medullary centers that receive input from the baroreceptor and mechanoreceptor pathways described in the preceding section.[32]

All of these neurally mediated control systems are subject to amplification or depression in the intact individual as a consequence of the continuously variable concentrations of circulating neurohumoral factors in plasma, especially the effect of catecholamines. The elements required for effective autonomic control of arterial blood pressure do not necessarily need to be fixed anatomic components of the system in order to exert a significant effect on the set-point for normal arterial blood pressure.

INCIDENTAL AND DELIBERATE DISTURBANCES OF BLOOD PRESSURE DURING ANESTHESIA

Reflex Hypertension

Impaired baroreflex responsiveness during general anesthesia implies not only relative arterial hypotension, if the set-point for cardiovascular homeostasis is shifted downward, but also a greater likelihood of hypertension after superimposed incidental sympathoadrenal stimulation. In effect, loss of baroreflex-mediated cardiodepressor activity during general anesthesia predisposes to underdamped autonomic activity, especially in lightly anesthetized patients.

Patients are at particular risk of hypertension and tachycardia during painful maneuvers such as laryngoscopy.[33] Underlying essential hypertension, which itself implies chronically impaired baroreceptor responsiveness, is associated both with a greater reduction in blood pressure after loss of consciousness and more severe hypertension and tachycardia in response to laryngoscopy than that seen in normotensive patients. Increases in blood pressure may be as great as 60 to 80 mm Hg, and heart rates as much as 50% above prelaryngoscopy control values.[34, 35]

The hypertensive cardiovascular response to laryngoscopy begins within 15 seconds[36] and is probably maximal after about 45 seconds of sustained stimulation of the hypopharynx and larynx.[37] Plasma epinephrine and norepinephrine levels simultaneously increase twofold to threefold,[38] suggesting that the cardiovascular changes are part of a larger, more generalized sympathoadrenal phenomenon. In fact, transient hypertension in response to the emotional stress of hospital admission may predict a subsequent severe pressor response to laryngoscopy[39]; this information may prompt incorporation of techniques into the anesthetic plan that anticipate and minimize intraoperative lability of hemodynamics.

Hypertension and tachycardia are major risk factors for patients with coronary artery disease because they predispose to acute myocardial ischemia. Electrocardiographic evidence of ischemia, arrhythmias, and other stigmata of coronary arterial insufficiency is frequent during laryngoscopy and may persist even after acute drug therapy has returned blood pressure to normotensive levels.[35] Consequently, a number of clinical strategies attempt to prevent or to minimize the pressor response to laryngoscopy and intubation.

The intense and specific analgesic properties of narcotics can make the nervous system indifferent to the acute barrage of afferent input generated by physical manipulation of the larynx and trachea. Fentanyl and other short-acting narcotics in intravenous dosages small enough to avoid postoperative respiratory depression may still provide effective suppression of hypertension and tachycardia during laryngoscopy and intubation.[40, 41] Deep inhalational anesthesia may also suppress autonomic responsiveness sufficiently to ablate reflex hypertension under these circumstances.[42]

Local anesthesia produced by sprayed or viscous lidocaine solutions blunts hypertension, but does not prevent tachycardia.[43] A similarly incomplete solution is afforded by intravenous lidocaine, even when given in doses of 1 to 3 mg/kg. Direct-acting vasodilators such as sodium nitroprusside may control blood pressure effectively but fail to prevent tachycardia.[44] Thiopental is a poor choice for suppression of laryngoscopy-induced hypertension and tachycardia, regardless of the dose employed, because it has minimal analgesic properties and shifts the baroreflex set-point in a direction that actually predisposes to tachycardia.[13] In general, neuroendocrine and reflex cardiovascular responses of any type can be virtually eliminated by intense pharmacologic sympathectomy produced either by epidural or by spinal anesthesia,[45] but the stimulus must originate at or below the level of sensory blockade, rarely practical for laryngoscopy.

Controlled Hypotension

The reduction of blood pressure set-points and the depression of baroreceptor responsiveness that occur during general anesthesia can be used effectively to minimize surgical hemorrhage. Blood pressure, not cardiac output, is the major determinant of intraoperative blood loss.[46] Mean arterial pressure can be safely reduced to two thirds of its normal value, producing a relatively dry surgical field without compromising tissue perfusion. "Deliberate," "induced," or "controlled" hypotension is of particular interest in contemporary anesthetic practice because it reduces the need for blood transfusion and may expedite surgery, reducing operating time and hospital costs.[47] In addition, controlled hypotension may facilitate specific difficult surgical maneuvers, such as the clipping of a cerebral aneurysm.

Anesthetic plans for controlled hypotension utilize high inspired concentrations of inhalational anesthetics or the intravenous administration of direct-acting vasodilator, ganglionic-blocking, or adrenergic-blocking drugs to effect a pharmacologically induced decrease in systemic vascular resistance. Generalized depression of baroreflex mechanisms allows maintenance of sustained arterial hypotension with minimal compensatory tachycardia, except in children or in young adults, in whom β-adrenergic blocking drugs may be required.[48]

Cardiac output during controlled hypotension is well maintained or may, in fact, be increased because vasodilator drugs produce a significant decrease in the impedance to ejection of cardiac stroke volume (see Chapter 6). Thus, despite a significant reduction in arterial blood pressure, there is normal metabolic homeostasis in peripheral tissues. Whereas hypotension due to hemorrhage or cardiac failure represents a state of low blood flow and high vascular resistance, controlled or deliberate hypotension is an induced state of low vascular resistance with normal or above-normal tissue blood flow,[49] provided that arterial pressures remain adequate to avoid vascular compression in critical tissue segments.[50]

The concept of controlled hypotension, less than 40 years old, is still controversial in regard to its risk/benefit ratio.[48] Risk is probably a function of the details of the technique employed. A transient state of increased baroreceptor responsiveness may occur in the immediate postoperative period after the use of nitroprusside for controlled hypotension,[51] placing patients with ischemic heart disease at some risk of tachycardia and myocardial ischemia. β-Adrenergic blocking drugs can be used to minimize residual baroreceptor responsiveness and may also increase the tolerance of patients with ischemic heart disease to decreased coronary perfusion pressures under these circumstances.[52]

Although most techniques for producing vasodilation or ganglionic blockade appear to be safe even when arterial hypotension is sustained, adenosine is associated with uneven distribution of cardiac output and a high likelihood of renal or cerebral ischemia.[53] Even when combined with isovolemic hemodilution, however, controlled hypotension accomplished with more conventional agents, such as nitroprusside or deep halothane, has been shown to be both safe and effective, reducing blood loss during total hip arthroplasty by 50% or more.[54]

The potential for metabolic injury during the autonomic depression and disruption of normal baroreceptor control of arterial blood pressure that occurs during controlled hypotension is sufficiently great that the skill and judgment of the anesthesiologist in manipulating blood pressure and setting acceptable lower limits is still an important determinant of the safety of this technique. Preexisting cerebral and myocardial disease, especially when of vascular origin, may affect both the degree of arterial hypotension selected and the duration of time it is sustained. Therefore, controlled hypotension may be appropriate only where the surgical procedure is clearly facilitated by a dry operative field, or where there is a demonstrable reduction of surgical bleeding or a relative or absolute limitation imposed on blood transfusion, such as occurs in the management of patients who are Jehovah's Witnesses.[55]

AUTONOMIC REFLEXES DURING ANESTHESIA

Despite generalized depression of baroreflex responsiveness, arterial blood pressure remains subject to some degree of autonomic control during general anesthesia. However, when the drugs used to produce anesthesia create a state of unconsciousness, they necessarily depress cortical and other higher centers, and thereby "disintegrate" autonomic homeostasis. The normal buffering of short-term autonomic responses is impaired, and both reflexly mediated cardiac excitation and cardiovascular depression are exaggerated. Unmodulated afferent input, the release of tonic inhibitory influences, or generalized disruption of central integrative functions may produce either hormonal or neurally mediated cardiovascular instability.

Neuroendocrine Responses

General anesthesia in the absence of surgical stimulation is associated with a decline in plasma catecholamine concentrations.[20, 21] Plasma norepinephrine rises perioperatively in proportion to the intensity and the extent of tissue injury. In contrast, epinephrine varies in a sporadic, unpredictable manner after surgical stress. Elevation of plasma cortisol and growth hormone occurs largely in response to tissue trauma. The hemodynamic effects of pituitary release of vaso-pressin (ADH) and enhanced renin-angiotensin activity may be suffi-cient to offset the generalized suppression of sympathoadrenal activity produced by halothane and enflurane.[22]

Spinal and epidural anesthesia also suppress the neuroendocrine response to stress. In fact, plasma norepinephrine demonstrates a lin-ear, inverse relationship to thoracic sensory level,[45] suggesting that the primary site of action is at the more diffuse afferent, or input, limb of this neuroendocrine reflex arc. The vasomotor paralysis produced si-multaneously by the effects of local anesthetics on the efferent limb of this autonomic pathway reduces systemic vascular resistance and in-creases venous capacity.[56] Although these events may cause relative arterial hypotension if venous return is not maintained, the blood pres-sure of most patients is effectively supported by stress-related release of ADH and renin-angiotensin.[57]

The neuroendocrine response to perioperative stress therefore ap-pears to make a major contribution to the maintenance of normal vital signs during anesthesia, but the benefit of assessing overall patient outcome on this basis alone has been challenged. Sustained salt and water retention, peripheral vasoconstriction, and suppression of im-mune competence may contribute negatively to longer-term outcome, especially in high-risk patients.[58] Selective adrenergic blockade, at least in patients at increased risk of myocardial ischemia, may be of value.

Limited neuroendocrine responsiveness appears, therefore, largely responsible for hemodynamic stability in the face of the direct cardio-vascular effects of most anesthetic techniques. Sustained sympathoad-renal activation, however, may be detrimental,[59] and can be eliminated intraoperatively by adequate inspired concentrations of inhalational an-esthetic agents[60] and subsequently by meticulous attention to perioper-ative analgesia, in particular, the use of regional anesthetic techniques to augment the anesthetic plan.

Cardiodepressor Reflexes

The removal of sympathoadrenal pathways from their modulation by higher centers during general anesthesia predisposes to tachycardia and hypertension. It may also increase the frequency and severity of cardiodepressor phenomena.[61] Although difficult to study, cardiode-pressor reflexes during anesthesia are sufficiently stereotyped to permit organization into three major categories: cranioautonomic reflexes, in which cranial nerves provide the afferent limb of the arc; visceroautonomic reflexes, in which the afferent limb consists of visceral autonomic fibers traveling along sympathetic or parasympathetic nerves into the spinal cord and, subsequently, up to brain stem level; and somatoautonomic reflexes, in which the afferent limb of the reflex arc is a classic somatic pain pathway. In all three types of pathways, the efferent limb is represented predominantly by the cardiodepressor influences of the vagus nerve, although there appears to be significant interaction between the various afferent limbs at a spinal cord level and between sympathetic and parasympathetic nuclei in medullary centers (Fig 4–4).

The prototype cranioautonomic cardiodepressor reflex is the carotid sinus baroreflex, already described. The oculocardiac reflex[62] is mediated via the trigeminal nerve and may be initiated during the stretch of extraocular muscles, especially during strabismus surgery. The vagus nerve provides a final common pathway for the efferent limb of all cranioautonomic reflex arcs, producing acute bradycardia—hence the persistent use of the synonym *vasovagal reflex* to describe a variety of cardiodepressor responses after stimulation of the carotid sinus, carotid body, aortic arch, as well as ventricular, pulmonary, and even pharyngeal receptors of various types.

All of these cardiodepressor responses tend to be exaggerated during light levels of anesthesia. They are both more frequent and more severe in the presence of mild central nervous system depression than in fully alert individuals. This phenomenon may reflect sensitization of peripheral receptors under these conditions[12, 15, 17] or the generalized depression of cortical and other modulating centers within the nervous system. Deeper levels of general anesthesia, by definition (Chapter 2), produce progressively more potent depression of reflex activity. Consequently, cranioautonomic cardiodepressor reflexes may become less apparent as the level of anesthesia becomes more profound, presumably because autonomic nuclei, efferent pathways, and the various effector functions are impaired directly by the effects of high concentrations of anesthetic agents.

Visceroautonomic reflexes are autonomic responses to afferent input from undifferentiated nerve endings in mesentery, or in intestine, urinary bladder, biliary tract, and other hollow organs.[63, 64] They are not triggered by the specialized baroreceptors or stretch receptors associated with the various types of cranioautonomic reflexes that utilize either the ninth or tenth cranial nerve as an afferent limb to complete a cranioautonomic reflex arc. In fact, the precise anatomic pathway by which the afferent impulses of visceroautonomic reflexes are transmit-

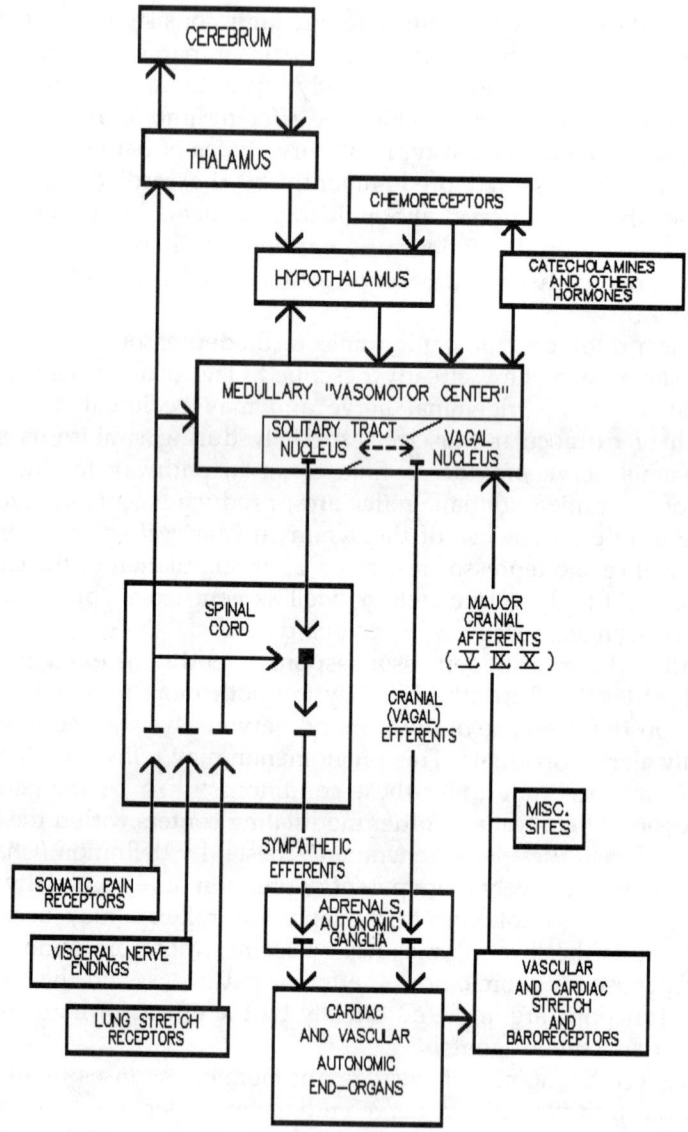

FIG 4-4.
Schematic diagram of the relationship between the components of various autonomic reflex arcs. Cranioautonomic, visceroautonomic, and somatoautonomic cardiodepressor reflexes all share a common efferent limb consisting of increased parasympathetic (vagal) outflow and reduced sympathetic tone. *Dashed arrow* represents reciprocal inhibition between sympathetic and parasympathetic centers in medulla.

ted along the spinal cord after they enter remains unknown. It is clear, however, that stimulation of these pathways produces an abrupt decrease in sympathetic tone, because of direct depression of sympathetic nuclei in the solitary tract of the medullary vasomotor center, as well as a simultaneous increase in vagal tone.

Because of wide variability in the initial balance between sympathetic and parasympathetic activity, the hemodynamic response to a visceroautonomic reflex may be hypotension either with or without simultaneous bradycardia. Reflex arterial hypotension occurs abruptly as a direct consequence of the withdrawal of sympathetic tone, with a marked reduction in systemic vascular resistance and an increase in venous capacity.[65] In contrast, hypotension of somewhat more gradual onset coincident with tachycardia, rather than bradycardia, especially if associated with cutaneous vasodilation, is more likely to be a nonreflexive systemic response to the release of prostacyclin from mesenteric or intestinal vascular structures after surgical manipulation.[66]

Bradycardia and hypotension produced by the third major type of cardiodepressor reflex appear to be paradoxical: they accompany surgical incision or other trauma to skin, skeletal muscle, or periosteum. These events are normally associated with the classic symptoms of acute somatic pain, arterial hypertension, and tachycardia. However, light levels of general anesthesia that fall short of those required for indifference to continuous surgical pain can disrupt autonomic integration sufficiently that there is net stimulation of the vagal nuclei in the course of a somatoautonomic reflex. Acute hypotension, bradycardia, and syncope in maximally stressed, unanesthetized individuals who have suffered significant soft tissue trauma without massive hemorrhage may occur by a similar mechanism.

In well-anesthetized patients, cardiodepressor reflexes, like all complex neural mechanisms, are effectively suppressed by the further deepening of anesthetic depth, or by the addition of drugs with specific analgesic properties to block the afferent pathways for somatic pain receptors or transmission through the spinal cord. Cardiodepressor reflexes may also be minimized by blockade of the efferent limb with use of atropine, but direct stimulation of sympathoadrenal pathways with adrenergic agonists may be simultaneously required to fully restore circulatory homeostasis. Because the mechanism common to all cardiopressor reflexes includes arteriolar vasodilation and reduced systemic vascular resistance, reflex hypotension under these circumstances is further exaggerated in patients with a preexisting circulating volume deficit, and may therefore respond to increased infusion rates of intravenous fluids.

THERMOREGULATION

Superficially, the regulation of body temperature in man appears to be a simple model for autonomic control systems. Central components in the hypothalamus act as comparators for afferent temperature-sensitive pathways and influence the output of both autonomic and somatic effector systems. The complexity of this system, however, is greater than had once been thought. Thermosensitive neurons appear, in fact, to be widely distributed not only in skin but also throughout the brain and spinal cord. Peripheral receptors respond both to warm and cold, and there may be specific central "deep-body" noncutaneous thermosensors (Fig 4–5). Thus thermoregulation is mediated not by one closed-loop pathway, but by a hierarchical complex of integrated reflex arcs that themselves conduct information at rates that are temperature dependent.[67]

Initial interest in temperature control during anesthesia focused on inadvertent hyperthermia caused by heat stress from heavy surgical draping in non–air-conditioned operating rooms, particularly in the summertime with use of "to-and-fro" breathing circuits.[68] However, the general principle that anesthetized patients lose their ability to remain homeothermic remains valid even in air-conditioned operating rooms with high rates of air flow, where they are frequently subject to inadvertent or incidental hypothermia ("core" body temperatures below 35° or 36° C). This phenomenon has also stimulated considerable interest in the mechanism, and the consequences, of hypothermia in the perioperative management of patients.[69]

Response to Hypothermia

Stimulation of cutaneous cold receptors initiates reflex peripheral vasoconstriction, activation of the metabolism of brown fat, and vigorous contraction of skeletal muscle. When cold stress is sustained, there may be a hormonally mediated increase in basal metabolic rate as well. These responses occur even without central hypothermia, although the intensity of the response to a given degree of cutaneous cold stress is enhanced by moderate reductions of core temperature (0.5° to 1.5° C), but eventually inhibited when patients become moderately hypothermic (core body temperatures less than 32° C).[70]

In effect, mild central hypothermia, such as commonly encountered postoperatively, increases the "gain" of thermoregulatory responsiveness and exaggerates shivering and other mechanisms by which

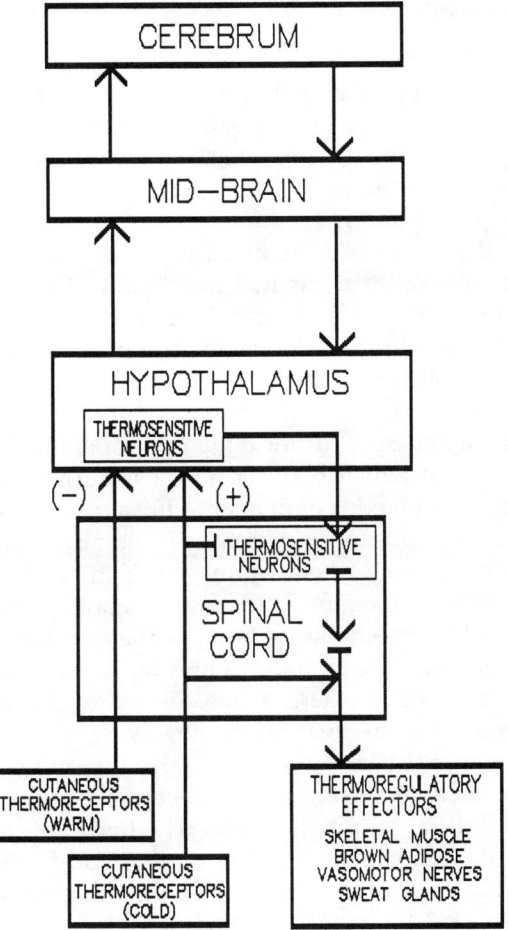

FIG 4–5.
Schematic diagram of the components of the autonomic thermoregulatory mechanism. Thermosensitivity is a property of both peripheral cutaneous and noncutaneous "deep-body" neurons. Hypothalamic neurons appear to act as central temperature-sensing receptors. Shivering and other forms of thermogenesis occur in response to stimulation of either peripheral or central thermosensors, with the magnitude of the response modulated by multiple factors, including the functional state of midbrain and higher centers.

the autonomic nervous system attempts to re-establish normal body temperature. When core body temperatures are reduced by 2° C or more, the gain of the system may be increased sufficiently that shivering is initiated even when cutaneous cold receptors are in environments as warm as 85° F.

Effects of Anesthesia

Anesthetized surgical patients consistently experience negative thermal balance, probably by multiple mechanisms: because the rate at which heat is generated by body tissues is less than that at which it is lost to the environment, the net effect, whatever the mechanism, is a fall in body temperature.

Body heat production is predominantly a function of skeletal muscle activity, and this is clearly reduced or, in the case of patients with neuromuscular blockade, eliminated during anesthesia. The change in the amount of heat produced by cardiac and other forms of metabolic activity varies depending on the specific anesthetic agents and techniques employed, although their contribution to overall thermal balance is relatively minor.

The predominant cause of incidental perioperative hypothermia is the increased rate at which body heat is lost during anesthesia. Four mechanisms are involved: conduction (direct contact with cold surfaces), convection (exposure to currents of cold air), radiation (continuous noncontact transfer of heat by means of infrared radiation), and evaporation (loss of moisture from skin, respiratory tract, and open body cavities). These mechanisms increase the rate at which body heat is lost as environmental temperatures and humidity are reduced.

It is unclear to what extent active thermoregulatory mechanisms minimize the rate of body heat loss and slow the fall in core temperature common in anesthetized patients. Active thermoregulation may be attenuated, delayed in onset, or completely abolished by anesthetic agents. There is also controversy as to whether the primary defect in intraoperative thermoregulation is the inactivation of the central components of autonomic responsiveness, or the more localized effects of anesthetic agents on the cutaneous and vascular effector components of the thermoregulatory control system.[71]

Some hypothermia-induced cutaneous vasoconstriction and a modest increase in nonshivering thermogenesis probably do occur under light levels of general anesthesia.[72] However, the generalized shivering that is a normal response to central hypothermia is sufficiently suppressed during general anesthesia to make these patients thermally passive in the typically hypothermic environment of the operating room.

Moderate and deeper levels of hypothermia (32°–26° C) are usually established intentionally. At these temperatures there is significant depression of cardiac output and cardiac electrical conduction, disrupted hemostasis, and diffuse and detrimental effects on hepatic, renal, and nervous system function.[73] Although once widely used to suspend metabolic activity and facilitate specialized cardiac and vascular surgery and neurosurgery,[74] induced hypothermia is now employed primarily as a component of extracorporeal perfusion.

Consequences of Hypothermia

Incidental hypothermia after routine surgery is of concern because, although not usually severe enough to have significant effects on most aspects of organ system function, there is an abrupt appearance of renewed thermoregulatory responsiveness during and immediately after emergence from general anesthesia. Even in healthy young patients, postoperative shivering is physically and psychologically uncomfortable. Vigorous stimulation of both shivering and nonshivering thermogenesis also requires significant increases in total body oxygen delivery and cardiac output. It may increase oxygen requirements as much as fivefold.[73, 75] Patients who are elderly, debilitated, or those with cardiac compromise may be unable to increase cardiac output in proportion to this enhanced demand, making them subject to postoperative hypoxemia and acidosis.

Given the virtually unavoidable situation of a mildly hypothermic patient emerging from anesthesia in an environment in which the ambient temperature is less than 30° C, vasoconstriction and shivering are routine features of anesthetic emergence. Some of the gross skeletal muscle contractions and exaggerated tremors seen before the return of a full level of consciousness, however, may not be simple expressions of a thermoregulatory response, but may represent the activation of unmodulated and uninhibited spinal reflex activity.[76]

In general, however, the rapidity and effectiveness with which application of warm blankets or the use of direct radiant heaters eliminates this phenomenon[77] suggest that it is an integral part of coordinated thermoregulatory reflex mechanisms. Local reflex input appears to augment the central response to stimulation of peripheral cold receptors. Initiation of shivering by epidural injection of local anesthetics stored at room temperature suggests that in addition to hypothalamic and cutaneous receptors, there are clinically important spinal cord or epidural thermosensitive areas involved in the complex scheme of thermoregulation.

Prevention of Hypothermia

Almost any form of intervention that reduces intraoperative heat loss can be shown to minimize the incidence or the severity of incidental hypothermia. Passive heat and moisture exchangers placed within the breathing circuit ("artificial noses"), thermoreflective drapes, and intravenous fluid warmers all delay or reduce, but do not reverse, the fall in core temperature usually seen in the first 2 to 3 hours of surgery.[78] Because of the inherent limitations in skin contact area available for the conduction of heat in adults as well as a large volume-to-surface ratio, supplementary active heating blankets placed on operating room tables appear to maintain body temperature effectively only in children who weigh less than 10 kg.[79]

Active heating and humidification of inspired gases may also prevent hypothermia and appear to be effective in all patients, regardless of size.[80] However, breathing circuit heating and humidification systems pose potential problems in the area of thermal and electrical safety, infection, and perioperative water balance. Routine elevation of operating room temperatures to values high enough to provide a neutral thermal environment has theoretic appeal but is generally impractical because it imposes working conditions unacceptable to most operating room personnel.

The anticholinergic properties of meperidine confer a unique ability to disrupt thermoregulation and suppress shivering, attenuating the associated increases in oxygen consumption and carbon dioxide production[81]; no similar antishivering effect is produced by other opioids.[82] Unfortunately, the ability of this drug to disrupt normal thermoregulatory mechanisms may also cause a rare but potentially lethal form of hyperpyrexia if the patient is also receiving pargyline or another monoamine oxidase inhibitor.[83]

MANAGEMENT OF PATIENTS WITH AUTONOMIC DISORDERS

Elderly Patients

The indications for, and the management of, techniques for general and regional anesthesia should reflect their known autonomic consequences. The greater the dependence of the patient on sympathoadrenal activation for maintenance of cardiovascular homeostasis, the more abrupt and profound the changes in blood pressure that follow generalized autonomic depression or pharmacologic sympathectomy.

Elderly patients, even those without established cardiovascular disease, have higher resting plasma concentrations of catecholamines than do young adults.[84] An increased catecholamine response to physical stress is also characteristic of the aging process. Higher levels of catecholamines appear to compensate, at least in part, for the reduced end-organ responsiveness that occurs in the effector components of the autonomic system of elderly patients.

As expected, however, elderly patients experience a greater fall in blood pressure after the catecholamine suppression associated with general or regional anesthesia than do their younger counterparts. Therapy for arterial hypotension under these circumstances includes intravenous fluid therapy combined, if necessary, with vasopressor drugs. Stimulation of both types of adrenergic receptors is needed to effectively reverse the simultaneous occurrence of arteriolar and venular dilation[56]; the increase in cardiac output produced by the chronotropic and inotropic effects of ephedrine or other pressors with both α- and β-adrenergic effects may also expedite the return of cardiovascular homeostasis. During regional anesthesia, repeated injections or continuous infusion of a pressor may be required, since true autonomic homeostasis cannot be reestablished until the pharmacologic sympathectomy is terminated.

Riley-Day Syndrome

There are nonphysiologic and nonpharmacologic forms of autonomic disruption that can also alter the design of the anesthetic plan. Riley-Day syndrome, a rare congenital disorder of peripheral autonomic development,[85] exaggerates many of the interactions between anesthetics and the autonomic nervous system that normally occur to a lesser extent. Children with this type of familial dysautonomia have such poorly arterial hypertension in response to emotional stress and such severe orthostatic and anesthetic-induced hypotension that they were once considered to be "at grave risk" for general anesthesia.[86] Predisposition to aspiration of gastric contents and unstable body temperatures also contributed to difficult anesthetic management.

More recently, however, fuller appreciation of the extent to which barbiturates disrupt baroreflex responsiveness and the degree to which inhalational anesthetics depress ganglionic and autonomic end-organ function has led to a revised, less dramatic assessment.[87] Currently, there is no absolute contraindication to general anesthesia for individuals with primary autonomic dysfunction; narcotic-based general anesthetic techniques are usually employed in conjunction with careful cardiovascular monitoring and the use of both active and passive measures to avoid aspiration or incidental hypothermia. Although this genetically transmitted disorder is rare, other dysautonomias of variable severity are frequently associated with metabolic diseases such as diabetes mellitus and essential hypertension.[88]

Spinal Cord Injury

In contrast to the reduced autonomic responsiveness seen with intrinsic dysautonomia, patients with mid- to upper-thoracic spinal cord transections are prone to increased autonomic responsiveness and hyperreflexia. If the cord transection is complete, surgical stimulation or manipulation of somatic or visceral autonomic pathways below the level of the injury may produce severe arterial hypertension.[89] Segmental reflex pathways are removed from the inhibitory influences of the medullary and higher centers that normally modulate their activity when the spinal cord and its pathways are intact (see Fig 4–4). Therefore, local vasoconstrictor activity is greatly exaggerated because it is disintegrated from overall autonomic homeostasis. Bradycardia and other compensatory adjustments by the rest of the autonomic nervous system cannot fully reestablish blood pressure homeostasis. In addition, segmental reflex adrenal activation may simultaneously release epinephrine, producing diaphoresis and the diffuse apprehension and anxiety associated with high plasma levels of epinephrine.[90]

The abruptness with which systolic blood pressures as high as 250 mm Hg can occur in patients with spinal cord injury suggests the importance of the contribution of local and segmental reflex mechanisms to the overall maintenance of cardiovascular homeostasis. All patients with mid to high thoracic cord transection levels are at risk, especially if the surgical site is innervated via sacral roots. Effective therapy can be achieved at afferent, efferent, or central sites. Although general and regional anesthesia have been advocated for these patients,[91] current approaches emphasize blockade at ganglionic sites,[92] since they rarely have conscious perception of pain or need analgesia.

Pheochromocytoma

It is equally important, but more difficult, to control hypertension in patients undergoing surgical resection of pheochromocytoma. The disruption of cardiovascular and arterial blood pressure homeostasis seen in these patients is attributable not to the subtle disintegration of autonomic mechanisms, but rather to the consequences of episodic massive release of catecholamines from tumor tissues. Extreme elevation of plasma norepinephrine and epinephrine and the urinary concentrations of their metabolites serve both to establish the diagnosis[93] and to explain the spectacular and abrupt hypertension and associated dysrhythmias that appear in response to tumor manipulation.[94] These extremely high concentrations of catecholamines also cause a functional contraction of circulating blood volume: chronic α- and β-adrenergic stimulation decreases venous capacity and elevates systemic vascular resistance.

The transient period of arterial hypotension that frequently occurs after tumor resection, even when there has been vigorous intravenous volume replacement therapy, may reflect adrenergic receptor desensitization ("down-regulation") in arteriolar smooth muscle due to prolonged exposure to abnormally high levels of plasma catecholamines.[95, 96] A reversible, rightward shift of the baroreceptor set-point may also occur, producing a persistent postoperative tachycardia that is unresponsive to restoration of circulating blood volume, but usually resolves within 48 to 72 hours.

The forbiddingly high perioperative mortality of surgical resection of pheochromocytoma in prior eras has been reduced to 1%, or less, in current practice, largely because of the practical application of an improved understanding of the pathophysiology of this disorder.[97] Priorities of anesthetic management include preoperative α-blockade[98] and aggressive expansion of contracted blood volume preoperatively, intraoperatively, and postoperatively.[99] Although halothane, unlike other inhalational anesthetics, may preferentially suppress catecholamine release from these tumors,[100] the tendency of this anesthetic agent to sensitize the myocardium to catecholamine-induced dysrhythmias has hastened its replacement with less arrhythmogenic agents such as enflurane and isoflurane.

Droperidol has been implicated in the precipitous release of catecholamines from pheochromocytomas[101] and should be avoided. The control of vascular resistance by sustained infusion of phentolamine has also been largely replaced by the use of nitroprusside infusion because of its rapid onset and offset and the potency of its vasodilator effects. Finally, recent investigation into the hemodynamic consequences of the paroxysmal elevations of systemic vascular resistance seen in patients with pheochromocytoma suggests that accurate assessment of their volume status requires pulmonary artery catheterization for continuous monitoring of left ventricular preload.[102]

SUMMARY

Impairment of cardiovascular and temperature homeostasis during anesthesia reflects, to some extent, drug-specific effects on end-organs. Fundamentally more important, however, anesthetics produce diffuse depression of autonomic mechanisms and the disintegration of their hierarchical control loops. Under all but the deepest levels of inhalational anesthesia, these homeostatic systems continue to function, although with progressively less efficacy than seen in the unanesthetized individual. The end-organ effects of specific anesthetic agents and techniques are most important in patients with preexisting disease in whom the capacity of effectors of the various autonomic reflex arcs is either impaired or is already driven to maximal levels of function by compensatory processes.

Simple conceptual models consisting of afferent, efferent, and central controlling components permit useful analysis of autonomic function. However, they do not reflect the true complexity of these control systems, nor do they convey the prioritized interaction between related autonomic and metabolic functions. Virtually all of these systems, although located to a large extent within the hypothalmus, are probably far less centralized than has been assumed. The "vasomotor center" and the "thermoregulatory" control areas appear to be only part of more widespread systems in which the spinal cord, in particular, modulates and processes visceral and somatic afferent input.

With the possible exception of nitrous oxide, cyclopropane, and ketamine, all anesthetic agents produce generalized depression of sympathoadrenal activity. Surgical injury to tissues, surgical pain, laryngoscopy, and other forms of perioperative stimulation produce the generalized release of neurohumoral and hormonal substances that characterize the neuroendocrine response to surgical stress. Pharmacologic sympathectomy produced by regional anesthesia, or deep levels of inhalational anesthesia, appears capable of suppressing both the neuroendocrine and the hemodynamic responses to surgical stimulation.

The desirability of "stress-free" anesthetic management remains controversial. Although hypertension, shivering, and other extremes of cardiovascular stress may be harmful to patients with a fragile balance between myocardial oxygen supply and demand, total elimination of the neuroendocrine response to tissue injury may leave uncompensated the direct end-organ effects of these agents themselves, producing the equally undesirable consequences of arterial hypotension and inadequate cardiac output.

REFERENCES

1. Bagshaw RJ: Systems theory and the anaesthetist. *Acta Anaesthesiol Scand* 1980; 24:379–392.
2. Bernard C: *Leçons sur les effets des substances toxiques et mèdicamenteuses.* Paris, Baillière, 1833.

3. Kirchheim HR: Systemic arterial baroreceptor reflexes. *Physiol Rev* 1976; 56:100–176.
4. Glick G, Braunwald E: Relative roles of the sympathetic and parasympathetic nervous systems in reflex control of heart rates. *Circ Res* 1965; 16:363–375.
5. Greene NM, Bachand RG: Vagal component of the chronotropic response to baroreceptor stimulation in man. *Am Heart J* 1971; 82:22–27.
6. Vatner SF, Braunwald E: Cardiovascular control mechanism in the conscious state. *N Engl J Med* 1975; 290:970–976.
7. Shepherd JT: Intrathoracic baroreflexes. *Mayo Clin Proc* 1973; 48:426–437.
8. Mancia G, Ferrari A, Gregorini L, Valentini R, Ludbrook J, Zanchetti A: Circulatory reflexes from carotid and extracarotid baroreceptor areas in man. *Circ Res* 1977; 41:309–315.
9. Higgins CB, Vatner SF, Braunwald E: Parasympathetic control of the heart. *Pharmacol Rev* 1973; 25:119–155.
10. Kidd C, Linden RJ: Recent advances in the physiology of cardiovascular reflexes, with special reference to hypotension. *Br J Anaesth* 1975; 47:767–776.
11. Price HL, Linde HW, Jones RE, Black GW, Price ML: Sympathoadrenal responses to general anesthesia in man and their relation to hemodynamics. *Anesthesiology* 1959; 20:563–575.
12. Millar RA: Some effects of inhalational anesthetics on neurocirculatory control. *Int Anesthesiol Clin* 1971; 9:69–90.
13. Price HL: The significance of catecholamine release during anaesthesia. *Br J Anaesth* 1966; 38:705–711.
14. Morton M, Duke PC, Ong B: Baroreflex control of heart rate in man awake and during enflurane and enflurane–nitrous oxide anesthesia. *Anesthesiology* 1980; 52:221–223.
15. Seagard JL, Elegbe EO, Hopp FA, Bosnjak ZJ, vonColditz JH, Kalbfleisch JH: Effects of isoflurane on the baroreceptor reflex. *Anesthesiology* 1983; 59:511–520.
16. Carter JA, Clarke TNS, Prys-Roberts C, Spelina KR: Restoration of baroreflex control of heart rate during recovery from anaesthesia. *Br J Anaesth* 1986; 58:415–421.
17. Seagard JL, Hopp FA, Donegan JH, Kalbfleisch JH, Kampine JP: Halothane and the carotid sinus reflex. *Anesthesiology* 1982; 57:191–202.
18. Fukunaga AF, Epstein RM: Sympathetic excitation during nitrous oxide–halothane anesthesia in the cat. *Anesthesiology* 1973; 39:23–36.
19. Roizen MF, Moss J, Henry DP, Kopin IJ: Effects of halothane on plasma catecholamines. *Anesthesiology* 1974; 41:432–439.
20. Skovsted P, Price HL: The effects of Ethrane on arterial pressure, preganglionic sympathetic activity, and barostatic reflexes. *Anesthesiology* 1972; 36:257–262.
21. Bosnjak ZJ, Seagard JL, Wu A, Kampine JP: The effects of halothane on sympathetic ganglionic transmission. *Anesthesiology* 1982; 57:473–479.
22. Perry LD, Van Dyke RA, Theye RA: Sympathoadrenal and hemody-

namic effects of isoflurane, halothane, and cyclopropane. *Anesthesiology* 1974; 40:465–570.

23. Cothert M, Wendt J: Inhibition of adrenal medullary catecholamine secretion by enflurane. *Anesthesiology* 1977; 46:400–403.
24. Skovsted P, Price HL: Central sympathetic excitation caused by diethyl ether. *Anesthesiology* 1970; 32:202–209.
25. Bristow JD, Prys-Roberts C, Fisher A, Pickering TG, Sleight P: Effects of anesthesia on baroreflex control of heart rate in man. *Anesthesiology* 1969; 31:422–428.
26. Duke PC, Fownes D, Wade JG: Halothane depresses baroreflex control of heart rate in man. *Anesthesiology* 1977; 46:184–187.
27. Hilton SM, Spyer KM: Central nervous regulation of vascular resistance. *Annu Rev Physiol* 1980; 42:399–411.
28. Korner PI: Integrative neural cardiovascular control. *Physiol Rev* 1971; 51:312–367.
29. Donald DE, Shepherd JT: Reflexes from the heart and lungs: Physiological curiosities or important regulatory mechanism. *Cardiovasc Res* 1978; 12:449–469.
30. Bosnjak ZJ, Dujic Z, Roerig DL, Kampine JP: Effects of halothane on acetylcholine release and sympathetic ganglionic transmission. *Anesthesiology* 1988; 69:500–506.
31. Donald DE, Shepherd JT: Autonomic regulation of the peripheral circulation. *Annu Rev Physiol* 1980; 42:429–439.
32. Coleridge HM, Coleridge JCG: Cardiovascular afferents involved in regulation of peripheral vessels. *Annu Rev Physiol* 1980; 42:413–427.
33. King BD, Harris LD Jr, Greifenstein FE, Elder JD, Dripps RD: Reflex circulatory responses to direct laryngoscopy and tracheal intubation performed during general anesthesia. *Anesthesiology* 1951; 12:556–566.
34. Prsy-Roberts C, Meloche R, Foex P: Studies of anaesthesia in relation to hypertension. I. Cardiovascular responses of treated and untreated patients. *Br J Anaesth* 1971; 43:122–137.
35. Foex P, Prys-Roberts C: Anaesthesia and the hypertensive patient. *Br J Anaesth* 1974; 46:575–588.
36. Wycoff CC: Endotracheal intubation: Effects on blood pressure and heart rate. *Anesthesiology* 1960; 21:153–158.
37. Stoelting RK: Circulatory changes during direct laryngoscopy and tracheal intubation. *Anesthesiology* 1977; 47:381–384.
38. Derbyshire DR, Chmielewski A, Fell D, Vater M, Achola K, Smith G: Plasma catecholamine response to tracheal intubation. *Br J Anaesth* 1983; 55:855–860.
39. Bedford RF, Feinstein B: Hospital admission blood pressure: A predictor for hypertension following endotracheal intubation. *Anesth Analg* 1980; 59:367–370.
40. Crawford DC, Fell D, Achola KJ, Smith G: Effects of alfentanil on the pressor and catecholamine responses to tracheal intubation. *Br J Anaesth* 1987; 59:707–712.

41. Martin DE, Rosenberg H, Aukburg SJ, et al: Low-dose fentanyl blunts circulatory responses to tracheal intubation. *Anesth Analg* 1982; 61:680–684.
42. Yakaitis RW, Blitt CD, Anguilo JP: End-tidal enflurane concentration for endotracheal intubation. *Anesthesiology* 1979; 50:59–61.
43. Denlinger JK, Ellison NE, Ominsky AJ: Effects of intratracheal lidocaine on circulatory responses to tracheal intubation. *Anesthesiology* 1979; 41:409–412.
44. Stoelting RK: Attenuation of blood pressure response to laryngoscopy and tracheal intubation with sodium nitroprusside. *Anesth Analg* 1979; 58:116–119.
45. Pflug AE, Halter JB: Effect of spinal anesthesia on adrenergic tone and the neuroendocrine responses to surgical stress in humans. *Anesthesiology* 1981; 55:120–126.
46. Sivarajan M, Amory DW, Everett GB, Buffington C: Blood pressure, not cardiac output, determines blood loss during induced hypotension. *Anesth Analg* 1980; 59:203–206.
47. Tinker JH, Cucchiara RF: Use of sodium nitroprusside during anesthesia and surgery. *Int Anesthesiol Clin* 1978; 16:89–112.
48. Leigh JM: The history of controlled hypotension. *Br J Anaesth* 1975; 47:745–749.
49. Wildsmith JAW, Marshall RL, Jenkinson JL, MacRae WR, Scott DB: Haemodynamic effects of sodium nitroprusside during nitrous oxide/halothane anaesthesia. *Br J Anaesth* 1975; 45:71–74.
50. Strunin L: Organ perfusion during controlled hypotension. *Br J Anaesth* 1975; 47:793–798.
51. Chen RYZ, Matteo RS, Chien S: Baroreflex sensitivity and induced hypotension. *Anesthesiology* 1979; 51:S76.
52. Salem MR, Ivankovic AD: Place of beta-adrenergic blocking drugs in the deliberate induction of hypotension. *Anesth Analg* 1970; 49:427–434.
53. Crystal GJ, Rooney MW, Salem MR: Regional hemodynamics and oxygen supply during isovolemic hemodilution alone and in combination with adenosine-induced controlled hypotension. *Anesth Analg* 1988; 67:211–218.
54. Thompson GE, Miller RD, Stevens WC, Murray WR: Hypotensive anesthesia for total hip arthroplasty. *Anesthesiology* 1978; 48:91–96.
55. Cunningham AJA: Controlled hypotension to minimize blood loss of anaemic Jehovah's Witness patient undergoing total hip and shoulder replacement. *Br J Anaesth* 1982; 54:895–897.
56. Butterworth JF, Piccione W, Berrizbeitia LD, Dance G, Shemin RJ, Conn LH: Augmentation of venous return by adrenergic agonists during spinal anesthesia. *Anesth Analg* 1986; 65:612–616.
57. Ecoffey C, Edouard A, Pruszczynski W, Taly E, Samil K: Effects of epidural anesthesia on catecholamines, renin activity, and vasopressin changes induced by tilt in elderly men. *Anesthesiology* 1985; 62:294–297.
58. Yeager MP, Glass DD, Neff RK, Brinck-Johnsen T: Epidural anesthesia

and analgesia in high-risk surgical patients. *Anesthesiology* 1987; 66:729–736.

59. Roizen MF: Should we all have a sympathectomy at birth? Or at least preoperatively? *Anesthesiology* 1988; 68:482–484.
60. Roizen MF, Horrigan RW, Frazer BM: Anesthetic doses blocking adrenergic (stress) and cardiovascular responses. *Anesthesiology* 1981; 54:390–398.
61. Price HL: *Circulation During Anesthesia and Operation.* Springfield, Ill., Charles C Thomas, 1967.
62. Karhunen U, Cozanitis DA, Brander P: The oculocardiac reflex in adults. *Anaesthesia* 1984; 39:524–528.
63. Rocco AG, Vandam LD: Changes in circulation consequent to manipulation during abdominal surgery. *JAMA* 1957; 164:14–18.
64. Seltzer JL, Ritter DE, Starsnic MA, Marr AT: The hemodynamic response to traction on the mesentery. *Anesthesiology* 1985; 63:96–99.
65. Ransohoff JL: Causes of sudden fall in blood pressure while exploring the common bile duct. *Ann Surg* 1908; 48:550–553.
66. Seltzer JL, Goldberg ME, Larijani GE, Ritter DE, Starsnic MA, Stahl GL: Prostacyclin mediation of vasodilation following mesenteric traction. *Anesthesiology* 1988; 68:514–518.
67. Simon E, Pierau F-K, Taylor DCM: Central and peripheral thermal control of effectors in homeothermic temperature regulation. *Physiol Rev* 1986; 66:235–300.
68. Wakim KG: Bodily reactions to high temperature. *Anesthesiology* 1964; 25:532–548.
69. Flacke JW, Flacke WE: Inadvertent hypothermia: Frequent, insidious, and often serious. *Semin Anesth* 1983; 2:183–196.
70. Vaughan MS, Vaughan RW, Cork RC: Postoperative hypothermia in adults: Relationship of age, anesthesia, and shivering to rewarming. *Anesth Analg* 1981; 60:746–751.
71. Hammel HT: Anesthetics and body temperature regulation. *Anesthesiology* 1988; 68:833–835.
72. Sessler DI, Olofsson CI, Rubinstein EH, Beebe JJ: The thermoregulatory threshold in humans during halothane anesthesia. *Anesthesiology* 1988; 68:836–842.
73. Sellick BA: Induced hypothermia. *Int Anesthesiol Clin* 1967; 5:118–131.
74. Zinn WJ, Warnock EH: Safe hypothermia: A report on the use of external ice baths in open heart surgery on one hundred patients. *JAMA* 1960; 174:146–148.
75. Roe CF, Goldberg MJ, Blair CS, Kinney JM: The influence of body temperature on early postoperative oxygen consumption. *Surgery* 1966; 60:85–92.
76. Sessler DI, Israel D, Pozos RS, Pozos M, Rubinstein EH: Spontaneous post-anesthetic tremor does not resemble thermoregulatory shivering. *Anesthesiology* 1988; 68:843–850.
77. Sharkey A, Lipton JM, Murphy MT, Giesecke AH: Inhibition of post-

anesthetic shivering with radiant heat. *Anesthesiology* 1987; 66:249–252.

78. Haslam KR, Nielsen CH: Do passive heat and moisture exchangers keep the patient warm? *Anesthesiology* 1986; 64:379–381.

79. Goudsouzian NG, Morris RH, Ryan JF: The effects of a warming blanket on the maintenance of body temperatures in anesthetized infants and children. *Anesthesiology* 1973; 39:351–353.

80. Stone DR, Downs JB, Paul WL, Perkins HM: Adult body temperature and heated humidification of anesthetic gases during general anesthesia. *Anesth Analg* 1981; 60:736–741.

81. MacIntyre PE, Pavlin EG, Dwersteg JF: Effect of meperidine on oxygen consumption, carbon dioxide production, and respiratory gas exchange in postanesthesia shivering. *Anesth Analg* 1987; 66:751–755.

82. Pauca AL, Savage RT, Simpson S, Roy RD: Effect of pethidine, fentanyl and morphine on post-operative shivering in man. *Acta Anaesthesiol Scand* 1984; 28:138–143.

83. Vigran IM: Dangerous potentiation of meperidine hydrochloride by pargyline hydrochloride. *JAMA* 1964; 187:953.

84. Ziegler MG, Lake CR, Kopin IJ: Plasma noradrenaline increases with age. *Nature* 1976; 261:333–334.

85. Riley CM, Day RL, Greeley DML, Langord WS: Central autonomic dysfunction with defective lacrimation: Report of five cases. *Pediatrics* 1949; 3:468–478.

86. Kritchman MM, Schwartz H, Papper EM: Experiences with general anesthesia in patients with familial dysautonomia. *JAMA* 1959; 170:529–533.

87. Meridy HW, Creighton RE: General anesthesia in eight patients with familial dysautonomia. *Can Anaesth Soc J* 1971; 18:563–570.

88. Rubenstein AE, Yahr MD: Adult onset autonomic dysfunction coexistent with familial dysautonomia in a consanguineous family. *Neurology* 1977; 27:168–170.

89. Shea JD, Gioffre R, Carrion H, Small MP: Autonomic hyperreflexia in spinal cord injury. *South Med J* 1973; 66:869–872.

90. Erickson RP: Autonomic hyperreflexia: Pathophysiology and medical management. *Arch Phys Med Rehabil* 1980; 61:431–440.

91. Rocco AG, Vandam LD: Problems in anesthesia for paraplegics. *Anesthesiology* 1959; 20:348–354.

92. Muravchick S, Brown BT, Carrion H, Politano VA, Pallares V: Pentolinium for control of reflex hypertension in spinal cord injured patients. *Paraplegia* 1978; 16:350–356.

93. Bravo EL, Gifford RW: Pheochromocytoma: Diagnosis, localization, and management. *N Engl J Med* 1984; 311:1298–1302.

94. Newell KA, Prinz RA, Brooks MH, Glisson SN, Barbato AL, Freeark RJ: Plasma catecholamine changes during excision of pheochromocytoma. *Surgery* 1988; 104:1064–1073.

95. Ahlquist RP: Adrenergic receptors and others. *Anesth Analg* 1979; 58:510–515.

96. Sibley DR, Lefkowitz RJ: Molecular mechanisms of receptor desensitiza-

tion: The beta-adrenergic receptor–coupled adenylate cyclase system as a model. *Nature* 1985; 317:124–129.

97. Desmonts JM, Marty J: Anaesthetic management of patients with pheochromocytoma. *Br J Anaesth* 1984; 56:781–787.
98. Crout JR, Brown BR: Anesthetic management of pheochromocytoma: The value of phenoxybenzamine and methoxyflurane. *Anesthesiology* 1969; 30:29–36.
99. Cooperman LH, Engelman K, Mann PEG: Anesthetic management of pheochromocytoma employing halothane and beta-adrenergic blockade. *Anesthesiology* 1967; 28:575–582.
100. Feldman JM, Blalock JA, Fagraeus L, Miller JN, Farrell RE, Wells SA: Alterations in plasma norepinephrine concentration during surgical resection of pheochromocytoma. *Ann Surg* 1978; 188:758–768.
101. Sumikawa K, Amakata Y: The pressor effect of droperidol on a patient with pheochromocytoma. *Anesthesiology* 1977; 46:359–361.
102. Mihm FG: Pulmonary artery pressure monitoring in patients with pheochromocytoma. *Anesth Analg* 1983; 62:1129–1133.

5

Neuromuscular Function and Blockade

In the earliest era of modern anesthesia, especially when nitrous oxide
was the sole anesthetic agent (Chapter 2), the tendency of anesthetized
patients to move away from the site of surgical stimulation was readily
apparent. Although useful as a guide to the assessment of depth of anesthesia, gross skeletal muscle movements were nevertheless a nui-
sance, even when the scope and the duration of a surgical procedure
were extremely limited. Deep levels of diethyl ether or chloroform anesthesia reliably minimized movement, but not infrequently also produced lethal cardiorespiratory depression.

In contemporary practice, even minor disturbances of the stability
of the surgical field during a microscopic vascular anastomosis or during retinal surgery can result in a failed procedure or irreversible injury
to the patient. Inadequate relaxation or unexpected movement can also
hinder visceral exposure, interfere with orthopedic repair, or make it
impossible to perform effective cosmetic surgery. In this chapter neuromuscular function and blockade in normal and abnormal states are discussed, and the factors that determine the selection of adjuvant drugs
used to provide skeletal muscle relaxation during general anesthesia
are reviewed.

MUSCLE TONE AND MOVEMENT DURING ANESTHESIA

Contraction of skeletal muscle may produce discrete muscle movements or more subtle changes such as sustained muscle tone. Drug-in-

duced loss of consciousness per se, even when produced by agents such as barbiturates that have no intrinsic relaxant properties, still produces a generalized reduction in muscle tone. This loss of tone may reflect the diffuse effects of anesthetics on the synapse-rich reticular formations, the basal ganglia, or the motor cortex. The effects are further potentiated by the action of some anesthetics on the spinal cord itself.[1] Even at moderate levels of anesthetic depth, however, a stimulus of adequate intensity may still provoke a clinically obvious evoked contraction of skeletal muscle.

Infiltration of local anesthetic at the surgical site or sensory blockade of the peripheral nerves that conduct afferent input from the point of stimulation abolishes these motor responses. At deeper levels of general anesthesia, movement in response to surgical stimulation is probably initiated through segmental spinal cord pathways which are simple polysynaptic reflex arcs. At lighter levels of anesthesia, however, these somatoreflexes are more likely to involve complex central integration, since they can be attenuated or abolished by coincident neural input, such as chest wall movement resulting from passive hyperventilation.[2]

Abolition of all overt skeletal muscle contraction can be accomplished with sufficient inspired concentrations of most inhalational general anesthetics. However, this strategy requires imposing a level of general anesthesia sufficiently profound that it not only blocks somatoreflex pathways but also suppresses autonomic pathways ("stage IV anesthesia"). The resultant disruption of autonomic homeostasis (Chapter 4) and the potential for compromise of organ perfusion at this level of anesthesia make this approach to the problem of "inadequate relaxation" practical only with agents such as diethyl ether and cyclopropane. They generate considerable sympathoadrenal stimulation, which largely offsets the depression of autonomic control mechanisms.

Curare

Since the evolution of modern surgery precluded the use of these agents because of their flammability, however, the goal of reconciling adequate muscle relaxation with cardiovascular stability required a new strategy of applied pharmacology. Although known to Western scientists for almost 400 years, the therapeutic use of curare in medical practice was limited to treatment of infection from *Clostridium tetani*, or to the modification of skeletal muscle activity during electroshock therapy until 1942, when its use to "provide rapid and complete muscular relaxation in resistant patients under general anesthesia" was described.[3] Incremental intravenous doses were added to a cyclopropane anesthetic, permitting reduction of inspired anesthetic concentrations while still producing transient relaxation of the abdominal musculature. Neither vital signs nor spontaneous respiration was grossly compromised, although monitoring of respiratory adequacy was limited to observation of diaphragmatic efforts.

Far more than just a novel application of an old drug, this clinical experiment became one of the great milestones in the application of pharmacologic principles to anesthetic practice: it suggested the use of a specific drug to produce a single desired component of anesthesia. The anesthetist, therefore, was no longer constrained to accept anesthetic effects and side effects in the degree and proportion dictated by the clinical pharmacology of the primary anesthetic agent. Instead, the administration of general anesthesia could now be rightly seen as an exercise in the application of pharmacologic principles to meet clinical requirements. In effect, the practice of anesthesia had moved from the realm of clinical art into the domain of applied science.

Like many important achievements in medicine, the use of curare did not receive immediate acceptance. Its molecular structure was not established until almost 6 years after its introduction into clinical practice. Nor was it, in fact, without hazard. Even in the United Kingdom, where curare-induced neuromuscular blockade was accepted in a relatively uncontroversial manner, the medical establishment gave practitioners "a grave and insistent warning to the inexperienced that we are dealing with one of the most potent poisons known."[4] In the United States a large-scale multi-institutional study was more specific, raising serious questions regarding the wisdom of the use of curare.[5]

The change in anesthetic practice was irreversible, however. The advantage of providing neuromuscular blockade as a separate component of the anesthetic routine, rather than as a useful side effect of deep levels of drug-induced unconsciousness, was obvious. Controversy regarding the safety of this practice did, however, stimulate far-reaching clinical and laboratory investigations into the pharmacology and physiology of drug-induced paralysis. Thus, rather than suppress the use of this drug, the concerns of conservative practitioners ultimately provided the basis for much of our current knowledge of the neuromuscular junction, neuromuscular blockade, respiration and ventilatory support, and the management of patients with neuromuscular disorders.

NEUROMUSCULAR FUNCTION

The neuromuscular junction is a complex anatomic structure that functions as an electrochemical transducer linking electrically excitable conducting and contracting elements. An evoked neural signal generates a change in conductance in the axonal membrane; transmembrane ion flux then generates an action potential that is propagated along the axon of the neuron to its terminal. There influx of calcium ions causes the release of membrane-bound vesicles containing acetylcholine.

The acetylcholine molecules diffuse into and across the synaptic gap, where they combine with highly specific cholinergic receptors (cholinoceptors) on the end-plate of the skeletal muscle membrane. Interaction between acetylcholine and cholinoceptors activates channels for ionic movement. Increased conductance for extracellular sodium generates a local depolarizing current; when the voltage across the membrane changes sufficiently, an end-plate potential (EPP) is produced that, in turn, triggers a propagated action potential (AP) across the surface of the skeletal muscle. This electrical event initiates the ionic flux within the muscle cell that initiates a mechanical skeletal muscle response.

Receptor Activation

At any moment a dynamic interaction of the factors involved in the release, receptor-binding, and subsequent hydrolysis of acetylcholine at the motor end-plate determines the number of receptor sites occupied and the number of adjacent ion channels activated. Simultaneous opening of about 20% of the approximately ten million ion channels will generate a voltage change large enough to reach the "threshold" value for transmembrane potential at which an EPP is spontaneously generated. The threefold to fourfold excess of cholinoceptors normally available represents the "margin of safety" for neuromuscular transmission.[6]

Two adjacent cholinoceptors must be activated simultaneously in order to open the shared ion channel to which they are physically attached.

The electrical consequences of widespread ion channel activation are generally "all-or-none" for skeletal muscle. If relatively few channels are activated, no EPP is generated. If, however, the end-plate is depolarized sufficiently, a subsequent skeletal muscle AP triggers the release of calcium ions from the sarcoplasmic reticulum (SR) within the muscle cell where it has been actively sequestered. The increase in myoplasmic calcium ion concentration that follows the release of calcium from the SR then initiates the formation of cross-linkages between the contractile proteins actin and myosin. This last event produces mechanical movement of the structural components of the muscle cell, and thus completes the complex process of excitation-contraction coupling.

Mechanical Contraction

Variations in the strength of a mechanical skeletal muscle response during partial neuromuscular blockade reflect a reduction in the number of muscle fibers that have been recruited and not a variable degree of responsiveness to the release of acetylcholine or to subsequent cholinoceptor stimulation. There is normally no mechanism for a graded contraction of a single skeletal muscle cell. Effective neuromuscular transmission can therefore be considered to be a phenomenon of probability: enhanced or reduced release of acetylcholine or altered availability of cholinoceptors at the end-plate simply change the likelihood that the end-plate threshold will be surpassed and a skeletal muscle AP subsequently generated. The overall force of gross skeletal muscle contraction, therefore, reflects the number of cells within the muscle group to participate in neuromuscular transmission in response to a particular episode of neural stimulation.

Neuromuscular Junction

Synaptic transmission at the neuromuscular junction has three main components: electrical propagation at presynaptic and at postsynaptic sites, as well as an intermediate step of cholinergic chemical transmission restricted to the highly specialized skeletal muscle motor end-plate. The capability of muscle cell membranes to respond electrically to the release of acetylcholine appears to be inhibited in non-end-plate areas of skeletal muscle by the continuing release of cyclic guanosine monophosphate from the nerve terminal.[7] Denervation injury, upper motor neuron disease, aging, disuse atrophy, or other causes of impaired proximodistal axonal transport result in the proliferation and thickening of the end-plate membrane. It is also associated with the appearance of extrajunctional cholinoceptors outside the end-plate area, in the perijunctional zone (Fig 5–1).

Cholinergic chemical transmission permits the amplification of the neuronal electrical stimulus and facilitates the modulation of overall synaptic transmission through mechanisms not available in purely electrical pathways.[8] Release of acetylcholine from the nerve terminal not

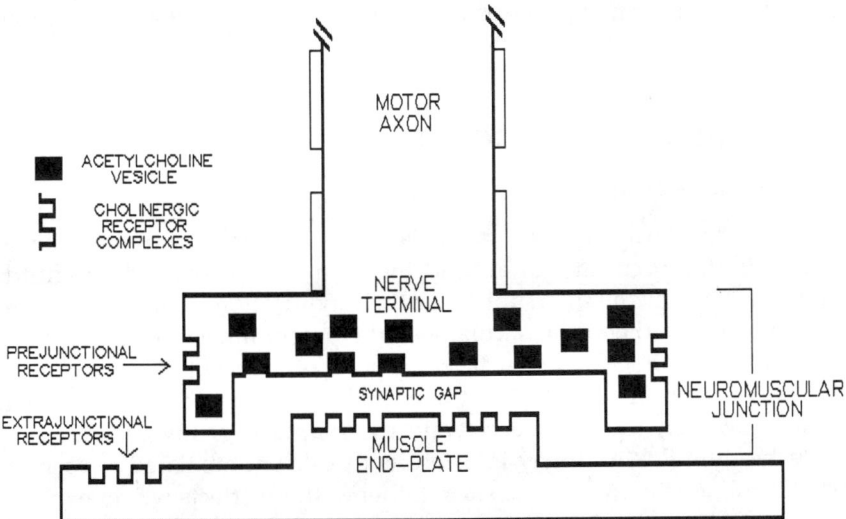

FIG 5–1.
Schematic anatomy of the mammalian neuromuscular junction. Acetylcholine is synthesized within, and released from, the motor nerve terminal in vesicular structures that merge into the terminal membrane. Cyclic guanosine monophosphate provides trophic support to the muscle and inhibits proliferation of cholinoceptors outside the immediate end-plate area. Extrajunctional receptors for acetylcholine may appear after pathologic or age-related denervation. Prejunctional receptors facilitate the synthesis and release of acetylcholine and may mediate posttetanic potentiation, fade, and other prejunctional phenomena seen during nondepolarizing neuromuscular blockade.

only activates end-plate receptors but also appears to facilitate the subsequent release of additional transmitter molecules by way of a positive feedback loop. Prejunctional cholinoceptors on the neuronal membrane accelerate the mobilization, and perhaps the synthesis, of acetylcholine.[9] The maintenance of a large releasable store of acetylcholine within the nerve terminal makes reliable transmission possible even during repeated or high-frequency stimulation, since the maximum rate of skeletal muscle contraction is therefore not limited by the speed with which the enzyme acetyltransferase can synthesize acetylcholine.

In fact, the mechanism by which curare and other nondepolarizing neuromuscular blocking drugs produce "fade," an inability to sustain contraction during repeated or tetanic stimulation, may reflect, at least in part, their presynaptic effects.[10] However, tetanic stimulation of motor nerves also augments the rate of acetylcholine synthesis by stimulating prejunctional cholinoceptors: repeated evoked neural stimulation produces a transient enhancement of neuromuscular transmission evident during incomplete competitive neuromuscular blockade, a clinical phenomenon known as posttetanic facilitation (PTF).

NEUROMUSCULAR BLOCKADE

Inhalational Anesthetics

The complexity of neuromuscular transmission and the sequence of events that occur at and around the neuromuscular junction afford multiple sites for the interruption or the modification of normal synaptic transmission (Fig 5–2). Virtually all the potent inhalational anesthetics produce indirect, nonspecific reductions of muscle tone as a consequence of their diffuse effects on neuronal synapses in brain and spinal cord. However, they also accelerate the reuptake of myoplasmic calcium by the SR,[11] and may interfere with calcium-mediated release of acetylcholine at prejunctional sites. Either of these effects would explain their ability to potentiate both the intensity and the duration of preexisting neuromuscular blockade. Only diethyl ether, however, has been shown to possess clinically significant intrinsic and specific neuromuscular blocking properties. This effect can be seen as a reduced magnitude of evoked neuromuscular response after direct nerve stimulation.[12]

When modern inhalational anesthetics are employed as part of the anesthetic plan, neuromuscular blockade is primarily a function of the relaxant drugs selected; rarely is it an essential quality of the primary anesthetic itself. The ability of potent inhalational anesthetics to reduce muscle tone may, however, be particularly important in infants[13] or in other patients with immature myoneural physiology, those with minimal muscle mass, or when used for patients in whom the effects of neuromuscular blocking drugs are unpredictable or contraindicated.

Metabolic Factors

Deficiencies of calcium effectively uncouple the electrical depolarization of the nerve terminal from the subsequent mobilization and release of acetylcholine. In addition, magnesium antagonizes the functions of ionized calcium within the nerve terminal. Therefore, pathologic or therapeutic hypermagnesemia can cause skeletal muscle weakness and potentiate drug-induced neuromuscular blockade. Much of the interaction between neuromuscular blocking drugs and aminoglycoside antibiotics, documented as reports of unexpected residual paralysis, probably reflects the ability of these "mycin" antibiotics to augment magnesium influx into electrically active nerve terminals. Predict-

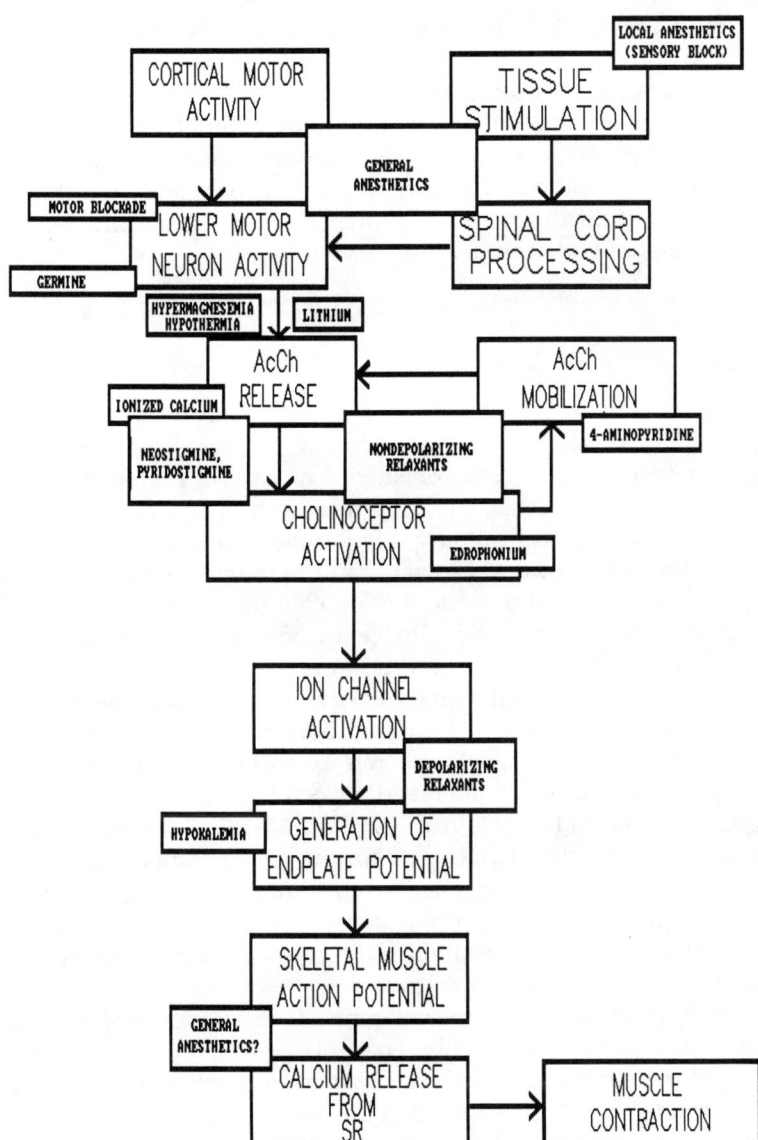

FIG 5–2.
Proposed sites of action for anesthetic agents, adjuvants, reversal drugs, and metabolic factors that modify the evoked mechanical responses of skeletal muscle. Each factor has been superimposed on the site or sequence of events responsible for neuromuscular transmission under normal circumstances at which it appears to exert its primary effect. *AcCh* = acetylcholine.

ably, their ability to potentiate neuromuscular blockade can be reversed, to some degree, by infusions of ionized calcium.[14]

Potentiation of neuromuscular blockade has also been reported after therapeutic use of another cation, lithium.[15] Similarly, mild-to-moderate hypothermia also potentiates neuromuscular blockade,[16] since the synthesis, mobilization, and release of acetylcholine from the nerve terminal constitute a metabolically intense process markedly depressed by reductions of body temperature.[17]

Nondepolarizing Blockade

Nondepolarizing relaxant drugs interrupt neuromuscular transmission on a physicochemical basis, reducing the access of acetylcholine molecules to end-plate receptor sites. The classic characterization of this type of neuromuscular blocking drug as a "pachycurare" conveys appropriately the concept of large, bulky molecules structured in such a way that they are attracted toward, and then overlie, end-plate cholinoceptors. They do not activate the ion channels that are separate but adjacent components of the cholinoceptor ion channel complex.

A similar hindrance to cholinoceptor access may occur at presynaptic sites as well. The specific qualities of nondepolarizing neuromuscular blockade probably are determined both by the dynamic, variable nature of presynaptic acetylcholine release and by the continuous competition between acetylcholine and relaxant molecules for access to end-plate cholinoceptors. Neuromuscular transmission is effectively interrupted by nondepolarizing relaxants even when near-normal amounts of acetylcholine are released by neural stimulation. Because of the competitive nature of the blockade, however, massive release of acetylcholine into the extracellular fluid of the synaptic gap may reestablish neuromuscular transmission.

Nondepolarizing neuromuscular blockade is therefore a relative, rather than an absolute, phenomenon. The end-plate machinery and the complex membrane-based system that both activate the release of calcium from the sarcoplasmic reticulum and initiate activation of contractile proteins in the skeletal muscle remain intact. Although the primary site of action for nondepolarizing relaxants appears to be postsynaptic, the neuromuscular margin of safety is sufficiently great that the concentrations of relaxant molecules needed to produce blockade are high enough to exert presynaptic effects. Changes in acetylcholine synthesis and release and the competitive nature of the antagonism produced at end-plate cholinoceptors distinguish nondepolarizing neuromuscular blockade clinically, as well as neurophysiologically, from other forms of reversible pharmacologic paralysis.

Depolarizing Blockade

Succinylcholine, the only depolarizing neuromuscular blocking drug currently in use in this country, produces skeletal muscle relaxation by a mechanism entirely different from that of the nondepolarizing relaxants. More precisely described as diacetylcholine or succinyldicholine (SDC), this drug is a duplex analog of acetylcholine[18] that produces neuromuscular blockade by stimulating end-plate cholinoceptors and activating adjacent ion channels. The end-plate repolarization that normally follows this sequence of events is markedly delayed.

Unlike nondepolarizing relaxants, SDC does not hinder the access of acetylcholine to cholinoceptors. In fact, it binds to cholinoceptors with a specificity and affinity sufficiently high to cause transient activation of the ion channel complexes at both presynaptic and postsynaptic sites. This phenomenon produces skeletal muscle fasciculations, tonic contractions of some types of smooth muscle,[19] and even ganglionic stimulation.[20]

Sustained end-plate depolarization and the loss of electrical potential at the muscle end-plate are the essential electrical characteristics of "depolarizing" neuromuscular blockade.[21] Repolarization is delayed because SDC produces persistent, rather than transient, activation of ion channels. The structure of SDC mimics acetylcholine at the receptor, yet it resists hydrolysis by the acetylcholinesterase subunits that are part of the cholinoceptor complex on the end-plate membrane.

The mechanism of SDC-induced depolarizing blockade may also involve sites other than the end-plate cholinoceptors. Molecules of SDC may become wedged within open ion channels, creating an "open channel blockade" that functionally deactivates the end-plate by allowing continuous ion flux even after SDC is no longer bound to cholinoceptors. In addition, molecules of SDC may subsequently infiltrate into the skeletal muscle cell, where they obstruct other ion channels and block the propagation of action potentials across the surface of the skeletal muscle cell.[14] The intracellular effects of SDC are sufficiently profound that even when the muscle end-plate itself is repolarized and reactivated, skeletal muscle AP may be abnormal. Unlike nondepolarizing agents, SDC-induced neuromuscular blockade is maintained even in the presence of massive release of acetylcholine. Classic depolarizing neuromuscular blockade is therefore noncompetitive.

Phase II Blockade

Initially, "phase I," or depolarizing blockade, the interruption of neuromuscular transmission, is virtually absolute, at least at an end-plate level. It is independent of the intensity or the frequency of nerve stimulation or other prejunctional events. These qualities of neuromuscular blockade may change if exposure to SDC is sustained, however.[22]

Although some descriptions imply that there is an abrupt transition to so-called "phase II," desensitization, or dual blockade,[23] other investigations describe a progressive transformation in the quality of SDC-induced paralysis to one that begins to resemble that produced by nondepolarizing drugs.[24] Characteristics referable to the altered release of acetylcholine from nerve terminals suggest that SDC can exert presynaptic effects: prolonged exposure of the nerve terminal may result in infiltration and inactivation of presynaptic ion channels. Under these circumstances, the elimination of positive feedback mechanisms that normally facilitate acetylcholine mobilization and release would produce fade in response to repetitive stimulation, at least across those neuromuscular junctions to which end plate function had returned.

In summary, it is now clear that pharmacologic neuromuscular blockade is produced by at least two distinct processes. Competitive, or nondepolarizing, relaxants act to interrupt the chemical phase of neuromuscular transmission: they prevent activation of the end-plate and possibly the presynaptic ion channels by hindering the access of acetylcholine molecules to cholinoceptors at these sites. These drugs produce a relative impairment of evoked responses, the extent of which varies with the frequency of stimulation. The neurophysiologic components needed for neuromuscular transmission remain intact.

In contrast, SDC is an acetylcholine analog that interrupts neuromuscular transmission by eliminating the normal sequence of postjunctional electrical events initiated by acetylcholine. It may also have effects at the surface of the skeletal muscle cell and at presynaptic nerve terminal cholinoceptors if exposure to this drug is prolonged. Unlike the nondepolarizing relaxants, SDC produces a brief initial period of ion channel activation and end-plate depolarization, presumably the mechanism that produces the skeletal muscle fasciculations and myalgias associated with its use.

TERMINATION OF DRUG-INDUCED
NEUROMUSCULAR BLOCKADE

Postsynaptic Effects

The process of antagonism or "reversal" of the effects of neuromuscular blocking drugs appears adequately explained by current concepts of neuromuscular physiology. Anticholinesterase drugs such as neostigmine, pyridostigmine, and edrophonium interfere with the enzymatic hydrolysis of acetylcholine, a process that normally occurs immediately after its combination with cholinoceptors on the skeletal muscle end-plate. Tissue or "true" acetylcholinesterase activity is membrane bound and highly concentrated within the end-plate complexes of cholinoceptors and their associated ion channel structures.

Drugs with anticholinesterase properties, in effect, enhance the life expectancy of acetylcholine molecules, allowing them to participate in repeated interactions with end-plate and presynaptic cholinoceptors. The effective local concentration of acetylcholine in the synaptic gap is therefore increased, a phenomenon that pushes the competitive balance between cholinergic agonist and neuromuscular blocking drug in a direction that favors ion channel activation and subsequent contraction of skeletal muscle.

Presynaptic Effects

Neostigmine and pyridostigmine may also have presynaptic effects that facilitate acetylcholine release and enhance the efficacy of these drugs in the antagonism or "reversal" of neuromuscular blockade. For any given frequency of neural stimulation, enhancement of the mobilization or of the release of acetylcholine increases the likelihood of successful neuromuscular transmission, even when a significant concentration of nondepolarizing relaxant molecules remains in the extracellular fluid of the synaptic gap. Some anticholinesterase drugs may also induce repetitive firing of nerve terminals in response to a single action potential.[25]

Unlike neostigmine and pyridostigmine, edrophonium has an electrostatic, rather than a covalent, attraction for acetylcholinesterase. Its predominant effect appears to be at postsynaptic cholinesterase sites, and it therefore has limited ability to enhance the release of acetylcholine. Very large doses of this drug overcome its normally short duration of interaction with acetylcholinesterase but do not alter its fundamental mode of action. Consequently, edrophonium may not antagonize profound levels of nondepolarizing neuromuscular blockade as effectively as the other two anticholinesterase drugs.[26]

Other approaches to antagonism of nondepolarizing neuromuscular blockade include augmentation of presynaptic acetylcholine mobilization with 4-aminopyridine.[27] Infusion of supplemental ionized calcium may also enhance the formation of acetylcholine vesicles and their exocytosis from the nerve terminal.[15] Germine monoacetate has also been used to induce repetitive firing at nerve terminals,[28] thus simulating tetanic stimulation pharmacologically.

Sustained Recovery

Anticholinesterase drugs transiently enhance neuromuscular transmission when given to patients with nondepolarizing neuromuscular blockade. Although this process is frequently called "reversal," implying a single, definitive action, return of neuromuscular transmission actually reflects two simultaneous processes. First, there is a short-term pharmacodynamic antagonism of the competitive effects of the relaxant molecules at the neuromuscular junction; second, there is a continuous pharmacokinetic process by which these molecules are cleared from plasma and from the extracellular fluid that surrounds the muscle endplate.

Plasma and extracellular fluid relaxant concentrations, at least under steady-state conditions, determine the prevailing degree of neuromuscular blockade.[29] With deep levels of paralysis, reversal and return of adequate neuromuscular transmission may require 30 to 45 minutes. If very high concentrations of relaxant produce a profound level of neuromuscular blockade, reversal with anticholinesterase may actually be impossible.[30] At clinically encountered levels of neuromuscular blockade, however, there appears to be an inverse relationship between the degree of preexisting neuromuscular blockade and the subsequent speed and completeness with which an anticholinesterase agent restores normal neuromuscular transmission.[31]

In anesthetic practice, spontaneous and timely return of some degree of evoked neuromuscular responsiveness before reversal provides objective evidence that the pharmacokinetic elimination of neuromuscular blocking drugs is proceeding at a reasonable rate. However, in patients with severe hepatic or renal disease, or in others in whom plasma concentrations of neuromuscular blocking drugs do not fall at normal rates, spontaneous recovery may be unusually slow, especially after multiple doses of nondepolarizing neuromuscular blocking drugs. Although neuromuscular transmission may improve briefly after the administration of large doses of anticholinesterase agents, this may be followed by "recurarization," the rapid return of drug-induced paralysis because of the persistent high concentrations of neuromuscular blocking drug.[32] The full and sustained return of adequate neuromuscular transmission, therefore, requires continuing relaxant elimination by pharmacokinetic processes, and is only secondarily influenced by the choice of anticholinesterase drug, or by its dosage.

Other Factors

Other processes that hinder neuromuscular transmission or prevent antagonism of neuromuscular blockade (Fig 5–2) include respiratory acidosis,[33] hypermagnesemia,[15] hypocalcemia, or hypokalemia.[34] Low serum potassium may, however, necessitate only a moderate increase in the dose of anticholinesterase drug.[35] Hypothermia, even to the moderate levels produced incidentally during the course of elective surgery, appears to potentiate nondepolarizing blockade by altering the dynamics of acetylcholine release from the nerve terminal and by delaying the elimination of the relaxant.[36] Quinidine, lidocaine, and local anesthetics also have potentiating effects on nondepolarizing neuromuscular blockade that are demonstrable in vitro[37] but that rarely assume clinical importance.

The termination of the depolarizing neuromuscular blockade produced by SDC occurs as a result of its eventual molecular destruction inside the end-plate, or by the diffusion of these molecules away from the surface of the skeletal muscle cell. The hydrolysis of SDC is then accomplished enzymatically by the action of endogenous plasma or "pseudo" cholinesterase. Enhancement of acetylcholine release has little effect on the restoration of neuromuscular transmission in SDC-induced blockade unless it has evolved into an early phase II phenomenon.

If sustained, however, phase II block ultimately becomes unresponsive to anticholinesterase agents or other pharmacologic techniques that simply increase acetylcholine activity within the synaptic gap.[38] Consequently, there is no process of reversal for depolarizing neuromuscular blockade that is comparable to that clinically employed after the use of nondepolarizing relaxant drugs. In fact, by interfering with plasma and tissue cholinesterase activity, anticholinesterase drugs may, in theory, prolong rather than terminate the effects of depolarizing relaxants such as SDC.

Persistence of depolarizing blockade beyond the usual period of 10 to 15 minutes after injection of SDC almost always reflects gross SDC overdosage or an intrinsic abnormality of the plasma cholinesterase enzyme responsible for its hydrolysis. If patients are genetically homozygous for an atypical genetic variant of normal plasma cholinesterase, SDC-induced paralysis may persist for an hour or more. There is no direct relationship, however, between the duration of SDC-induced paralysis and the "dibucaine number" that has been used to quantify plasma cholinesterase activity in vitro.[39]

Only the administration of purified, normal human plasma cholinesterase terminates depolarizing block promptly in patients with severe enzymatic abnormalities.[40] If heterozygous for an abnormal configuration of plasma cholinesterase that retains some residual cholinesterase activity, patients usually recover from SDC-induced blockade spontaneously, but in a somewhat variable and unpredictable manner. Reduced cholinesterase activity may also be acquired: it has been reported after exposure to organophosphate-type insecticides or the use of echothiophate eyedrops,[41] as a consequence of liver failure, or as a manifestation of aging.[42] Although this enzyme has no established physiologic function, it is of unique interest to the anesthesiologist because it is responsible for the hydrolysis and inactivation not only of SDC but also of ester-type local anesthetics. Plasma cholinesterase does not, however, inactivate trimethaphan, as had once been assumed.[43]

AUTONOMIC SIDE EFFECTS

Although relatively specific for agonist molecules, cholinoceptors at different sites in the peripheral nervous system vary in their affinity and in their selectivity for acetylcholine analogs. The extent to which a neuromuscular blocking drug activates or inhibits muscarinic and nicotinic cholinoceptor complexes determines both the characteristics and the severity of the autonomic side effects with which it is associated. For the nondepolarizing neuromuscular blocking drugs currently available, the quality and duration of neuromuscular blockade are sufficiently similar that the selection of a neuromuscular blocking drug has been based largely on its anticipated effects on arterial blood pressure and heart rate.[44]

A ratio of median-effective autonomic dose (AD_{50}) to clinically effective neuromuscular blocking dose (ED_{95}) quantitates the "autonomic margin of safety" for each of these agents and permits anticipation of the cardiovascular effects that will follow their intravenous injection. A unique parameter must be calculated for ganglionic blockade, for vagal blockade, and for histamine release, however. Some of these data require isolation of autonomic reflex arcs, and therefore can be obtained only from animal studies. Consequently, conclusions regarding the clinical application of these drugs based on comparisons of the degree of separation between their neuromuscular and autonomic effects (Table 5–1) must acknowledge differences in autonomic responsiveness between human and laboratory species.

Curare (*d*-tubocurarine) is the original "prototype" nondepolarizing neuromuscular blocking drug. It also produces ganglionic blockade by interrupting cholinergic transmission at ganglionic sites, and therefore can attenuate significantly the sympathetic and parasympathetic responses that occur during anesthesia. This property can be used to clinical advantage when it is part of a minimalist anesthetic approach such as the "Liverpool technique" because the ganglionic blockade decreases overall anesthetic requirement by attenuating cardiovascular responses to surgical stimulation.[45] However, the net sympatholysis produced by this relaxant appears to be somewhat greater than its interruption of parasympathetic efferent activity; in many applications, therefore, large doses of *d*-tubocurarine produce a significant reduction in both blood pressure and heart rate. The tendency of this drug to release histamine also can reduce systemic vascular resistance, and may contribute to abrupt arterial hypotension.

Methylation of the molecular structure of *d*-tubocurarine lowers the likelihood of histamine release and increases its potency. These effects separate more widely the dosages that produce neuromuscular blockade from those associated with autonomic side effects, and thus improve the autonomic margin of safety. The resultant semisynthetic neuromuscular blocking drug, metocurine (originally called dimethyl tubocurarine, but subsequently shown to have three methyl groups), displays a clinically obvious increase in selectivity for skeletal muscle nicotinic receptors.[46] The cardiovascular stability associated with the

TABLE 5–1.

Estimated Relative Margins of Safety for the Autonomic Effects of Nondepolarizing Relaxant Drugs

Drug	For Ganglionic Blockade	For Vagal Blockade	For Histamine Release
d-Tubocurarine	1	1	1
Metocurine	6	5	2
Atracurium	12	15	3
Vecuronium	30	65	"High"
Pancuronium	110	5	"High"

use of this drug was the primary factor responsible for its displacement of *d*-tubocurarine in patients with cardiovascular disease or others at particular risk of arterial hypotension.

Completely synthetic nondepolarizing neuromuscular blocking drugs can be "chemically engineered" to avoid both ganglionic blockade and histamine release. They may, however, have equally problematic side effects when they produce blockade at cardiac muscarinic cholinoceptors. Gallamine produces dose-dependent vagal blockade and marked tachycardia. Pancuronium has similar, but less dramatic, atropine-like effects that nevertheless cause tachycardia if large intravenous doses are administered rapidly.[47] Pancuronium may also precipitate the release of catecholamines from adrenergic nerve terminals by a mechanism similar to that of tyramine,[48] further increasing cardiac stimulation, cardiac output, and, in some cases, arterial blood pressure.

Further modification of the steroidal molecular structure of pancuronium has produced a configuration that is virtually free of cardiovascular side effects, yet one that retains the ability to produce potent neuromuscular blockade. Vecuronium does not stimulate the release of histamine, nor does it produce significant effects in autonomic ganglia or blockade of cardiac muscarinic sites.[49] Consequently, it produces no change in cardiac or hemodynamic status even when multiples of ED_{95} are used by rapid intravenous injection to speed the onset of the neuromuscular blocking effect of this drug.[50]

Pancuronium, vecuronium, and the newest member of this group, pipecuronium, all require organ-dependent biotransformation, however. Therefore the duration of the neuromuscular blockade that they produce may be unacceptably prolonged in patients with severe renal or hepatic disease. A similar problem occurs with alcuronium and fazadinium, two agents that also retain sufficient histamine-releasing and autonomic-blocking properties to make their clinical utility questionable, although they remain available in Europe.

Similarly succinyldicholine can act as a cholinergic agonist at ganglionic and at muscarinic autonomic sites. Marked changes in heart rate, either tachycardia or bradycardia, occur, depending on the net balance between the sympathetic and parasympathetic activity within the autonomic nervous system. In patients with atropine-produced vagal blockade, ganglionic stimulation by SDC produces tachycardia and hypertension, especially if the drug is given by sustained infusion.[51] In contrast, stimulation of muscarinic cholinoceptors at the sinoatrial node may induce sinus bradycardia in patients with low residual levels of sympathetic tone, or in those who have not received atropine, especially after repeated doses of SDC.

The mechanism of SDC-induced bradycardia and its relationship to the production of succinylmonocholine, a metabolite of SDC, remain unclear despite widespread agreement that this phenomenon occurs.[52] There are also a wide variety of cardiac dysrhythmias associated with the use of SDC, including nodal rhythms and ventricular dysrhythmias. SDC may also lower the ventricular threshold for ectopy during laryngoscopy, tracheal intubation, or other situations of intense autonomic stimulation.[53]

Atracurium is a nondepolarizing relaxant that undergoes spontaneous hydrolysis in plasma by a mechanism independent of the plasma activity of cholinesterase. Consequently it has a predictable and consistent duration of clinical effect in patients of all ages, even those with end-stage hepatic or renal dysfunction. The cardiovascular and autonomic side effects of this drug, however, are more pronounced than those of the steroidal relaxant molecules, comparable with those already described for older "curariform" agents such as curare and metocurine.[54] Although it has a reasonably wide autonomic margin of safety, some degree of hypotension or bradycardia is not uncommon after the injection of a large intravenous dose of atracurium. Histamine release can also produce cardiovascular instability if atracurium is given by rapid bolus during anesthetic induction.[55]

A new benzylisoquinolinium diester, doxacurium, is a longer-acting nondepolarizing neuromuscular blocking drug that, like atracurium, has a reliable, organ-independent mechanism responsible for the termination of its action. Rapid intravenous injection may produce some histamine release, although it appears to have little effect on blood pressure or heart rate.[56] Mivacurium, another new agent, has both reliable pharmacokinetics and a minimal degree of autonomic side effects, provided that plasma cholinesterase activity, essential for its elimination, is near normal.[57]

MONITORING OF NEUROMUSCULAR BLOCKADE

The complexities of neuromuscular blockade and the danger of unrecognized residual respiratory paralysis are sufficiently great that monitoring of neuromuscular blockade is an essential part of contemporary anesthetic practice. Although described almost a half-century ago,[58] direct electrical stimulation of a peripheral nerve to evoke a skeletal muscle response has been used to guide the administration of neuromuscular blocking drugs during anesthesia for only the past few decades. Correlating the various forms of electrical and mechanical evoked responses with the clinical adequacy of surgical relaxation or recovery of neuromuscular function has been accomplished even more recently.

Single Twitch

Few anesthesiologists would argue with the contention that "the only satisfactory method of monitoring neuromuscular function is stimulation of an accessible peripheral motor nerve and observation or measurement of the response of the skeletal muscles supplied by this nerve."[21] The force of evoked muscle contractions is observed or measured in response to three basic patterns of peripheral nerve stimulation: single twitch, "train-of-four," and tetanus (Fig 5–3).

Single evoked muscle twitches produced by supramaximal stimuli no more frequent than one per second can be used to quantitate the reductions in the magnitude of neuromuscular response by direct com-

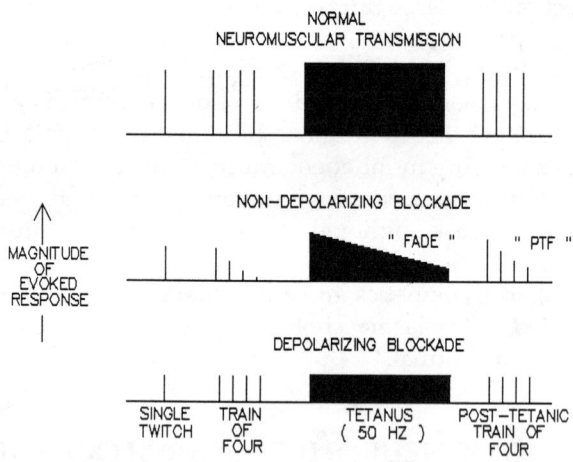

FIG 5–3.
Typical evoked response patterns for normal neuromuscular transmission and for nondepolarizing and depolarizing neuromuscular blockade. Prejunctional limitations of acetylcholine release become apparent during nondepolarizing blockade as "fade" because the neuromuscular margin of safety is reduced. With SDC-induced depolarizing blockade, evoked responses are reduced in direct proportion to the number of motor units that have been inactivated.

parison with an initial, unparalyzed control value. Twitch height, the force of an evoked response, is reduced by both depolarizing and nondepolarizing blockade. Since there is adequate time between stimuli to permit the nerve terminals to mobilize normal quantities of acetylcholine for subsequent release, this technique does not stress the presynaptic components of the neuromuscular junction, and therefore is useful primarily for monitoring postsynaptic events.

At a molecular level, no reduction in single-twitch height is usually seen until at least 75% of the end-plate cholinoceptors are inactivated by competitive, nondepolarizing neuromuscular blocking drugs.[6] The number of receptor-activated ion channels that must open simultaneously in order to produce an EPP is far less than the total number of receptor-channel complexes normally available at the end-plate. Because of this "margin of safety," tests of evoked single twitch rarely reveal the full extent to which neuromuscular blocking drugs have altered end-plate dynamics.

Tetanic Stimuli

Tetanic stimulation (stimulus frequencies of 30 Hz or greater) initially mobilizes, and then depletes, the nerve terminal of releasable stores of acetylcholine. Progressively fewer molecules of this neurotransmitter are released as the tetanic stimulus is sustained. Therefore, when the cholinoceptor redundancy that normally characterizes neuromuscular transmission is reduced by nondepolarizing blockade, the force of an evoked tetanic response "fades" dramatically as acetylcholine release declines. By exaggerating presynaptic and postsynaptic events, tetanic stimulation reveals relatively subtle deficiencies of neuromuscular transmission that cannot be observed with single twitch alone.[21] The degree of fade increases with higher frequency stimulation and with more prolonged duration of stimulus.[59] Tetanic fade does not occur during classic depolarizing (phase I) blockade because SDC disables muscle fiber motor end-plates in a noncompetitive, "all-or-none" manner that does not vary depending on local acetylcholine concentrations.

Tetanic stimulation also facilitates the synthesis of acetylcholine within the motor nerve terminal. Although depleted by continued rapid release during tetanic stimulation, subsequent acetylcholine release will be enhanced after a short period of neuronal inactivity. During nondepolarizing blockade, competition between acetylcholine and relaxant molecules for cholinoceptors limits ion channel activation. After a tetanically augmented barrage of acetylcholine molecules, however, some end-plate areas with limited channel activation may now reach their threshold for an EPP and for propagation of a skeletal muscle. The contractile response of that skeletal muscle cell can then be added to the response of those that are still functioning, thus transiently augmenting the total force of the gross evoked response. This phenomenon of posttetanic facilitation (PTF) is, in effect, a stimulation artifact useful in distinguishing nondepolarizing from depolarizing neuromuscular blockade. However, it alters the dynamics of acetylcholine synthesis and release sufficiently to make interpretation of subsequent evoked responses extremely difficult.

Train-of-Four

The introduction of the use of a train-of-four (TOF) stimulation pattern, consisting of four stimuli equally spaced within 2 seconds, has become the general standard for clinical monitoring of nondepolarizing blockade.[60] Unlike single twitch, the interval between stimuli in TOF is short enough to partially deplete prejunctional acetylcholine stores. Like tetanic stimulation, therefore, TOF can demonstrate limited availability of cholinoceptors at the end-plate and loss of the "margin of safety" by producing a progressive reduction in the magnitude of evoked response. The presence of this "fade" distinguishes between nondepolarizing and depolarizing blockade.[10]

Unlike tetanic stimulation patterns, TOF is not disruptive of the normal dynamic balance between acetylcholine synthesis and release. It does not produce PTF or confuse interpretation of subsequent evoked responses, unless applied more frequently than every 10 seconds. In addition, the comparison of the relative magnitude of the fourth to the first twitch response within the train-of-four yields a TOF ratio that provides a quantitative measure of the depth of nondepolarizing neuromuscular blockade even without an unparalyzed control value.[61]

An analogous but less precise technique requires only a gross "count" of the number of visible evoked components produced by TOF stimulation. TOF also appears to correlate reliably with clinical signs (Table 5–2) of adequate respiratory muscle strength.[62–64] Although this technique provides no more information regarding SDC-induced phase I depolarizing blockade than does single twitch, it does provide an early warning that transition to phase II depolarizing blockade has begun.

TABLE 5–2.

Correlation Between Evoked Neuromuscular Responses and Clinical Parameters After Nondepolarizing Neuromuscular Blockade

Control Twitch (%)	Typical Train-of-Four Count and Ratio	Surgical Relaxation	Sustained Headlift?	Maximum Inspired Pressure (cm H_2O)	Maintain Patent Airway?
100	4/4, 100%	—	Yes	−100	Yes
90	4/4, 75%	—	Yes	−90	Yes
80	4/4, 60%	—	Yes	−60	Yes
70	4/4, 40%	Minimal	Variable	−40	Variable
60	4/4, 20%	Minimal	No	−30	No
40	4/4, 10%	Poor	No	−20	No
25	3/4	Poor	No	< −20	No
20	2/4	Adequate	No	Minimal	—
10	1/4	Good	No	Minimal	—
0	0/4	Maximal	No	—	—

Other Techniques

For practical reasons, the monitoring of neuromuscular blockade during anesthesia is generally done by stimulating the ulnar nerve with surface or needle electrodes and by measuring subsequent evoked responses of the adductor pollicis or first interosseus muscles of the hand. Both mechanical (mechanomyogram) and electrical (unprocessed compound electromyogram [EMG], or integrated electromyogram [IEMG]) systems using TOF stimulation patterns are available.

IEMG is essentially equivalent to measurements of evoked force of thumb adduction if nondepolarizing neuromuscular blockade is used.[65] IEMG is also more quantitative and precise than gross visible or tactile assessment of the evoked response to TOF stimulation. The assessment of SDC-induced neuromuscular blockade using the IEMG is, however, severely compromised by the process of depolarization and by subsequent alteration of skeletal muscle electrical characteristics.[66] For profound nondepolarizing neuromuscular blockade, when there may be no initial evoked response to either single-twitch or TOF stimulation, tetanic stimulation can provide an alternative form of objective assessment of the degree of neuromuscular blockade through the technique of "posttetanic count."[67]

The results of studies using many different systems for monitoring neuromuscular transmission suggest a wide and dramatic variability of the intrinsic sensitivity of different types of skeletal muscles to relaxant drugs, especially those that produce nondepolarizing blockade. Monitoring neuromuscular blockade at sites other than those that utilize the ulnar nerve and the intrinsic muscles of the hand cannot be assumed to provide equivalent responses.[68] An exceptionally large margin of safety for neuromuscular transmission in the motor units of the respiratory diaphragm[69] explains the classic observation that *d*-tubocurarine has a "diaphragm-sparing effect."

More recent measurements confirm that a threefold larger dose of atracurium is required to accomplish diaphragmatic paralysis than that needed for comparable relaxation of peripheral skeletal muscle.[70] Because the mechanism by which it produces neuromuscular blockade is noncompetitive and does not reflect a balance between prejunctional and postjunctional events, there appears to be no comparable difference in sensitivity for SDC-induced depolarizing blockade in the diaphragm compared with paralysis of other types of skeletal muscle.

MANAGEMENT OF PATIENTS WITH NEUROMUSCULAR DISORDERS

Presynaptic Disorders

The response of patients with neuromuscular disorders to neuromuscular blockade is generally predictable once the pathophysiology is known (Table 5–3). Prejunctional disorders such as the Eaton-Lambert "myasthenic syndrome"[71] are characterized by skeletal muscle weakness due to inadequate acetylcholine release.[27] These patients are unusually sensitive to both nondepolarizing and depolarizing neuromuscular blockade. Neuromuscular transmission does not improve after the use of anticholinesterases such as neostigmine because their effect is predominantly postsynaptic, while the lesion responsible for the disorder is presynaptic. Aminoglycoside antibiotics further impair the release of acetylcholine, and therefore may aggravate weakness or residual paralysis in these patients. Many require postoperative mechanical ventilation until even minimal residual plasma concentrations of neuromuscular blocking drugs are pharmacokinetically dissipated.

A similar clinical strategy is employed for the management of acute adult botulism, or the more recently understood syndrome of infant botulism.[72] The bacterial toxin responsible for skeletal muscle weakness in both varieties of this disease impairs acetylcholine release from nicotinic neuronal sites. This mechanism makes even more dramatic the reduced capacity for acetylcholine release seen in normal infants during the first 2 years of life.[13]

TABLE 5–3.

Summary of Responses to Neuromuscular Blocking Drugs in Patients
With Nervous System and Muscle Disorders

Lesion/Disease	Response to Succinylcholine	Sensitivity to Nondepolarizers
Central nervous system		
Cerebral infarction	Hyperkalemia	Decreased
Parkinsonism	Normal	Normal
Multiple sclerosis	Hyperkalemia	Normal
Spinal cord		
Amyotrophic lateral sclerosis (ALS)	Contracture	Increased
Poliomyelitis	?	Increased
Traumatic paraplegia	Hyperkalemia	Variable
Peripheral nerve		
Neuropathies	?	Decreased
Denervation injury	Contracture, hyperkalemia	Variable
Neuromuscular junction		
Myasthenia gravis	Reduced sensitivity	Increased
Myasthenic syndrome	Increased sensitivity	Increased
Muscle		
Myotonias and muscular dystrophies	Contracture, hyperkalemia, myoglobinuria, hyperthermia, normal or increased sensitivity	Variable: Normal or increased

Postsynaptic Disorders

Postsynaptic abnormalities of neuromuscular transmission can be produced by a wide variety of disorders. Either direct end-plate pathology or injury to the motor neurons that provide trophic support for the end-plate may change cholinoceptor function at these sites. Myasthenia gravis is now known to be an autoimmune disease producing loss of functional motor end-plate cholinoceptors.[73] Consequently, these patients have enhanced sensitivity to nondepolarizing relaxant drugs, since the effect of these drugs potentiates underlying cholinoceptor deficiency.[74] Unlike patients with myasthenic syndrome, however, patients with myasthenia gravis respond dramatically to anticholinesterase agents, and the use of anticholinesterase agents plays an important role in both the therapeutic and the anesthetic management of these patients.

The duration and intensity of nondepolarizing neuromuscular blockade are sufficiently variable in patients with myasthenia gravis that many clinicians continue to avoid the use of all neuromuscular blocking drugs in these patients. In fact, patients with myasthenia gravis are not sensitive to SDC but are resistant to depolarizing block-ade,[75] perhaps because loss of muscle end-plate receptors or changes in cholinoceptor configuration reduce the affinity of these highly specialized sites for SDC. The onset of a phase II depolarizing blockade after the use of SDC, however, may be even more rapid and less predictable than in normal patients.[76]

Some postjunctional neuromuscular disorders are characterized by an increase, rather than a decrease, in skeletal muscle cholinoceptors. Injuries or diseases producing denervation and muscle atrophy are associated with end-plate proliferation across the skeletal muscle surface and the generation of additional extrajunctional cholinoceptors. Normally myotrophic influences from neurons modulate skeletal muscle metabolism, maintain cellular integrity, and provide inhibitory substances that limit the formation of cholinoceptors to the immediate area under the nerve terminal.[77] Stroke, spinal cord transection, amyotrophic lateral sclerosis (ALS), syringomyelia, poliomyelitis, disuse atrophy, and, to some extent, aging all produce a relative state of denervation hypersensitivity to acetylcholine that appears to be mediated by an increase in postjunctional cholinoceptors.

Cholinoceptor proliferation, in general, increases the neuromuscular margin of safety for competitive blockade. It therefore reduces sensitivity (and increases the dose requirement) for nondepolarizing drugs.[78, 79] Monitoring neuromuscular blockade in a relaxant-resistant paretic or paralyzed limb will obviously lead to gross overdosage of normal musculature. In addition, it may put the patient at risk of residual paralysis sufficient to compromise spontaneous postoperative ventilation.[80] A similar phenomenon of resistance to nondepolarizers has been described after extensive soft tissue thermal injury[81]; however, the underlying mechanism for this phenomenon may involve exaggerated acetylcholine release,[82] a prejunctional effect. Despite receptor proliferation, ALS may also be associated with an additional myasthenic-like syndrome that ultimately produces an increase in sensitivity to nondepolarizing blockade.[83]

Proliferation of the motor end-plate and the appearance of extrajunctional receptors on the skeletal muscle surface after anatomic or functional denervation also change the neuromuscular response to SDC. This drug exerts its effects primarily at end-plate receptors and ion channels, but may have a more generalized and disruptive effect on skeletal muscle membranes.

The use of SDC in patients with generalized muscle atrophy or in individuals who have suffered massive trauma may precipitate the release of sufficient quantities of intracellular potassium to produce ventricular fibrillation and cardiac arrest.[84] The period of risk begins several weeks after initial injury[85]; it appears, therefore, that injured skeletal muscle undergoes a process of atrophy with a change in membrane characteristics. Consequently, any patient with a chronic muscle-wasting process should be considered at risk for massive potassium release after the administration of SDC.[86] Although patients with renal failure when first seen in the operating room may have an already elevated serum potassium level, these patients do not appear subject to more dramatic release of potassium after the administration of SDC than do normal individuals, about 0.1 to 0.3 mEq/L.[87]

Dystrophies and Myotonias

Muscular dystrophies and myotonias are associated, as are other syndromes of intrinsic skeletal muscle pathology, with abnormal contractile responses to SDC.[88] Depolarization by SDC also causes significant muscle fiber injury: potassium efflux, release of intracellular creatinine phosphokinase, and transient myoglobinemia are common.[89] SDC-induced contractures in myotonia may be so severe and sustained that patients are difficult to ventilate.[90] Triggered by events within skeletal muscle cells themselves, these contractures are beyond the influence of events occurring at the neuromuscular junction, and therefore do not respond to subsequent administration of nondepolarizing relaxants. These agents have, however, been used to produce surgical relaxation, with variable results.[91] Increased sensitivity to nondepolarizing relaxants has been most frequently reported; the likelihood of postoperative ventilation is, therefore, usually underestimated.[92]

Malignant Hyperthermia

Some forms of muscular dystrophy and myotonia predispose to malignant hyperthermia (MH). In susceptible patients with or without muscular disorders, MH may be initiated or "triggered" by SDC or by trace amounts of any of the potent inhalational anesthetics.[93] Halothane is a particularly potent and reliable stimulus, at least in the animal model for this disorder.

The fundamental mechanism responsible for this abrupt and violent hypermetabolic crisis remains unknown; virtually all trigger agents and predisposing situations appear to alter membrane-mediated movement of calcium ions.[11] Cardiac glycosides, neostigmine, belladonna alkaloids, procainamide, and, of course, ionized calcium are contraindicated in susceptible patients.[94] Skeletal muscle contraction can be sufficiently intense that it produces direct mechanical tissue injury. Potentially lethal systemic hyperthermia, hypercarbia, metabolic acidosis, and hypoxemia are due to abrupt and massive increases in oxygen consumption and metabolic activity that exceed the aerobic capacities of the cardiovascular and respiratory systems.

MH is not just an idiosyncratic skeletal muscle response to anesthetic drugs. It is a fundamental, genetically determined neuromuscular disorder in which intracellular control of skeletal muscle metabolism is impaired. The similarity of the severe hyperthermic responses to generalized sympathoadrenal stimulation and stress that occur in elk, deer, and other mammals suggests that MH may be a vestigial remnant of metabolic evolution. Now known to appear during emotional or physical stress as well as in response to exposure to anesthetic agents, MH may occur hours after anesthetic induction,[95] or long after exposure to anesthetic agents is terminated, well into the recovery phase.[96]

Other forms of induced skeletal muscle hyperactivity may be less fundamental and more iatrogenic. Neuroleptic malignant syndrome represents an abnormal central nervous system response to butyrophenones or other drugs that alter dopaminergic metabolism in the brain stem and in the basal ganglia.[97] Although this disorder, like MH, is characterized by hyperthermia and skeletal muscle rigidity, the pathology is central, not peripheral. Hyperthermia occurs as a consequence of the disruption of normal thermoregulation and the loss of normal inhibition of motor activity. Intrinsic control of skeletal muscle metabolism and the neuromuscular junction is normal. Unlike MH, therefore, skeletal muscle contractions associated with the neuroleptic malignant syndrome respond promptly to neuromuscular blockade.

The probability of uncomplicated survival after anesthesia-induced MH, once less than 50%,[98] has improved dramatically with better understanding of the underlying disease and more extensive experience with the management of this disorder. The anesthetic plan for MH-susceptible patients usually includes a narcotic-based anesthetic utilizing pancuronium for relaxation; inspired gases are delivered through an anesthetic breathing circuit flushed free of traces of volatile agents. Dantrolene sodium has been used to treat overt MH, or may be given prophylactically to prevent its occurrence. This drug also appears to work as well when given intravenously immediately before anesthesia as when administered over a period of several days before anesthetic induction.

Although a personal or family history of anesthetic or stress-related hyperthermia is obviously important, unremarkable prior anesthetic experiences may precede a subsequent full-blown hyperthermic response in susceptible patients.[94] Masseter spasm or other signs of sustained skeletal muscle contraction in response to SDC may represent less severe and variant forms of hypermetabolic muscular derangement, but they should be considered evidence of MH susceptibility until proved otherwise.[99] For elective surgery in patients with an equivocal family history, muscle biopsy and subsequent abnormal responsiveness to caffeine may establish the diagnosis more clearly. Regional anesthesia with either amide-type or ester-type local anesthetics, once controversial, now appears to be an appropriate alternative to general anesthesia if this anesthetic plan is compatible with the surgical procedure.[100]

CLINICAL PHARMACOLOGY OF RELAXANTS

Side Effects

Neuromuscular blocking drugs are small, polar molecules. A quaternary ammonium center of positive charge confers special affinity for those cholinoceptors accessible from the extracellular space, mostly in the peripheral nervous system. These qualities of polarity and charge also make these molecules hydrophilic and hinder their diffusion across the blood-brain barrier, minimizing central nervous system side effects.

Nevertheless, pancuronium, perhaps because of its intrinsically lipid-soluble steroidal structure, may produce sufficient blockade of central nervous system cholinoceptors to reduce anesthetic requirements.[101] An analogous form of central nervous system cholinoceptor blockade, that produced by atropine, is well known to cause delayed anesthetic emergence.[102] The uteroplacental barrier similarly restricts, but does not completely prevent, transplacental transfer of neuromuscular blocking drugs from mother to fetus. Concentrations of these drugs in fetal blood are about 10% or less of maternal levels, even when relatively lipid-soluble neuromuscular blocking drugs such as vecuronium are used.[103]

In general, the clinically important side effects produced by neuromuscular blocking drugs reflect differences in the intensity and specificity with which they antagonize or stimulate various synaptic mechanisms in the peripheral nervous system. Neuromuscular blocking drugs such as curare, metocurine, and atracurium produce ganglionic blockade; therefore they are associated with hypotension and, to a lesser extent, bradycardia. An affinity for vagal muscarinic sites, such as exhibited by gallamine or pancuronium, will produce tachycardia.[104]

Although the mechanism of neuromuscular blockade for the various nondepolarizing relaxants is generally believed to be quite similar, curariform and steroidal agents each bring a unique combination of presynaptic neuronal and postsynaptic end-plate effects to this process. The synergism noted when nondepolarizing relaxants are combined in both laboratory[105] and clinical investigations[106] suggests that they actually each exert what appears clinically to be a uniform effect through diverse actions at both presynaptic and postsynaptic sites,[107, 108] in varying degrees, which may reflect interactions between adjacent receptor sites.

When used alone, all the nondepolarizers are capable of producing adequate surgical relaxation if twitch height is reduced to 20% of its initial control value in the presence of a potent inhalational anesthetic, or to 10% of its initial value when used as part of a narcotic-based technique.[109] At this degree of twitch height depression, the TOF response is reduced to two twitches. Although inhalational anesthetics potentiate the less-than-complete suppression of evoked responses by nondepolarizing relaxants, there is no evidence that the addition of inhalational anesthetics to an anesthetic technique in which evoked neuromuscular response has already been abolished will produce a greater degree of surgical relaxation.

The speed of onset and the profound degree of relaxation characteristic of SDC-induced depolarizing blockade remain unequaled. Various pharmacologic manipulations, including intentional overdosage and the injection of subclinical "priming" doses before anesthetic induction, have been advocated to accelerate the onset of nondepolarizing blockade.[110] None are so effective, reliable, or practical, however, that nondepolarizers have completely replaced SDC for rapid intravenous anesthetic induction sequences.

There is persistent concern, however, regarding the side effects of SDC because of its ubiquitous agonist activity and its resultant tendency to increase intracranial, intraocular, and intragastric pressures.[111, 112] None of the cardiovascular side effects of SDC are either significant or persistent enough to dictate the conditions under which this drug is to be used or avoided. Fasciculations, myalgias, and other signs or symptoms of skeletal muscle injury also commonly follow the use of SDC. The pattern of muscle pain and its high frequency of occurrence in patients who ambulate a short time after emerging from general anesthesia suggest that SDC may damage the gamma-efferent muscle spindle system that normally prevents overstretch of skeletal muscle.[20] Although the frequency and the severity of this side effect appear to be reduced when visible fasciculations are suppressed, there is no completely effective way to eliminate myalgias when SDC is used for neuromuscular blockade.

Pharmacokinetics

Differences in the time required for spontaneous recovery of neuromuscular transmission after the use of a single intubating dose of currently available nondepolarizing relaxant drugs are relatively small. From equal levels of twitch height depression, spontaneous recovery can usually be expected in 15 to 45 minutes.[109] Pharmacokinetic parameters such as elimination half-time cannot be used to predict directly the clinical duration of neuromuscular blockade, although there is a consistent and linear correlation between changes in plasma concentration and the time required for return of neuromuscular transmission

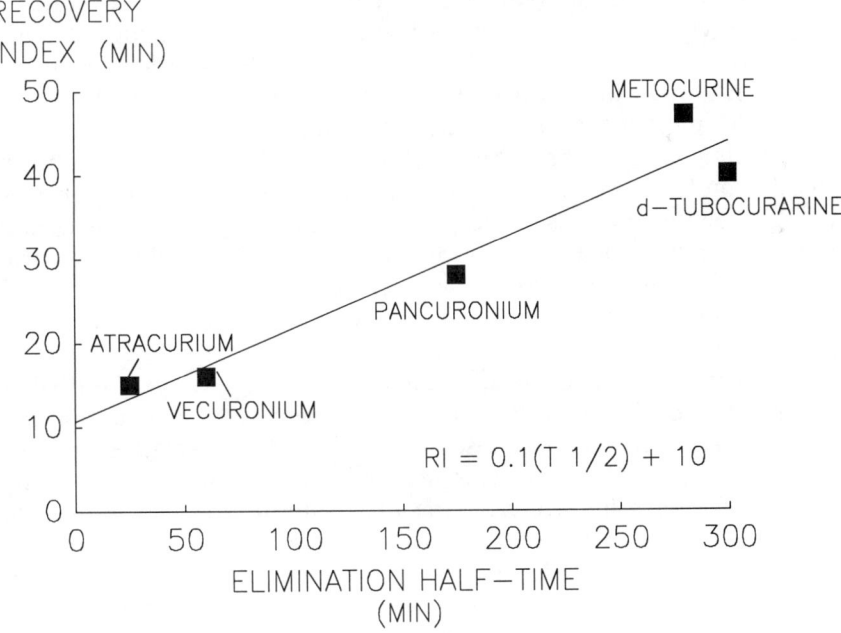

FIG 5–4.
The relationship between time required to return spontaneously from 75% to 25% twitch height depression (*recovery index;* RI) and the half-time of plasma concentrations of nondepolarizing relaxant drugs is direct and linear.

(Fig 5–4). Therefore, nondepolarizing relaxants that require elimination or excretion by organ- or enzyme-specific pathways have prolonged effects in patients with significant impairment of those organ systems.

Current strategies for the synthesis of new nondepolarizing relaxant drugs emphasize use of a molecular structure that is subject to hydrolysis or can be biodegraded by other spontaneous processes in human plasma. Finding agents of this type that are significantly shorter acting or longer acting than those nondepolarizers currently available also appears to be a high priority.[113] Recent emphasis on the virtues of the administration of these drugs by continuous infusion, rather than by intermittent bolus injection, may also make their clinical effects more predictable and practical, especially for surgery of short duration.[114]

SUMMARY

Neuromuscular blockade permits maintenance of adequate surgical relaxation virtually independent of the overall degree of depth of anesthesia. Although drug-induced neuromuscular blockade has been employed routinely to produce skeletal muscle paralysis for almost 50 years, the mechanisms by which the neuromuscular transmission is transiently disrupted and then restored are still not entirely understood. Nondepolarizing neuromuscular blockade appears to be primarily a competitive process of receptor inactivation at postjunctional, and perhaps prejunctional, cholinoceptors. Depolarizing blockade produced by SDC is characterized by a brief period of direct agonism and ion channel activation followed by inactivation of both receptors and ion channels.

Abnormal responses to neuromuscular blocking drugs are becoming better reconciled with the mechanisms of the various neuromuscular disorders. Prejunctional diseases reflect reduced ability to release acetylcholine; they therefore respond well to anticholinesterase therapy because it allows the acetylcholine that is released to be utilized to maximal effect. Postjunctional disorders such as denervation myopathy may produce a decreased sensitivity to nondepolarizing neuromuscular blockade if there has been a proliferation of cholinoceptors at extrajunctional sites. Conversely, myasthenia gravis is characterized by increased sensitivity to nondepolarizing neuromuscular blockade: changes in configuration or loss of end-plate cholinoceptors reduce opportunities for ion channel activation.

The goals of pharmacologists working to design new neuromuscular blocking drugs include avoidance of the phenomenon of depolarization, with its attendant side effects, and synthesis of new nondepolarizing neuromuscular blocking drugs with rapid onset and a high autonomic margin of safety. In addition, there appears to be considerable interest in those molecular configurations that do not require enzyme-specific pathways for the termination of their action.

REFERENCES

1. Austin GM, Pask EA: Effect of ether inhalation upon spinal cord and root action potentials. *J Physiol* 1952; 118:405–411.
2. Katz RL: Comparison of electrical and mechanical recording of spontaneous and evoked muscle activity. *Anesthesiology* 1965; 26:204–211.
3. Griffith HR, Johnson GE: The use of curare in general anesthesia. *Anesthesiology* 1942; 3:418–420.
4. Gray TC, Halton J: A milestone in anaesthesia (*d*-tubocurarine chloride)? *Proc R Soc Med* 1946; 39:400–410.
5. Beecher HK, Todd DP: A study of the deaths associated with anesthesia and surgery: Based on a study of 599,548 anesthesia in ten institutions 1948–1952, inclusive. *Ann Surg* 1954; 140:2–34.
6. Paton WDM, Waud DR: The margin of safety of neuromuscular transmission. *J Physiol* 1967; 191:59–90.
7. Kallo JR, Steinhardt RA: The regulation of extrajunctional acetylcholine receptors in the denervated rat diaphragm muscle in culture. *J Physiol* 1967; 191:59–90.
8. Hubbard JI: Microphysiology of vertebrate neuromuscular transmission. *Physiol Rev* 1973; 53:674–714.
9. Standaert FG: Release of transmitter at the neuromuscular junction. *Br J Anaesth* 1982; 54:131–145.
10. Bowman WC: Prejunctional and postjunctional cholinoceptors at the neuromuscular junction. *Anesth Analg* 1980; 59:935–943.
11. Nelson TE, Sweo T: Calcium uptake and calcium release by skeletal muscle sarcoplasmic reticulum. *Anesthesiology* 1988; 69:571–577.
12. Watland DC, Long JP, Pittinger CB, Cullen SC: Neuromuscular effects of ether, cyclopropane, chloroform and Fluothane. *Anesthesiology* 1957; 18:883–890.
13. Goudsouzian NG: Maturation of neuromuscular transmission in the infant. *Br J Anaesth* 1980; 52:205–214.
14. Durant NN: The physiology of neuromuscular transmission, in Katz RL (ed): *Muscle Relaxants: Basic and Clinical Aspects.* Orlando, Fla., Grune & Stratton, 1985, pp 19–38.
15. Havdala HS, Borison RL, Diamond BI: Potential hazards and applications of lithium in anesthesiology. *Anesthesiology* 1979; 50:534–537.

16. Ham J, Miller RD, Bennet LZ, Matteo R: Pharmacokinetics and pharmacodynamics of *d*-tubocurarine during hypothermia in the cat. *Anesthesiology* 1978; 49:324–329.

17. Hubbard JI, Jones SF, Landau EM: The effect of temperature change upon transmitter release, facilitation, and posttetanic potentiation. *J Physiol* 1971; 216:591–609.

18. Castillo JC, DeBeer EJ: The neuromuscular blocking action of succinylcholine (diacetylcholine). *J Pharmacol Exp Ther* 1950; 99:458–464.

19. Eakins KE, Katz RL: The action of succinylcholine on the tension of extraocular muscles. *Br J Pharmacol* 1966; 26:205–211.

20. Paton WDM: The effects of muscle relaxants other than muscle relaxation. *Anesthesiology* 1959; 20:453–463.

21. Ali HH, Savarese JJ: Monitoring of neuromuscular function. *Anesthesiology* 1976; 45:216–249.

22. Katz RL, Wolf CE, Papper EM: The non-depolarizing neuromuscular blocking action of succinylcholine in man. *Anesthesiology* 1963; 24:784–789.

23. Lee C: Dose relationship of phase II, tachyphylaxis, and train-of-four fade in suxamethonium-induced dual neuromuscular block in man. *Br J Anaesth* 1975; 47:841–845.

24. Churchill-Davidson HC, Katz RL: Dual, phase II, or desensitization block? *Anesthesiology* 1966; 27:536–538.

25. Cronnely R: Muscle relaxant antagonists. *Semin Anesth* 1985; 4:31–40.

26. Kopman AF: Edrophonium antagonism of pancuronium-induced neuromuscular blockade in man: A reappraisal. *Anesthesiology* 1979; 51:139–142.

27. Agoston S, vanWeerden T, Westra P, Broekert A: Effects of 4-aminopyridine in Eaton-Lambert syndrome. *Br J Anaesth* 1978; 50:383–385.

28. Higashi H, Yonemura K, Shimoji K: Antagonism of neuromuscular block by germine monoacetate. *Anesthesiology* 1973; 38:145–152.

29. Shanks CA, Somogyi AA, Triggs EJ: Dose-response and plasma concentration–response relationships of pancuronium in man. *Anesthesiology* 1979; 51:111–118.

30. Feldman SA, Agoston S: Failure of neostigmine to prevent tubocurarine neuromuscular block. *Br J Anaesth* 1980; 52:1199–1203.

31. Katz RL: Clinical neuromuscular pharmacology of pancuronium. *Anesthesiology* 1971; 34:550–556.

32. Walts LF, Thorpe WK, Dillon JF: Recurarization—fact or fiction? *Anesth Analg* 1971; 50:879–885.

33. Miller RD, VanNyhuis LS, Eger EI II, Way WL: The effect of acid-base balance on neostigmine antagonism of *d*-tubocurarine–induced neuromuscular blockade. *Anesthesiology* 1975; 42:377–383.

34. Miller RD, Roderick L: The effect of hypokalemia on a pancuronium neuromuscular blockade and its antagonism by neostigmine. *Br J Anaesth* 1978; 50:541–544.

35. Waud BE, Mookerjee A, Waud DR: Chronic potassium depletion and sensitivity to tubocurarine. *Anesthesiology* 1982; 57:111–115.
36. Miller RD, Roderick LL: Pancuronium-induced neuromuscular blockade, and its antagonism by neostigmine, at 29, 37, and 41°C. *Anesthesiology* 1977; 46:333–335.
37. Usubiaga JE: Potentiation of muscle relaxants by quinidine. *Anesthesiology* 1968; 29:1068–1069.
38. Lee C: Succinylcholine: Its past, present, and future, in Katz RL (ed): *Muscle Relaxants, Basic and Clinical Aspects.* Orlando, Fla., Grune & Stratton, 1985, pp 69–85.
39. King J, Griffin D: Relationship between suxamethonium apnea, serum cholinesterase activity and inhibitor numbers. *Br J Anaesth* 1974; 46:908–911.
40. Viby-Mogensen J: Succinylcholine neuromuscular blockade in subjects homozygous for atypical plasma cholinesterase. *Anesthesiology* 1981; 55:429–434.
41. Pantuck EJ: Echothiopate eye drops and prolonged response to suxamethonium. *Br J Anaesth* 1966; 38:406–407.
42. Shanor SP, VanHees GR, Baart N, Erdos EG, Foldes FF: The influence of age and sex on human plasma and red cell cholinesterase. *Am J Med Sci* 1961; 242:357–361.
43. Alston TA, deBros FM: Trimethaphan is not inactivated by pseudocholinesterase (abstract). *Anesthesiology* 1989; 71:A268.
44. Scott RPF, Savarese JJ: The cardiovascular and autonomic effects of neuromuscular blocking agents, in Katz RL (ed): *Muscle Relaxants: Basic and Clinical Aspects.* Orlando, Fla., Grune & Stratton, 1985, pp 117–141.
45. Burstein CL, Jackson A, Bishop HR: Curare in the management of autonomic reflexes. *Anesthesiology* 1950; 11:409–421.
46. Savarese JJ, Ali HH, Antonio RP: The clinical pharmacology of metocurine: Dimethyltubocurarine revisited. *Anesthesiology* 1977; 47:277–284.
47. Miller RD, Eger EI II, Stevens WC: Pancuronium-induced tachycardia in relation to alveolar halothane, dose of pancuronium and prior atropine. *Anesthesiology* 1975; 43:352–355.
48. Nana A, Cardan E, Domokos M: Blood catecholamine changes after pancuronium. *Acta Anaesthesiol Scand* 1973; 17:83–87.
49. Engbaek J, Ording H, Sorensen B: Cardiac effects of vecuronium and pancuronium during halothane anesthesia. *Br J Anaesth* 1983; 55:501–505.
50. Casson WR, Jones RM: Vecuronium-induced neuromuscular blockade: The effect of increasing dose on speed of onset. *Anaesthesia* 1986; 41:354–357.
51. William CH, Deutsch S, Linde HW, Bullough JW, Dripps RD: Effects of intravenously administered succinyldicholine on cardiac rate, rhythm, and arterial blood pressure in man. *Anesthesiology* 1961; 22:947–954.
52. Yasuda I, Hirano T, Amaha K, Fudeta H, Obara S: Chronotropic effects

of succinylcholine and succinylmonocholine on the sinoatrial node. *Anesthesiology* 1982; 57:289–292.

53. Galindo AH, Davis TB: Succinylcholine and cardiac excitability. *Anesthesiology* 1962; 23:32–40.
54. Basta SJ, Savarese JJ, Ali HH, Moss J, Giofrioddo M: Histamine releasing potencies of atracurium, dimethyl tubocurarine and tubocurarine. *Br J Anaesth* 1983; 55:1055–1065.
55. Hughes R, Chapple DJ: The pharmacology of atracurium, a new competitive neuromuscular blocking agent. *Br J Anaesth* 1981; 53:31–44.
56. Basta SJ, Savarese JJ, Ali HH, et al: Clinical pharmacology of doxacurium chloride. *Anesthesiology* 1988; 69:478–486.
57. Ali HH, Savarese JJ, Embree PB, et al: Clinical pharmacology of mivacurium chloride (BW 109OU) infusion: Comparison with vecuronium and atracurium. *Br J Anaesth* 1988; 61:541–546.
58. Harvey AH, Masland RL: A method of study of neuromuscular transmission in humans. *Bull Johns Hopkins Hosp* 1941; 68:81–93.
59. Gissen AJ, Katz RL: Twitch, tetanus and post-tetanic potentiation as indices of nerve-muscle block in man. *Anesthesiology* 1969; 30:481–487.
60. Ali HH, Utting JE, Gray TC: Stimulus frequency in the detection of neuromuscular block in humans. *Br J Anaesth* 1970; 42:967–978.
61. Ali HH, Savarese JJ, Lebowitz PW, Ramsey FM: Twitch, tetanus and train-of-four as indices of recovery from non-depolarizing neuromuscular blockade. *Anesthesiology* 1981; 54:294–297.
62. Ali HH, Wilson RS, Savarese JJ, et al: The effect of tubocurarine on indirectly elicited train-of-four response and respiratory measurements in humans. *Br J Anaesth* 1975; 47:570–574.
63. Beemer GH, Rozenthal P: Postoperative neuromuscular function. *Anaesth Intensive Care* 1986; 14:41–45.
64. Pavlin EG, Holler H, Schoene RB: Recovery of airway protection compared with ventilation in humans after paralysis with curare. *Anesthesiology* 1989; 70:381–385.
65. Weber S, Muravchick S: Correlation of electrical and mechanical evoked responses during onset and recovery for non-depolarizing neuromuscular blockade. *Anesth Analg* 1986; 65:771–776.
66. Weber S, Muravchick S: Monitoring technique affects measurement of recovery from succinylcholine. *J Clin Monit* 1987; 3:1–5.
67. Bonsu AK, Viby-Mogensen J, Fernando PUE, Muschhal K, Tamilarasan A, Lambourne A: Relationship of post-tetanic count and train-of-four response during intense neuromuscular blockade caused by atracurium. *Br J Anaesth* 1987; 59:1089–1092.
68. Caffrey RR, Warren ML, Becker KE: Neuromuscular blockade monitoring comparing the orbicularis oculi and adductor pollicis muscles. *Anesthesiology* 1986; 65:95–97.
69. Waud BE, Waud DR: The margin of safety of neuromuscular transmission in the muscle of the diaphragm. *Anesthesiology* 1972; 37:417–422.
70. Pansard J-L, Chauvin M, Lebraut C, Bauneau P, Duvaldestin P: Effect of

an intubating dose of succinylcholine and atracurium on the diaphragm and the adductor pollicis muscle in humans. *Anesthesiology* 1987; 67:326–330.

71. Lambert EH, Eaton LM, Rooke ED: Defect of neuromuscular conduction associated with malignant neoplasms. *Am J Physiol* 1956; 187:612–613.

72. Dowell VR: Infant botulism: New guise for an old disease. *Hosp Pract* 1978; 13:67–72.

73. Drachman DB: Myasthenia gravis (first of two parts). *N Engl J Med* 1978; 298:136–143.

74. Buzello W, Noeldge G, Krieg N, Brobmann GF: Vecuronium for muscle relaxation in patients with myasthenia gravis. *Anesthesiology* 1986; 64:507–509.

75. Eisenkraft JB, Book WJ, Mann SM, Papatestas AE, Hubbard M: Resistance to succinylcholine on myasthenia gravis: A dose-response study. *Anesthesiology* 1988; 69:760–763.

76. Wainwright AP, Brodrick PM: Suxamethonium in myasthenia gravis. *Anaesthesia* 1987; 42:950–957.

77. Fambrough DM: Control of acetylcholine receptors in skeletal muscle. *Physiol Rev* 1979; 59:164–227.

78. Shayevitz JR, Mateo RS: Decreased sensitivity to metocurine in patients with upper motor neuron disease. *Anesth Analg* 1985; 64:767–772.

79. Gronert GA: Disuse atrophy with resistance to pancuronium. *Anesthesiology* 1981; 55:547–549.

80. Moorthy SS, Hilgenberg JC: Resistance to non-depolarizing muscle relaxants in paretic upper extremities of patients with residual hemiplegia. *Anesth Analg* 1980; 59:624–627.

81. Dwersteg JF, Pavlin EG, Heimbach DM: Patients with burns are resistant to atracurium. *Anesthesiology* 1986; 65:517–520.

82. Brown TCK, Bell B: Electromyographic responses to small doses of suxamethonium in children. *Br J Anaesth* 1987; 59:1017–1021.

83. Rosenbaum KJ, Neigh JL, Strobel GE: Sensitivity to non-depolarizing muscle relaxants in amyotrophic lateral sclerosis: Report of two cases. *Anesthesiology* 1971; 35:638–641.

84. McLeskey CH, McLoed DS, Hough TL, Stallworth JM: Prolonged asystole after succinylcholine administration. *Anesthesiology* 1978; 49:208–210.

85. Mazze RI, Escue HM, Houston JB: Hyperkalemia and cardiovascular collapse following administration of succinylcholine to the traumatized patient. *Anesthesiology* 1969; 31:540–547.

86. Tobey RE, Jacobsen PM, Kahle CT: The serum potassium response to muscle relaxants in neural injury. *Anesthesiology* 1972; 37:332–337.

87. Koide M, Waud BE: Serum potassium concentrations after succinylcholine in patients with renal failure. *Anesthesiology* 1972; 36:142–145.

88. Azar I: The response of patients with neuromuscular disorders to muscle relaxants: A review. *Anesthesiology* 1984; 61:173–187.

89. Miller ED, Sanders DB, Rowlingson JC, Berry FA Jr, Sussman MD, Ep-

stein RM: Anesthesia-induced rhabdomyolysis in a patient with Duchenne's muscular dystrophy. *Anesthesiology* 1978; 48:146–148.

90. Mitchell MM, Ali HH, Savarese JJ: Myotonia and neuromuscular blocking agents. *Anesthesiology* 1978; 49:44–48.

91. Mudge BJ, Taylor PB, Vanderspek AFL: Perioperative hazards in myotonic dystrophy. *Anaesthesia* 1980; 35:492–495.

92. Aldridge LM: Anaesthetic problems in myotonic dystrophy. *Br J Anaesth* 1985; 57:1119–1130.

93. Gronert GA: Malignant hyperthermia. *Anesthesiology* 1980; 53:395–423.

94. Britt BA: Malignant hyperthermia. *Can Anaesth Soc J* 1985; 32:666–677.

95. Murphy AL, Conlay L, Ryan JF, Roberts JT: Malignant hyperthermia during a prolonged anesthetic for reattachment of a limb. *Anesthesiology* 1984; 60:149–150.

96. Grinberg R, Edelist G, Gordin A: Postoperative malignant hyperthermia episodes in patients who received safe anaesthetics. *Can Anaesth Soc J* 1983; 30:273–276.

97. Smego RA, Durack DT: The neuroleptic malignant syndrome. *Arch Intern Med* 1982; 142:1183–1185.

98. Arens JF, McKinnon WMP: Malignant hyperpyrexia during anesthesia. *JAMA* 1971; 215:919–922.

99. Donlon JV, Newfield P, Sreter F, Ryan JF: Implications of masseter spasm after succinylcholine. *Anesthesiology* 1978; 49:298–301.

100. Paasuke RT, Brownell AKW: Amide local anaesthetics and malignant hyperthermia (editorial). *Can Anaesth Soc J* 1986; 33:126–129.

101. Forbes AR, Cohen NH, Eger EI II: Pancuronium reduces halothane requirement in man. *Anesth Analg* 1979; 58:497–499.

102. Baraka A, Yared J-P, Karam A-M, Winnie A: Glycopyrrolate-neostigmine and atropine-neostigmine mixtures affect postanesthetic arousal times differently. *Anesth Analg* 1980; 59:431–434.

103. Demetriou M, Depoix J-P, Diakite B, Fromentin M, Duvaldestin P: Placental transfer of ORG NC 45 in women undergoing caesarean section. *Br J Anaesth* 1982; 54:643–645.

104. Riker WF, Wescoe WC: The pharmacology of Flaxedil with observations on certain analogs. *NY Acad Sci* 1951; 54:573.

105. Waud BE, Waud DR: Interaction among agents that block end-plate depolarization competitively. *Anesthesiology* 1985; 63:4–15.

106. Lebowitz PW, Ramsey FM, Savarese JJ, Ali HH: Potentiation of neuromuscular blockade in man produced by combination of pancuronium and metocurine or pancuronium and *d*-tubocurarine. *Anesth Analg* 1980; 59:604–609.

107. Galindo A: The role of prejunctional effects in myoneural transmission. *Anesthesiology* 1972; 36:598–608.

108. Blaber LC: The prejunctional actions of some non-depolarizing blocking drugs. *Br J Pharmacol* 1973; 47:109–116.

109. Donlon JV, Ali HH, Savarese JJ: A new approach to the study of four non-depolarizing relaxants in man. *Anesth Analg* 1974; 53:924–939.

110. Martin C, Bonneru J-J, Brun J-P, Albanese J, Gouin F: Vecuronium or suxamethonium for rapid sequence intubation: Which is better? *Br J Anaesth* 1987; 59:1240–1244.
111. Craythorne NWB, Rohenstein HS, Dripps RD: Effects of succinylcholine on intraocular pressure in adults, infants, and children during general anesthesia. *Anesthesiology* 1960; 21:59–65.
112. Miller ED, Way WI: Inhibition of succinylcholine-induced increased intragastric pressure by non-depolarizing muscle relaxants and lidocaine. *Anesthesiology* 1971; 34:185–188.
113. Savarese JJ, Wastila WB: Current research in relaxant development. *Semin Anesth* 1986; 5:304–311.
114. Shanks CA: Pharmacokinetics of the non-depolarizing neuromuscular relaxants applied to calculation of bolus and infusion of dosage regimens. *Anesthesiology* 1986; 64:72–86.

6

Cardiovascular Function

The contraction of cardiac muscle is mediated by subcellular components similar to those required for neuromuscular function. Actin and myosin are the contractile proteins found in both systems, and calcium appears to play a ubiquitous and crucial role in the coupling of electrical excitation to mechanical contraction. Relaxation in both systems is an active process requiring calcium-ion resequestration into intracellular membrane-bound compartments. Unlike skeletal muscle, however, cardiac muscle is electrically self-activating. Consequently there is no need for the elaborate prejunctional mechanisms that mediate and modulate the release of acetylcholine in skeletal muscle.

The structure of the cardiac chambers and of myocardial tissues imposes characteristics unique to the process of contraction in the heart. Although the quality and the quantity of skeletal muscle activity during anesthesia are rarely of interest unless they interfere with the surgical procedure, cardiovascular performance is essential to the maintenance of all vital functions. Therefore a working knowledge of the mechanism of cardiac contraction and its application to the understanding of the effects of anesthetic agents in various acute and chronic disease states will be discussed in the sections that follow.

PHYSIOLOGY OF CARDIAC CONTRACTION

Cellular Organization

Skeletal muscle is anatomically and physiologically divided into "motor units," each consisting of an efferent motor nerve fiber and the various skeletal muscle cells upon which it applies specialized nerve endings. Each skeletal muscle motor unit is capable only of an all-or-none (quantal) evoked response; consequently variations in the intensity of skeletal muscle contractions reflect the recruitment of more, or fewer, motor units in response to efferent electrical activity of different frequency and amplitude. Stretch and loading of skeletal muscle modify the tension that is generated, but the overall evoked force of skeletal muscle contraction reflects primarily the number of participating motor units.

In contrast, cardiac muscle cells are mechanically and electrically interconnected into a "functional syncytium" that requires the participation of all subunits in each contractile event.[1] There are no motor units or analogous structures in the myocardium. After endogenous electrical activation by "pacemaker" cells, a wave of depolarization spreads across the cardiac muscle mass; complete propagation is facilitated by its internal electrical conducting system. Recruitment of myocardial cells is therefore complete following each wave of electrical activity.

With the exception of the acutely ischemic or severely depressed heart, any variability in the evoked force of contraction in cardiac muscle represents an altered level of cardiac muscle cell function. Incomplete recruitment of cardiac contractile elements under these circumstances produces the alternating large and small stroke volumes responsible for the pulsus alternans arterial wave-form pattern characteristic of the failing myocardium.

Force of Contraction

An exceedingly complex interaction of intrinsic and extrinsic factors, many of which are just now becoming well defined, determines the tension developed by individual myocardial cells after electrical activation. The classic observations of Frank and Starling[2] established the fundamental relationship between end-diastolic ventricular pressure or volume at the beginning of cardiac contraction and the amount of blood subsequently ejected during the course of the cardiac contraction cycle. Since cardiac output is the product of stroke volume and heart rate, at any given heart rate cardiac output was therefore shown to be a function of the pressures within the cardiac chambers.

If a ventricle became more distended by larger-than-usual amounts of returning venous blood, the Frank-Starling relationship dictated that increasing stretch of cardiac muscle fibers would augment the subsequent contractile response. A greater force of contraction in the following cardiac cycles would enhance the fraction of blood volume subsequently ejected from the ventricle. Increased stroke volume, in turn, lowered end-systolic volume before the next contraction. By this mechanism, heart size was restored to its original "equilibrium" value within a few heartbeats. Since variation of cardiac chamber size appeared to alter directly the length of cardiac muscle fibers, regulation of stroke volume by variations in muscle fiber length was considered a "heterometric" control system for force of ventricular contraction.

Observations of the fine structure of skeletal muscle provided the initial model for the physiology of cardiac contraction. In particular, the "sliding-filament" hypothesis, in which the force of evoked mechanical contraction reflected the number of microscopic cross-linkages between contractile proteins, was easily reconciled with the characteristics of intact ventricular function.[3] Both skeletal muscle and cardiac muscle demonstrated a length-tension relationship with a broad area of positive slope, a phenomenon implying that ultimate contractile tension was sensitive to increased initial stretch or "preloading." If forcibly lengthened past the displacement associated with maximal force of contraction, however, these two muscle tissues also demonstrated a reduced force of contraction that presumably reflected a state of over-stretch, with loss of the overlap of contractile elements needed to establish effective cross-linkages and generate maximal evoked tensions.

In fact, this simple analogy between skeletal and cardiac muscle has failed to withstand continuing scrutiny. An assessment of ventricular function with use of input/output analysis suggests that the "Starling curve" probably has no descending limb. Ventricular function is, in fact, more accurately described as a family of curves,[4] each curve representing a length-tension relationship produced by a different level of intrinsic contractility (Fig 6–1).

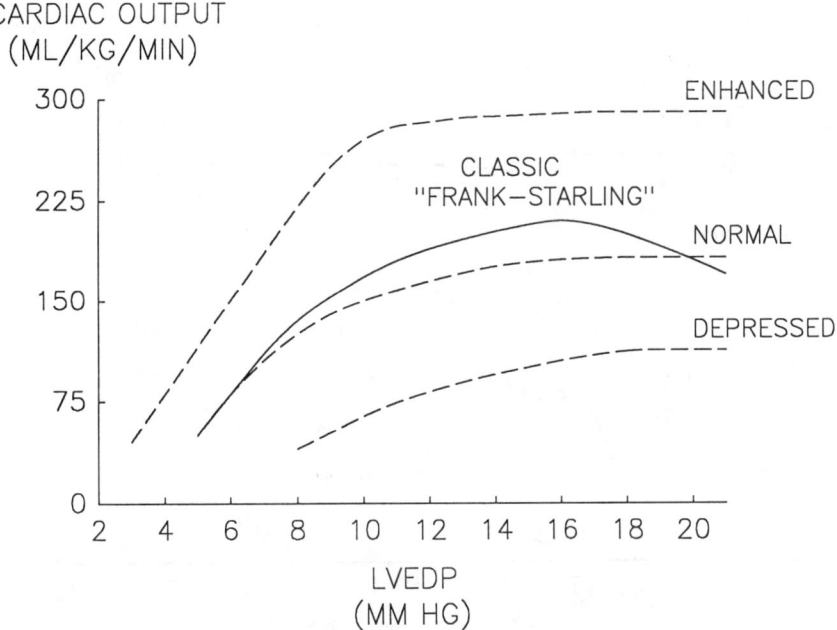

FIG 6–1.
Ventricular function curves showing typical relationships between "preload" (left ventricular end-diastolic pressure, or LVEDP) and cardiac output, assuming constant heart rate. The classic concept that declining cardiac output due to heart failure reflects an extreme rightward placement on the Frank-Starling relationship *(solid line)* has been replaced by representations of a spectrum of ventricular function states *(dashed lines)* ranging from inotropically stimulated ("enhanced") to overt cardiomyopathy ("depressed"). Myocardial failure is a progressive transition from a normal to a depressed ventricular function curve. Inadequate cardiac function or failure is therefore rarely caused by high LVEDP; rather, increased preload is symptomatic of an integrated, partially compensatory cardiovascular response to inadequate cardiac output.

More intense studies of the relationship between initial muscle fiber length and subsequent evoked contractile tension have also revealed that when viewed at the level of the basic subcellular contractile unit, the sarcomere, skeletal muscle is far more compliant than cardiac muscle, developing tension at graded, but near-normal, levels despite variations in sarcomere length as great as 25%.[5] Cardiac muscle, in contrast, generates adequate tensions only over an extremely narrow span of initial sarcomere length, and developed tension in this tissue also falls abruptly if fiber length is reduced by as little as 20%. Unlike skeletal muscle, cardiac muscle tissues have no plateau for the development of maximal force of contraction (Fig 6–2).

Cardiac muscle, unlike skeletal muscle, is subject to powerful, nonheterometric control of contractile force. In fact, tension can increase tenfold with virtually no change in initial fiber length.[6] Cardiac muscle

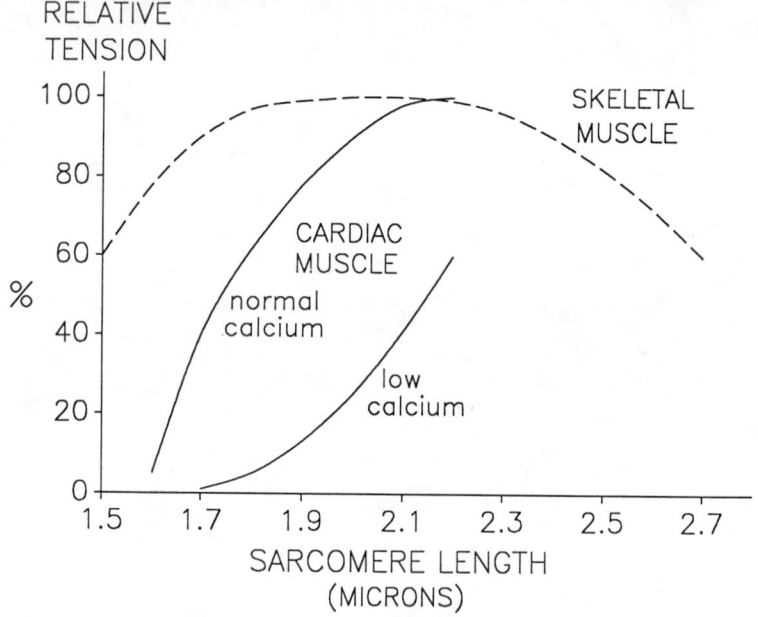

FIG 6–2.
Relative contractile tensions produced by isolated cardiac *(solid lines)* and skeletal muscle *(dashed line)* contractile units (sarcomeres) at different degrees of stretch. Skeletal muscle fibers produce consistent mechanical responses over a wide range of sarcomere length, and they are relatively independent of the availability of extracellular calcium. Cardiac muscle, in contrast, develops peak tension only at optimal fiber length, and tension is exquisitely sensitive to the concentration of extracellular calcium. The microarchitecture of the myocardial syncytium virtually eliminates the possibility of "overstretch" of cardiac sarcomeres beyond 2.2 μm.

fibers are enmeshed in an extremely rigid extracellular connective tissue matrix that provides an absolute limit to sarcomere length. Collagen fiber "struts" align and interconnect adjacent cardiac sarcomeres, preventing overstretch. These struts also tether the myocardial capillaries, preventing their collapse during the external mechanical compression associated with cardiac contraction.[7] The stiff "cytoskeleton" of myocardial tissues may also provide sufficient elastic recoil during diastole that a negative pressure is generated within cardiac chambers, augmenting venous return and improving significantly the mechanical efficiency of the heart as a pump.[8]

Excitation-Contraction Coupling

The mechanism by which cardiac muscle sarcomeres develop their tension over a very limited range of fiber length is suggested by recent studies of the cellular physiology of contractile mechanisms. Variation in the force of cardiac contraction may largely reflect a unique form of excitation-contraction coupling provided by myoplasmic calcium. Calcium appears not only to serve as the chemical link between electrical depolarization and subsequent mechanical response but also to modulate the magnitude of contractile force. In cardiac muscle, the peak developed tension is directly proportional to intramyoplasmic calcium concentrations.[9]

The release of intracellular calcium stores from the sarcoplasmic reticulum (SR) of cardiac muscle initiates contraction, as it does in skeletal muscle. In addition, however, the magnitude of a transmembrane calcium current generated by influx of extracellular calcium determines the tensions developed by subsequent cardiac contraction (Fig 6–3). Changes in cardiac fiber length too small to alter the amount of contact between the sliding filaments of the contractile proteins nevertheless modulate contractile force by altering calcium influx through ion-specific channels, or may alter the sensitivity of the contractile proteins to local concentrations of calcium.[10, 11] Length-dependent activation of contractile proteins is already well established as an important feature of the mechanism of vascular smooth muscle contraction, a tissue that also exhibits a strong relationship between degree of stretch and subsequent force of contractile response.[12]

Calcium

Length-dependent calcium activation of cardiac contraction may also explain the dramatic, if transient, enhancement of stroke volume

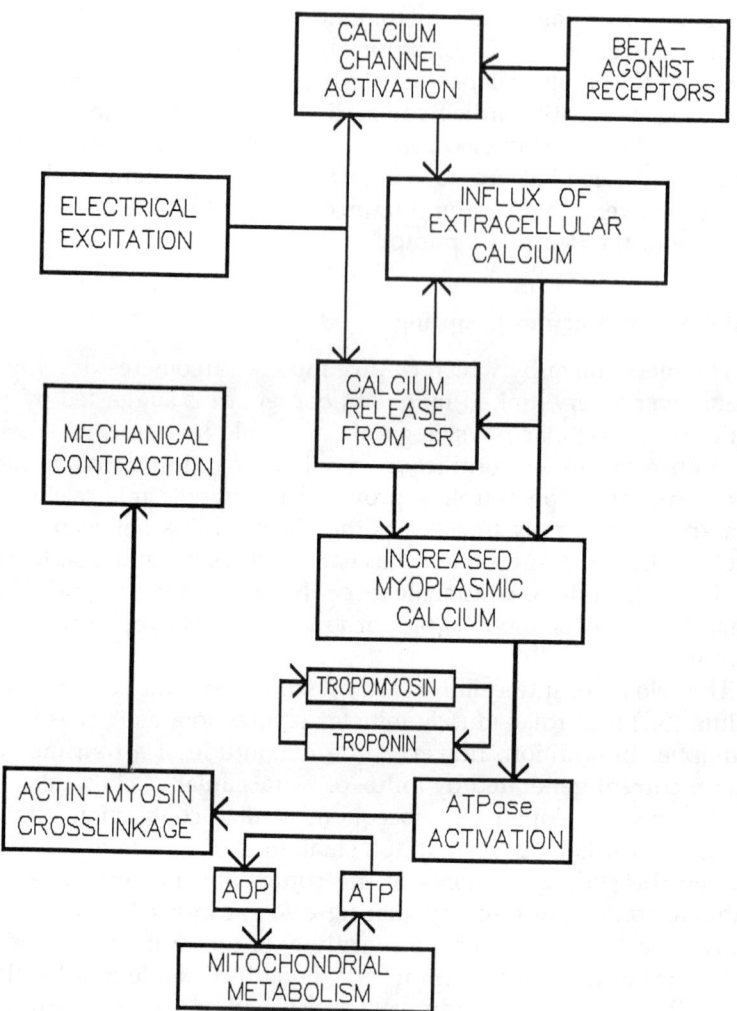

FIG 6–3.
Sequence of events in excitation-contraction coupling of cardiac muscle. Release of calcium from the cardiac sarcoplasmic reticulum *(SR)* facilitates the influx of extracellular calcium needed to develop a full contractile response. Relaxation requires resequestration of
calcium into the SR and the extrusion of calcium back to extracellular sites; these are en-
ergy-requiring, active processes. *ADP* = adenosine diphosphate; *ATP* = adenosine
triphosphate.

that follows infusions of ionized calcium in patients with failing or depressed myocardial function. Improved ventricular function occurs, even in the absence of generalized hypocalcemia, in response to augmented transmembrane calcium currents, not to the restoration of depleted total body calcium stores. Similarly, there is evidence that catecholamines enhance contractile performance by generating more of the high-energy phosphates needed to energize contraction, and by facilitating myocardial calcium influx and enhancing the participation of this ion in the contractile process.[6]

The relaxation of cardiac muscle, like its contraction, is an energy-consuming process. Active resequestration of calcium ions into the transverse tubules of the SR restores the supply of readily releasable calcium for the next contraction. Calcium that has entered the cell through transmembrane channels must also be exchanged for extracellular sodium by a process of active transport. This process lowers myoplasmic calcium sufficiently to inhibit contraction and permit relaxation to occur.[13] Sufficient depletion of high-energy compounds can therefore lead to generalized failure of myocardial relaxation, a phenomenon seen clinically after conditions of inadequate myocardial preservation during cardiopulmonary bypass as ischemic contracture or "stone heart."

The cellular mechanism of myocardial failure appears, similarly, to involve impaired dynamics of calcium release, uptake, and resequestration into the SR.[14] Digitalis and other cardiac glycosides are metabolic poisons that interfere with this process of sodium and calcium-ion exchange. By limiting calcium extrusion, these drugs allow gradual increases in intramyoplasmic calcium concentration, and in this manner they improve the contractile performance of cardiac muscle in failing hearts. Similar improvements in contractile performance are not produced by digitalis or similar drugs in the healthy heart, since under these circumstances calcium dynamics are already optimal and coupled appropriately to sarcomere length.

Metabolic Requirements

Excitation-contraction coupling and the contractile process itself thus appear to be more complex in cardiac than in skeletal muscle. The energy required to maintain a two-step system of calcium-ion flux is significantly greater than for the single process that occurs in skeletal muscle; oxygen consumption is, indeed, almost tenfold higher in noncontracting cardiac muscle than in similarly inactive skeletal muscle cells. Twenty percent of total myocardial oxygen demand is required simply for the maintenance of these ionic transport systems and for the generation of the subcellular components needed for cellular integrity. The balance of myocardial oxygen consumption is used to fuel the process of cardiac contraction itself.[15]

The myocardium can generate sufficient adenosine triphosphate (ATP) for both tissue maintenance and mechanical contraction by metabolizing lactate, glucose, ketones, or amino acids, although fatty acids are the preferred substrate if sufficient oxygen is available to the myocardial cell.[16] Under conditions of myocardial ischemia or hypoxemia, however, glucose is preferentially metabolized, and the myocardium therefore produces, rather than consumes, lactate. Sustained anaerobic glycolysis does not produce a sufficient amount of high-energy phosphates for continuing contraction, however, and this metabolic environment eventually produces local acidosis and myocardial tissue damage.

Other Control Mechanisms

Mechanical Frank-Starling considerations and length-dependent activation are the coarse and fine heterometric mechanisms, respectively, that are the most important intrinsic systems regulating the contractile force of cardiac muscle. There are other mechanisms, however, that do not require changes in muscle cell or sarcomere length. Peak myocardial tension may increase with stimulation frequency itself. The treppe, or "staircase," force-frequency relationship is also demonstrable in isolated mammalian heart muscle: decreased diastolic time associated with increased heart rate appears to limit the amount of calcium that can be extruded from the cell between heartbeats. This leads to a progressive but transient increase in myoplasmic calcium and enhancement of cardiac contractile state without measurable change of sarcomere length.[6]

Another "homeometric" or constant-length phenomenon is pressure-induced regulation, the Anrep effect.[4] If, as is believed, this phenomenon represents the release of catecholamines from intramyocardial stores, it is actually an extrinsic control mechanism and not an intrinsic property of cardiac muscle. The term *flow-induced regulation* has also been used to describe the slow, secondary increase in peak contractile cardiac muscle tension that follows acute ventricular distention even after there are no further measurable increases in fiber length.[17] Similarly, decline in contractile force occurs after acute cardiac decompression or unloading. Both responses appear to occur as a result of delayed changes in the rate of calcium release from the SR. They may be a result of the alteration of the sensitivity of contractile proteins to myoplasmic calcium, a phenomenon that occurs during the preceding heterometric responses mediated by length-dependent activation. Neither pressure- nor flow-induced regulation is apparent in intact subjects with normal hearts, but both may have some clinical relevance in patients with myocardial failure.

Contractility

The physiologic implications of the details of excitation-contraction coupling in cardiac muscle are substantial. The length-tension relationship of cardiac tissues and the classic concept of heterometric control of cardiac contraction can no longer be isolated from concepts of inotropic state or "contractility." All changes in cardiac muscle fiber length alter both the mechanical advantage and the efficiency of excitation-contraction coupling, and therefore effect developed tension and contractility. In effect, length-dependent activation of the contractile process provides constant adjustment of intrinsic contractility in response to variations in muscle fiber length and heart size by modulating the rate of calcium-ion movement from extracellular sites into cardiac muscle cells.

Heterometric regulation apparently does not reflect any structural limitations of the contractile apparatus, since changes in sarcomere length are relatively limited. Nevertheless, it is of importance in both normal and in failing hearts. It makes possible the constant adjustments of cardiac chamber size needed for dynamic mechanical equilibrium between right and left ventricular stroke volumes, which inevitably must differ because transient fluctuations of venous return occur with ventilation, orthostasis, or imposed increases in intrathoracic pressure.

HEMODYNAMIC CONCEPTS

General Descriptors

Hemodynamics is a descriptive discipline requiring measurements of the movement of blood through the heart and vasculature. It is not an adequate conceptual framework for understanding the total integration of systems as complex as the autonomic and cardiovascular systems. Instead, hemodynamics provides numerical tools that can then be used to study the factors that determine, regulate, or disrupt cardiac output. Hemodynamic concepts are, in effect, working definitions that quantify blood pressures, volumes, flow rates, resistive elements, frequencies, and the known physical relationships between these quantities.

Cardiac output describes total system volumetric blood flow, measured, estimated, or calculated as the product of heart rate (or pulse rate) and the average amount of blood ejected from the left ventricle with each contraction (stroke volume). Pulse, heart rates, and stroke volume can be measured as either instantaneous, or averaged, values. Cardiac output and stroke volume may be individually adjusted for body surface area, as cardiac index or as stroke volume index, respectively. These variables fluctuate on a beat-to-beat basis, since they reflect the interplay of the extremely complex system of internal and external regulatory mechanisms that ultimately determine cardiac output.

Mean arterial [blood] pressure (MAP) is an estimate of the amount of hydraulic energy available for overall organ perfusion. It is derived from the geometric mean of systolic and diastolic arterial blood pressures that are, respectively, the upper and lower limits of the pulsatile arterial pressure wave. The overall "driving pressure" across the circulation as a whole is determined by subtracting central venous pressure (CVP) from MAP. The ratio of driving pressure and cardiac output provides the basis for estimates of flow resistance expressed as total peripheral resistance (TPR) or systemic vascular resistance (SVR).

Analogous estimates of pulmonary vascular resistance (PVR) utilize the ratio of cardiac output and the driving pressure across the pulmonary circuit, which is mean pulmonary artery pressure (PAP) less left atrial pressure (LAP). All of these calculations are based on assumptions that the rheology of blood is independent of frequency and essentially the same as that of a pure newtonian fluid of low viscosity. None of these conditions are, in fact, entirely satisfied, but these assumptions nevertheless permit reasonably accurate measurements useful for most clinical and laboratory situations.[18]

Inotropic State and Myocardial Performance

Contractility and other concepts of cardiovascular function not directly referable to the pumping action of the heart are difficult to verify clinically. Both cellular microarchitecture and the overall geometry of the large, thick-walled ventricular chamber are sufficiently complex that few conclusions regarding the contractile state of myocardial fibers can be drawn from measurements that have been made in the intact heart. Physiologically, contractility, or "inotropic state," describes the level of metabolic activation, or the potential, of the myocardial sarcomere to contract rapidly and forcefully. As a cellular function, it can be quantified only by in vitro estimates of the maximal velocity of cardiac fiber shortening at zero-loading (V_{max}), a theoretic situation determined by extrapolation.

Contractility is not, strictly speaking, a hemodynamic measurement because it cannot be determined directly from measurements of integrated cardiovascular function or quantified from the circulatory movement of blood. Changes in contractility can, however, be inferred clinically either from serial measurements of the rate at which pressure is generated within the left ventricle (dP/dT) during isovolumetric cardiac contraction, immediately before the ejection of stroke volume, or from the changes in ventricular work or power that occur at constant cardiac volume. However, these techniques actually measure myocardial function, a tissue-level phenomenon, and not contractility itself (Fig 6–4).

Cardiovascular Function

Myocardial function reflects the general level of activation of cardiac muscle tissues, and not the maximal capacity of individual sarcomeres. Ballistocardiographic indices, such as the IJ-wave systolic time intervals and even more recently developed echocardiographic and radiographic techniques, may also provide reasonable estimates of myocardial performance by determining the rate at which ventricular volume changes (dV/dT). Ventricular function is an organ level assessment determined by both cellular and tissue elements, and is altered by mechanical and geometric factors such as heart size and chamber wall thickness.[19] At the uppermost level of this hierarchy of factors is integrated cardiovascular function, in some cases limited by the performance of cardiac muscle, but largely modulated by systemic demands and autonomic nervous system activity.

Preload and Afterload

The performance of the intact cardiovascular system is judged hemodynamically by the analysis of the characteristics of systolic ejection. The volume of blood ejected with each contraction reflects primarily the extent of initial cardiac fiber stretch produced by blood returning to the heart (preload) and the maximum ventricular wall tension that must be overcome during systolic contraction (afterload). Length-dependent activation of calcium-ion flux increases in proportion to preload. At any given fiber length, however, myocardial contractile state may be further enhanced or depressed by variations in the availability

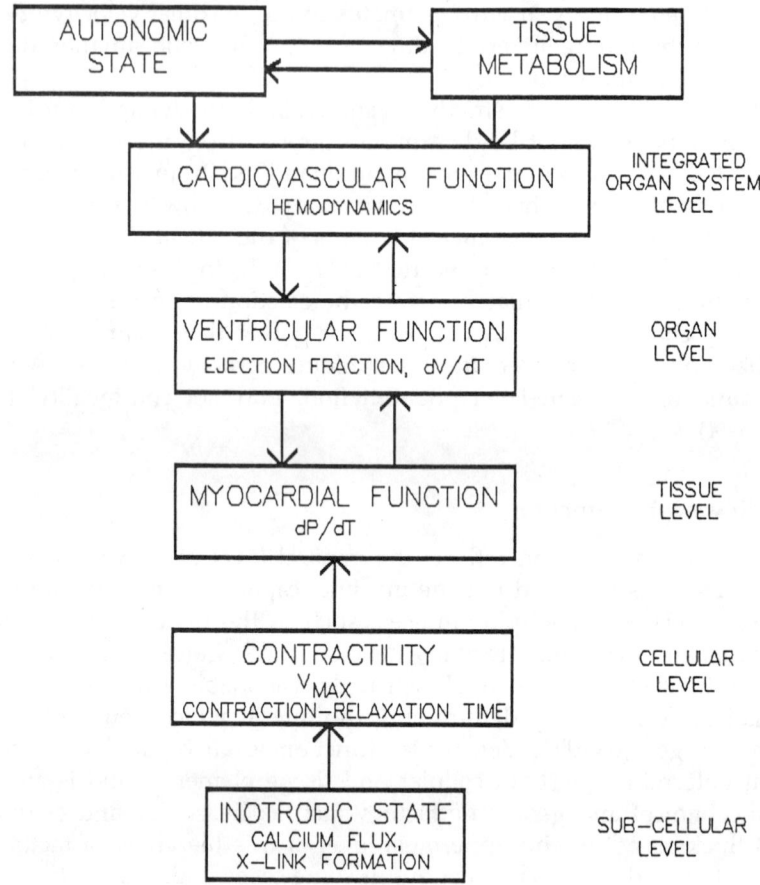

FIG 6–4.
Hierarchy for assessment of circulatory function from integrated organ system analysis down to the level of subcellular components. The physiologic parameters used to assess each level of function are shown within boxes. Integrated cardiovascular and ventricular function are modified by, but in turn influence, functions at lower levels down to that of the myocardium. Cellular and subcellular functional states are relatively autonomous unless local metabolic environment is severely disrupted. V_{max} = maximum velocity of fiber shortening; dP/dT = rate of pressure change; dV/dT = rate of volume change.

of calcium ions, local concentrations of catecholamines, changes in temperature, or other metabolic factors.

Intrinsic contractility or inotropic state does not dictate or limit stroke volume or cardiac output unless the heart is failing. Similarly, the augmentation of contractile state itself by inotropic agents does not increase cardiac output in the normal heart because inotropy is but one element within the physiologic control systems that normally determine cardiovascular function.[20] Stroke volume may also vary to some degree in response to changes in intracardiac tissue resistance, blood viscosity, and the inertia of blood itself.

Fiber stretch from ventricular filling immediately before systole is a function of end-diastolic ventricular wall tension and ventricular wall compliance. The actual degree of preload is difficult to quantitate directly, however, since it is determined by the simultaneous interaction of diastolic ventricular pressure, end-diastolic volume, and ventricular wall thickness. Useful clinical correlates for ventricular preload do exist, however, in measurements of central venous (or right ventricular) pressures and left atrial (or pulmonary capillary wedge pressures [PCWP]) for the right and left ventricles, respectively. The validity of any of these clinical instruments assumes no significant change in cardiac size and no cardiac septal defects or valvular dysfunction, since these factors disrupt normal filling patterns from atrial to ventricular chambers.

In the intact heart, afterload is conceptualized as the ventricular wall tension against which myocardial fibers contract to generate the pressures that open the aortic valve and eject stroke volume against the hydraulic resistance provided by the peripheral circulation. Although determined largely by intra-aortic blood pressure, afterload is further increased by cardiac chamber enlargement, but reduced by ventricular hypertrophy or other mechanisms that increase wall thickness.[21]

The dynamic characteristics of systolic ejection further complicate analysis of afterload and hinder attempts at precise quantification. Because the resistive qualities of aortic blood flow are frequency dependent, neither systolic ventricular wall tension, aortic pressure, TPR, nor SVR adequately defines what is more appropriately described as impedance to ventricular ejection.[22] To some extent, the actual volume of blood ejected with each stroke reflects the frequency with which contraction occurs, and the velocity with which blood flows from the left ventricle into the aorta and the peripheral circulation. Afterload, therefore, remains a largely conceptual, nonmeasurable hemodynamic parameter.[23]

REGULATION OF CARDIAC OUTPUT

Contemporary concepts of the control of cardiac output emphasize that the heart plays a "permissive" role in circulatory homeostasis.[24] Under normal conditions, cardiac output is neither limited by ventricular function nor increased by inotropic intervention. The heart, in effect, functions as both a load- and a demand-sensitive pump. Unless the cardiovascular system is failing or is maximally stressed, cardiac output is ultimately regulated by the peripheral circulation in response to tissue requirements for oxygen and for metabolic substrates.

The Peripheral Circulation

Variations in SVR produced by changes in the caliber of peripheral arteries, arterioles, and perhaps even smaller vessels regulate cardiac output directly. They increase the impedance to circulatory blood flow and alter the rate of venous return.[25] TPR reflects both SVR and the additional resistive qualities imposed by blood viscosity that, under normal circumstances, change little on a moment-to-moment basis.

Larger elements of the circulation may also be subject to tonic vasoconstrictor influences from the sympathetic nervous system. Autonomic denervation usually produces generalized vasodilation at this level. Vascular smooth muscle in the smallest segments (terminal arterioles, capillaries, and venules) responds primarily to the local metabolic environment, however, and does not appear to be under central neural control.[26] Intense metabolically induced local vasodilation, perhaps mediated by adenosine, may, however, precipitate retrograde vasodilation back to the level of the small arteries, significantly altering systemic vascular resistance under conditions of generalized ischemia.[27] This observation suggests the possibility that local metabolic or electrical mechanisms can augment the integrated control of blood flow. Exercise and stress can generate a superimposed anticipatory or secondary sympathetic vasoconstriction sufficiently powerful to overcome local metabolic control. However, the pattern of blood flow distribution, rather than the amount of cardiac output itself, is usually altered under these circumstances.

Precise metabolic autoregulation of regional blood flow appears to predominate in organs such as skeletal muscle and the heart,[28] where metabolic requirements vary greatly with activity level; oxygen requirements can increase tenfold or more above resting levels. In contrast, myogenic autoregulation provided by pressure-sensitive vascular smooth muscle units assures constancy of local perfusion pressures in brain and kidney, organs with consistent metabolic requirements and a relative intolerance of ischemia. In these tissues, metabolic factors appear to function secondarily: they become potent vasodilators when the primary, pressure-based microcirculatory control systems fail to provide adequate tissue perfusion.[29]

Splanchnic vascular beds and the microcirculation of the skin appear to have the least well-developed autoregulatory control. These tissues are perfused in direct proportion to mean arterial pressure, at least at low levels of sympathetic activity. They can become markedly ischemic during periods of arterial hypotension associated with intense vasoconstriction. The splanchnic circulation is an important source of functional blood volume reserve, however. An active component of baroreceptor and cardiopulmonary stretch receptor reflex arcs (Chapter 4), this vascular bed is also highly responsive to circulating vasoconstrictor substances. Although a significant degree of venomotor tone is maintained even under basal conditions, acute increases in sympathetic outflow or in plasma catecholamines produce both arteriolar vasoconstriction and enhanced venomotor tone. Subsequently active contraction of splanchnic capacity for blood volume augments venous return and increases cardiac filling and stroke volume.

Because of its large capacity for blood, the venous segments of the splanchnic circulation also allow effective short-term adjustments of cardiac output, dampening or smoothing the effect of postural change on hemodynamics.[30] In fact, the role of the postarteriolar segments of the circulation in most vascular beds is to provide active, adjustable vascular capacitance. At any moment, two thirds of blood volume in transit through the circulation can be found, between capillaries and the right atrium.

CVP, or right atrial pressure, does not quantitate volumetric venous return directly. Instead, it reflects the interaction between volumetric blood flow and the physical compliance of the right side of the heart and the circulation. Therefore the central hemodynamic pressure measurements used in clinical practice to estimate cardiac preload are not so much the determinants of cardiac output as they are parameters that describe the conditions under which cardiac output is provided.[31]

Other Factors

Reflex adjustments of venomotor tone alter venous blood volume acutely, compensating for transient interruption of venous return or for overall deficiencies of circulating blood volume. Systemic vascular resistance, in contrast, is largely determined by the local metabolic adjustments of arteriolar vasomotor tone that generate the impedance to ejection, which determines stroke volume and, in turn, defines the steady-state value of cardiac output in the normal heart. These interactions between the arterial and venous segments of the peripheral circulation and the heart itself are further complicated, but also buffered, by the autonomic reflex arcs that ensure homeostasis of blood pressure and central blood volume (Fig 6–5).

Continuous interplay between preload and afterload also mediates the regulation of longer-term variations in cardiac output. Acute changes in cardiac chamber size and the length-dependent activation of myocardial contraction reconcile the inevitable discrepancies between right and left ventricular performance produced by cyclic variations in pulmonary blood volume and pressure.[32] The physical constraints of the pericardium may also provide some additional mechanical coordination between right- and left-sided cardiac output.

Afterload itself limits the output of either ventricle only at maximum myocardial fiber length, or in the presence of myocardial failure. Rapid reduction of afterload may enhance stroke volume temporarily in the healthy heart, however, because it produces an accelerated velocity of myocardial contraction. Velocity, as opposed to force, of contraction is an important determinant of stroke volume since it sustains

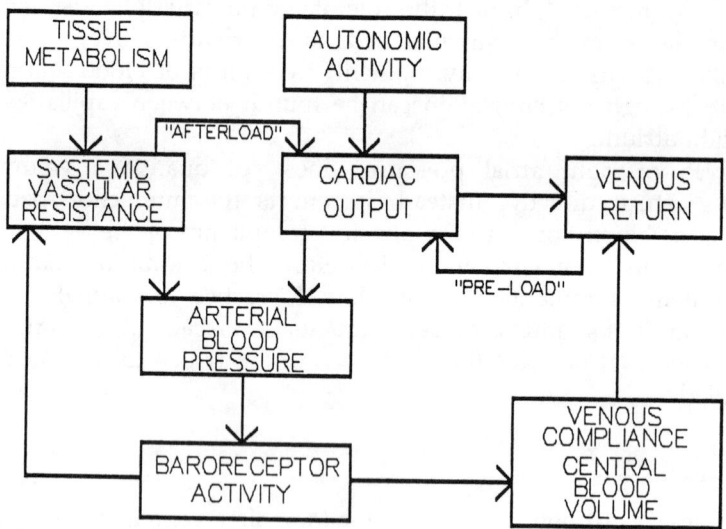

FIG 6–5.
Interrelationship between the major hemodynamic factors that determine cardiac output under physiologic conditions. Cardiac output is modulated by the state of the peripheral circulation, which, in turn, reflects body tissue metabolism and the general level of autonomic activation. Intrinsic factors such as myocardial contractility determine cardiac output only when ventricular function is severely compromised.

ventricular emptying: once the inertia of the mass of blood comprising stroke volume has been overcome, forward aortic flow may occur even when ventricular pressures have fallen below those within the proximal aorta.[33]

CARDIOVASCULAR FUNCTION DURING ANESTHESIA

In the unanesthetized subject, therefore, cardiac output is determined primarily by the state of the peripheral circulation. The effects of anesthetic agents on cardiac output reflect not only changes in myocardial function itself but also the influence of these drugs on the other components of the cardiovascular system and on autonomic activity, which is mediated by many sources of input.

With few exceptions, surgical patients arrive in the operating room with a high level of sympathoadrenal activity. Apprehension, pain, tissue injury, or, in some cases, autonomic responses that are compensating for end-organ failure produce neurally and humorally mediated arteriolar vasoconstriction and venoconstriction. Anesthetic induction then becomes an abrupt transition from a nonbasal state of autonomic activity to one of acute autonomic "disintegration" (Chapter 4).

Further alterations in cardiovascular function are subsequently produced acutely by mechanical stimulation, alteration, or disruption of autonomic reflex arcs intraoperatively. Some anesthetic agents have additional direct effects on cardiac and vascular structures that explain their effect on cardiac output. The interplay between primary, compensatory, and coincidental cardiovascular events may be so complex, however, that it is impossible to distinguish between drug- and process-related changes during anesthesia and surgery. Nevertheless, a consideration of the ability of anesthesia and anesthetic agents to alter cardiac output, ventricular function, and the homeostasis of arterial blood pressure and volume is essential to the design of a rational anesthetic plan.

Nonspecific Circulatory Effects

The induction of general anesthesia is a process usually associated with a fall in arterial blood pressure, due largely to transient reduction of venous return. Venous distensibility increases rapidly with the suppression of preinduction levels of sympathoadrenal activity because of the short plasma half-lives of catecholamines.[34] Epidural and spinal anesthesia produce a more localized regional sympathectomy, but may be associated with a similar fall in blood pressure. Both situations respond promptly to the augmentation of venous return by increased rates of intravenous fluid administration, the use of postural tilt, or both. Arterial hypotension immediately after induction, in most cases, reflects anesthesia-related changes in autonomic tone and the peripheral circulation, and not drug-specific cardiac effects. Patients with impaired myocardial function, however, may exhibit an additional element of cardiovascular decompensation if drugs with direct myocardial-depressant properties are used for anesthetic induction.

Generalized depression of baroreceptor sensitivity and the shifts in autonomic set-points produced by anesthetic agents also make spontaneous recovery of arterial blood pressure to preinduction levels unlikely during sustained general anesthesia. Under these circumstances, cardiovascular function no longer reflects the net interaction of a tightly controlled complex of neural, humoral, and mechanical elements. The cardiovascular system begins behaving as if it were the simple sum of its components. During general anesthesia, the physiologic equilibrium for preload, afterload, and cardiac output is achieved largely on the basis of physical, flow-dependent factors, in particular the adequacy of venous blood return.

The sympathoadrenal-stimulating properties of some obsolete inhalational anesthetics, such as diethyl ether, fluroxene, and cyclopropane, and of other agents still in use, such as ketamine and nitrous oxide, may support, or even increase, venomotor tone, preload, and cardiac output during anesthetic induction.[35-37] Arterial hypotension is avoided, however, only if the patient has sufficient autonomic reserve to permit function at a higher level of sympathoadrenal activation. If used in patients with severe cardiac failure, or for those already utilizing maximal sympathoadrenal drive to compensate for hemorrhagic shock or other underlying pathology, the direct myocardial-depressant effects of these drugs may nevertheless produce hypotension.[38, 39]

Narcotics, especially the newer, potent synthetics such as fentanyl and alfentanil, have effects highly specific for opiate receptors and analgesic centers. This characteristic minimizes the production of more diffuse effects on nervous system structures. Consequently, anesthetic plans utilizing a combination of nitrous oxide and intravenous narcotics are associated with higher plasma levels of catecholamines and more neuroendocrine responsiveness to pain and surgical stimulation than are usually seen with the potent inhalational anesthetics.[40]

Even the use of very high doses of narcotics for anesthesia may not, however, completely suppress the cardiovascular responses to surgical stress.[41, 42] Addition of benzodiazepines to establish a "stress-free" anesthetic under these circumstances,[43] or to minimize the risk of recall during surgery,[44] may produce significant generalized depression of autonomic centers. Ultimately arterial hypotension and decreases in cardiac output under these circumstances may differ little from those associated with the use of potent inhalational anesthetics.[45, 46]

Cardiac Effects

Many intraoperative changes in cardiac function and hemodynamics do, in fact, reflect drug-specific effects, even in healthy patients. Morphine has intrinsic venodilator effects that may be centrally mediated; reduced venous return and arterial hypotension commonly follow its use in large doses, even without signs of the histamine release that this drug also may produce.[47] Synthetic opioids are less problematic. Fentanyl has virtually no direct effect on myocardial or peripheral vascular function, but sufentanil may be associated with arterial hypotension on induction because of arteriolar vasodilation by a mechanism that is, at present, poorly understood.[48]

Droperidol has some direct venodilator activity in addition to transient arteriolar relaxation mediated by α-adrenergic blockade, but appears to have no direct effect on myocardial or ventricular function itself.[49] The ability of thiopental to produce direct myocardial depression in proportion to its administered concentration is widely accepted. Each of the potent inhalational agents in current use also depresses the contractility of myocardial tissues directly, but to varying degrees, and perhaps by somewhat different mechanisms.[50]

To be represented in a manner consistent with clinical observations, the effects of these drugs on cardiac output must be explained in the context of their overall effects on the peripheral circulation and on the hemodynamics of the intact subject. Halothane produces a direct, dose-related depression of ventricular function and slows heart rate. Hypercarbia associated with spontaneous ventilation during halothane anesthesia produces the arteriolar vasodilation that contributes to the relative arterial hypotension seen under these circumstances.[51] With controlled ventilation and normocarbia, however, halothane decreases myocardial performance and stroke volume in a dose-dependent manner; arterial blood pressure declines in direct proportion to cardiac output, since systemic vascular resistance remains virtually unchanged.[52]

Halothane appears to reduce the vigor, but does not disrupt the normal synchrony, of ventricular contraction.[53] Myocardial depression becomes less profound as the duration of halothane anesthesia exceeds several hours: progressive improvement in cardiac output over time is associated with reduced systemic vascular resistance, a phenomenon that may be mediated by somewhat attenuated, but still functional, baroreflex pathways.[52] The use of nitrous oxide as a carrier gas and as a coanesthetic minimizes the myocardial depressant properties of halothane, which are more obvious when this drug is used in oxygen alone.[54] Like chloroform and other halogenated hydrocarbons, halothane predisposes the myocardium to catecholamine-induced dysrhythmias, and must be used with caution when aminophylline or exogenous catecholamines are required.

The cardiovascular characteristics of enflurane are more complex than those of halothane. At equipotent inspired concentrations, enflurane produces equal or greater direct myocardial depression than does halothane.[55] The effect of this myocardial depression on stroke volume is further aggravated by venodilation, since it simultaneously reduces venous return and ventricular preload. Thus, enflurane-induced depression of cardiac output and simultaneous reduction of systemic vascular resistance[56] produce marked arterial hypotension. Arterial blood pressure may be as low as 60% of the values obtained in awake subjects, even at alveolar concentrations less than 2 times the minimum alveolar concentration (MAC) in unstimulated subjects.[57] The hypercarbia that occurs during spontaneous ventilation with enflurane does not produce an increase in sympathoadrenal activity sufficient to compensate for these cardiovascular effects.[58] Unlike halothane, the addition of nitrous oxide to the anesthetic plan also fails to improve the hemodynamic environment produced by enflurane alone in oxygen.[59]

Isoflurane produces a more modest degree of myocardial depression than does halothane or enflurane.[50] Clinically, the reduction in stroke volume produced by isoflurane is offset by increased heart rate in most patients; thus there may be little change in cardiac output under those circumstances.[60] Isoflurane is a potent vasodilator in skin and skeletal muscle, however. Consequently, reduced systemic vascular resistance may still produce significant arterial hypotension relative to the values obtained before anesthetic induction.[61]

Hypercarbia-induced sympathoadrenal activity during spontaneous ventilation with isoflurane anesthesia further stimulates heart rate and increases cardiac output. The direct vasodilator effect of carbon dioxide on other vascular beds reduces systemic resistance even further, however, so that there is rarely a return to normal arteriolar blood pressure levels.[60] Almost all of these cardiovascular effects are dose related, and they appear to be attenuated during prolonged exposure to isoflurane. Isoflurane, like enflurane, produces sinus tachycardia, but neither of these halogenated ethers potentiates catecholamine-induced dysrhythmias in a manner analogous to that of halothane.

The effects of general anesthetics on the electrical characteristics of the heart are quite complex and difficult to study. Intravenous agents rarely alter the automaticity of cardiac depolarization or the intramyocardial conduction of electrical impulses. Their effects on heart rate, if any, usually are mediated by muscarinic actions, the release of vasoactive agents such as histamine, or they reflect changes in autonomic reflex activity mediated by diffuse central nervous system effects. Isoflurane and enflurane must increase heart rate indirectly: they have been shown to produce direct depression of the sinoatrial node and of atrial and atrioventricular conduction pathways.[62] Halothane exhibits similar properties and, in addition, also depresses ventricular conduction.[63] This allows additional time for electrical reentry phenomena, and may explain the ability of halothane to potentiate catecholamine-induced ventricular dysrhythmias.

ANESTHETIC IMPLICATIONS OF CARDIAC DISEASE

General Principles

General considerations of the cardiovascular effects of anesthetic agents are derived from studies of patients without disease. Relative arterial hypotension under these circumstances is of interest primarily because it identifies and quantifies the applied pharmacology of these drugs. The ubiquitous depression of ventricular performance produced by the potent inhalational anesthetics becomes far more significant in the design of an anesthetic plan for patients with failing, ischemic, or damaged hearts when the adequacy of tissue perfusion itself is in question (Table 6–1).

The opioids, whether naturally occurring or synthetic, appear to produce little or no direct depression of myocardial function. Their intraoperative effects on the arteriolar and venous circulations are usually the result of reflexly mediated and neuroendocrine cardiovascular responses to pain; these drugs are therefore generally characterized by the maintenance of arterial blood pressure and little change in cardiac output. Thus where ventricular "pump" function is sufficiently impaired by disease to be the limiting factor in integrated cardiovascular function, these drugs have been the traditional anesthetic agents of choice. A similar rationale has been applied to the selection of intravenous agents such as etomidate, propranidid, propofol, high-dose benzodiazepines, and ketamine.[64–67]

TABLE 6–1.
Management Priorities for Various Categories of Cardiovascular Dysfunction

Disorder	Major Lesions	Pathophysiology	Management Priorities
Cardiomyopathies			
Nonobstructive	Impaired ventricular function	Inadequate CO; pulmonary congestion	Optimize LVEDP; inotropic support; avoid myocardial depressants; afterload reduction with vasodilators
Obstructive	Outflow tract obstruction	Inadequate SV with cardiac stimulation	Controlled myocardial depression; maintain adequate pre-, afterload to avoid outflow tract collapse
Ischemic	Inadequate myocardial perfusion	Ischemia, infarction; myopathy; dysrhythmia	Minimize m_{vo_2} by avoiding hypertension and tachycardia; adequate diastolic time and pressure; other therapy as needed
Shock states			
Hemorrhagic	Circulating hypovolemia	Inadequate CO, low BP; high SVR, tissue hypoxia	Volume replacement, surgical control of bleeding
Cardiogenic	Inadequate ventricular function	Inadequate CO, low BP; high SVR; tissue hypoxia	Afterload reduction, inotropes and pressors; no myocardial depression
Septic	Cardiovascular toxins	Low SVR; low BP; high CO; high Vo_2, fever	Volume therapy, antibiotics, fever control, abscess drainage
Traumatic	Tissue damage, edema circulating hypovolemia	Low BP; variable CO; variable Vo_2	Debridement, transfusion, fluid therapy; avoid vasodilators

Common cardiac valvular disorders

Disorder	Pathophysiology	Characteristics	Management goals
Aortic stenosis	Ventricular outflow obstruction; concentric ventricular hypertrophy	Small stroke volume; high SVR; ischemia; noncompliant ventricle	Maintain adequate SVR but avoid systemic hypertension or tachycardia; maintain sinus rhythm
Aortic insufficiency	Regurgitation of stroke volume; eccentric hypertrophy	Low forward CO; left ventricular distention	Minimize impedance to ventricular ejection with vasodilators; avoid bradycardia or myocardial depression
Mitral stenosis	Obstructed ventricular filling	Low, "fixed" CO; atrial enlargement; pulmonary congestion and hypertension	Maintain adequate preload but avoid tachycardia or pulmonary congestion; high $F_{I}O_2$ to avoid hypoxemia
Mitral insufficiency	Regurgitation of ventricular volume	Left atrial and ventricular distention; dysrhythmias; pulmonary hypertension	Minimize afterload, avoid pulmonary congestion; antiarrhythmics as needed; high $F_{I}O_2$ to avoid hypoxemia

CO = cardiac output; BP = blood pressure; $F_{I}O_2$ = fractional concentration of oxygen in inspired gas. LVEDP = left ventricular end-diastolic pressure; mVO_2 = myocardial oxygen consumption; SV = stroke volume; SVR = systemic vascular resistance; VO_2 = total body oxygen consumption.

Few of the intravenous agents, however, provide all the necessary components required for general anesthesia (Chapter 2). The addition of adjuvant drugs to the anesthetic routine frequently compromises the basic goals of a "nondepressant" anesthetic approach. Although nitrous oxide stimulates overall cardiovascular function[37] and may offset anesthetic-induced depression of healthy hearts, it nevertheless can produce significant further impairment of ventricular function when the myocardium is ischemic or otherwise compromised.[46] Maintenance of ventricular function at levels that will ensure adequate cardiac output intraoperatively, assumed in normal hearts, may then require active intervention in patients with left ventricular dysfunction. Although less common, depression of right ventricular function may also limit cardiac output if significantly impaired by disease or by trauma.[68]

Ischemic Heart Disease

A different pharmacologic strategy is required for patients with good ventricular function but inadequate coronary artery blood flow. Under these circumstances, myocardial ischemia, rather than ventricular dysfunction, becomes the primary factor that compromises cardiovascular homeostasis. Assuming adequate respiratory function and full arterial oxygen saturation, patients with coronary artery disease benefit from anesthetic techniques designed to minimize myocardial oxygen demand while maintaining myocardial blood flow.

The depressed contractility and altered hemodynamic characteristics produced by halothane, enflurane, and isoflurane anesthesia actually reduce myocardial oxygen demand in proportion to the lesser amount of myocardial work performed under these circumstances.[69] The myocardial oxygen required for each cardiac contraction is reduced as stroke volume and ventricular wall tension, the major determinants of ventricular stroke work, decline. Lowering the contractile state itself may also reduce myocardial oxygen demand if ventricular chamber size and wall geometry remain unchanged.[66] Total myocardial work, and thus total myocardial oxygen requirement, also varies in direct proportion to heart rate, which is simply the number of working strokes required each minute.

There is no evidence that anesthetic agents themselves disrupt myocardial oxidative metabolism at a cellular level or reduce the stores of high-energy phosphates normally maintained within myocardial tissues. The extremely sensitive and precise vascular mechanisms that provide metabolic autoregulation of coronary blood flow, probably mediated by adenosine,[28] appear to remain largely undisturbed during general anesthesia. Coronary blood flow is therefore distributed in direct proportion to local metabolic activity within the limitations of coronary artery patency, arterial pressure, and local mechanical compressive forces generated during cardiac contraction.[70] Coronary artery vasospasm[71] during light general anesthesia, or a unique isoflurane-induced maldistribution or "steal" of intramyocardial blood flow from one area to another, may, however, produce intraoperative electrocardiographic and metabolic evidence of ischemia in some patients with coronary artery disease.[72, 73]

Myocardial ischemia during general anesthesia, therefore, usually reflects an unfavorable balance between myocardial oxygen supply and demand, largely determined by externally imposed hemodynamic conditions. The primary factors producing myocardial ischemia or infarction during general anesthesia appear to be tachycardia, increased ventricular wall tension, or diastolic arterial blood pressure inadequate to meet left ventricular perfusion requirements.[74] Arterial hypertension, especially when associated with tachycardia, can create subendocardial ischemia even when coronary autoregulatory mechanisms are well maintained.[75] Therefore the agent chosen for management of patients with ischemic heart disease may be an essential element of the anesthetic plan largely because it permits or hinders rapid and precise control of the hemodynamic environment in which the myocardium is expected to function.[76]

None of the anesthetic agents currently available has cardiovascular characteristics ideal for patients predisposed to myocardial ischemia. The inhalational agents produce vasodilation and reduced venous return and usually depress cardiac output. They reduce cardiac work and oxygen demand, but also may produce significant arterial diastolic hypotension. Enflurane and isoflurane also stimulate tachycardia, doubly disadvantageous because it shortens diastolic perfusion time and simultaneously increases oxygen demand. The potent inhalational anesthetic agents may also be difficult to use without an unacceptable degree of arterial hypotension if ischemic disease is sufficiently severe that it produces cardiomyopathy.

When used in doses sufficient to block reflex arterial hypertension, narcotics cause postoperative respiratory depression and problems with delayed extubation. They may not reliably suppress intraoperative awareness unless used with other nervous system depressants.[44] Consequently, many clinicians utilize hybrid, combined techniques for general anesthesia that take advantage of some of the desirable characteristics of each of these major anesthetic groups, relying on the lower doses of each type of drug to minimize their unwanted side effects.[46]

The same principles and priorities of intraoperative management apply whether patients with ischemic heart disease undergo cardiac or noncardiac surgery. Similar guidelines are applicable to most patients with hypertension as well, since both coronary artery disease and hypertension of nonrenal origin represent different points in a common pathophysiologic spectrum of autonomic hyperreactivity, contracted blood volume, and pathologically elevated arteriolar resistance. End-organ compromise due to vascular insufficiency of heart, brain, and kidney is great enough to increase mortality in these patients eightfold to tenfold compared with healthy, normal individuals of the same age.[77]

Lack of preoperative antihypertensive therapy may greatly increase the probability of intraoperative myocardial ischemia and infarction. Unfavorable hemodynamics associated with abrupt arterial hypertension or hypotension disrupt the balance between myocardial oxygen supply and demand.[78] Arbitrary standards for "safe" or ischemia-free levels of heart rate and systolic blood pressure are more consistent in awake than in anesthetized individuals,[79] primarily because the rate-pressure-product (RPP) and similar derived indices[80] do not take into account the variations in heart size and contractile state that occur during general anesthesia. Neither the addition of left ventricular end-diastolic pressure to RPP to produce a "triple product" nor other attempts to predict "endocardial viability"[81] generate reliable hemodynamic predictors of ischemia in anesthetized patients with coronary artery disease.

Preoperatively, exercise electrocardiography may be of value in identifying ischemic foci and in provoking ischemia-induced dysrhythmias. Dipyridamole mimics the effects of hemodynamic stress on uneven myocardial perfusion during thallium scan. Therapy with antihypertensive drugs, vasodilators, β-blocking agents, antiarrhythmic drugs, and, most recently, calcium channel antagonists should be continued up to the time of surgery if they successfully maintain a favorable hemodynamic environment.[82, 83]

Aortic Valve Disease

The principles of an anesthetic plan for patients with valvular heart disease are derived directly from an understanding of the specific mechanical constraints that limit cardiac function in each disorder.[84] The universal goal is to maintain a benign hemodynamic environment that is consistent with adequate ventricular "pump" function and cardiac output, usually done by maintaining or even augmenting endogenous compensatory mechanisms.

In patients with stenosis of the aortic valve, chronic mechanical obstruction to ejection of stroke volume produces a hypertrophic, noncompliant left ventricle that empties slowly through a restrictive orifice at relatively high pressures, and with elevated ventricular wall tensions.[85] Energy-consuming "pressure work" is therefore high, and the diastolic time available for coronary perfusion is compromised by the additional time required for completion of systole. The balance between myocardial oxygen supply and demand is therefore frequently unfavorable and the risk of ischemia high.

Intraoperatively, stroke volume is maintained and myocardial ischemia minimized if tachycardia is avoided and there are no abrupt changes in systemic vascular resistance or other factors that alter the impedance to ventricular ejection. Stroke volume, and thus cardiac output, may fall precipitously if the patient is allowed to have periods of inadequate ventricular preload, or if dysrhythmias produce a loss of the atrial "kick" associated with normal sinus rhythm. Abrupt pharmacologic sympathectomy, such as produced by spinal anesthesia, lowers both systemic vascular resistance and venous return. In patients with aortic stenosis, this may produce protracted and potentially catastrophic arterial hypotension.

Aortic valvular insufficiency or regurgitation, on the other hand, produces retrograde blood flow from the aorta into the left ventricle during diastole, normally offset by a compensatory increase in heart rate. A large stroke volume is ejected from a distended, compliant ventricular chamber that functions at relatively normal filling and ejection pressures. Total cardiac output is high, but net "forward" cardiac output is only at near-normal levels, at least until volume overload eventually precipitates left ventricular failure.

Because the increase in ventricular workload is "volume work" rather than "pressure work," myocardial balance in patients with aortic insufficiency tends to be well maintained, and ischemia is therefore less common than in patients with stenotic aortic lesions. Moderate increases in heart rate improve pump function because they limit the diastolic time during which regurgitant flow can occur. Peripheral vasodilation may lower the impedance to ventricular ejection and enhance ventricular emptying.[86] Intraoperative bradycardia or large, abrupt increases in systemic resistance may precipitate acute left ventricular volume overload and abrupt cardiopulmonary collapse.

Mitral Valve Disease

The obstruction to blood flow produced by a stenotic mitral valve restricts left ventricular filling and thus compromises stroke volume and cardiac output. Cardiac pump function is thus limited mechanically, and will be further compromised if congestion of blood volume within the left atrium produces atrial dilation and chronic electrical fibrillation, a dysrhythmia that eliminates the normal augmentation of ventricular filling provided by sinus rhythm. In patients with mitral stenosis, tachycardia or atrial fibrillation with rapid ventricular response may impair cardiac output severely,[87] and predisposes to myocardial ischemia in patients with coexisting coronary artery disease.[88]

Sustained pulmonary congestion and hypertension in patients with mitral stenosis may also produce right ventricular failure, which occasionally responds to pulmonary vasodilator therapy.[89] However, fundamental priorities of anesthetic management include avoidance of tachycardia or tachyarrhythmias to allow maximum time for left ventricular filling, and meticulous monitoring of right ventricular preload and afterload to minimize pulmonary congestion or the possibility of right ventricular failure. However, extremes of bradycardia may also produce profound hypotension resulting from inadequate cardiac output, since stroke volume in mitral stenosis is small and relatively fixed.

Chronic mitral regurgitation or insufficiency, unlike mitral stenosis, is a cardiac valvular disorder characterized by volume overload of both left ventricle and atrium. Left ventricular stroke volume is ejected simultaneously in both a forward and a retrograde direction[90]; cardiac enlargement may be severe, although the ventricular wall exhibits a compliant, low-pressure form of hypertrophy that is not frequently associated with myocardial ischemia. Increased pulmonary vascular pressures and volumes from chronic regurgitant flow eventually produce right ventricular failure. This may result in a leftward shift of the intraventricular septum that impairs left ventricular filling, compromising the generous left ventricular end-diastolic volumes needed to maintain adequate left ventricular "forward" stroke volume.[91]

Maintenance of adequate left ventricular preload and avoidance of extremes of heart rate ensure ample left ventricular stroke volume and prevent dysrhythmias produced by prolapse of mitral valve leaflets.[92] Reduction of impedance to left ventricular ejection with arteriolar vasodilators may also improve overall hemodynamics.[86] Among patients seen at initial presentation with isolated symptoms of mitral valve prolapse, only those with thickened leaflets and hemodynamic disruption require antibiotic prophylaxis; only some of these require eventual valve replacement,[93] although all are prone to dysrhythmias if preload or afterload is inadequate.

Cardiomyopathies

Careful fluid management augmented by the judicious use of inotropes can reduce heart size and improve ventricular function in patients who have poor pump function, with or without valvular disease. The use of vasodilators to achieve left ventricular "unloading" has also assumed an increasingly prominent role in the therapy of congestive heart failure, valvular disorders, cardiomyopathies, or other hemodynamic situations in which impedance to ventricular ejection limits cardiac output.

In hypertrophic obstructive cardiomyopathy, classically described as idiopathic hypertrophic subaortic stenosis (IHSS), however, stroke volume is compromised by vigorous myocardial contraction. Ventricular hypertrophy and physical outflow tract obstruction, rather than diminished ventricular function, characterizes this disorder.[94] Patients with hypertrophic obstructive cardiomyopathy are also at increased risk of dysrhythmias[95] and may experience acute reduction of stroke volume and profound hypotension if cardiac chamber size or outflow tract diameter is reduced because of inadequate venous return, abrupt reduction in impedance to systolic ejection,[96] tachycardia, or the use of inotropic rather than vasoconstrictor agents to support arterial blood pressure.

Most approaches to anesthetic management of hypertrophic obstructive cardiomyopathy include the use of halothane or other anesthetic agents that produce dose-related, generalized depression of ventricular function and heart rate. Additional principles include maintenance of generous ventricular preload. Arterial hypotension, if it occurs, is usually treated not with inotropes but with volume infusion and α-adrenergic agonists to increase systemic vascular resistance.[97]

For patients with depressed ventricular pump function, regardless of etiology, the anesthetic plan must include provisions for monitoring right or left ventricular filling pressures to ensure adequate stroke volume and favorable hemodynamics. Central venous pressure may be used as an estimate of right ventricular preload if there is no significant discrepancy between right and left ventricular function. However, measurements of pulmonary capillary wedge pressure provide more accurate estimates of preload of the left side of the heart if there is a significant degree of left ventricular dysfunction,[98, 99] at least in the absence of gross pulmonary hypertension.

Although, like all invasive devices, insertion of a pulmonary artery catheter is associated with both morbidity and mortality,[100, 101] this device has also been of unique and extraordinary value in the management of patients with grossly altered hemodynamics. It permits measurements of cardiac output and the calculation of systemic vascular and pulmonary vascular resistances, hemodynamic parameters that quantify the severity of the disease process and provide a guide to subsequent intervention and anesthetic management.[102]

Conduction Defects

Although cardiac dysrhythmias are common during and after anesthesia in patients with preexisting cardiac conduction defects, electrical pathways within the heart are left largely undisturbed by almost all anesthetic agents. There is little evidence that general anesthesia itself can precipitate complete heart block in asymptomatic patients, even those with preexisting bifascicular conduction defects.[103] Nor is it clear that anesthetic agents change the threshold for endogenous dysrhythmias.[104] Wolff-Parkinson-White syndrome and other "preexcitation syndromes," however, do appear to be aggravated by the episodes of tachycardia commonly encountered in the course of anesthesia, mostly by the sympathoadrenal stimulation produced in response to painful stimuli and surgical stress.[105]

Direct surgical manipulation of the carotid sinus may also produce acute and severe intraoperative conduction defects.[106] Cardiac conduction disturbances also occur as a manifestation of congenital conduction abnormalities.[107] However, artificial pacemaker insertion is rarely indicated other than for the management of patients with established syncopal episodes. Children with congenital heart block respond more promptly and more effectively than adults to noninvasive therapies such as intravenous atropine.[108]

SUMMARY

Cardiac muscle is distinguished from other contractile tissues by its intrinsic electrical automaticity and a complex system of length-dependent excitation-contraction coupling. Myocardial contractility is continually modified by variable influx of calcium ions from extracellular sites, and extrinsically by neural and humoral factors. Because of the various mechanisms for heterometric regulation of contractility, the complex architecture of the myocardial cytoskeleton, and the geometry of the cardiac chambers, assessment of contractility or ventricular function in vivo is largely an implication derived from measurements of pressures, stroke volume, cardiac output, and systemic vascular resistance.

Clinically, integrated cardiovascular function is a more relevant concept than inotropic state or contractility itself, since the heart usually functions as a demand pump. In the normal heart, inhalational anesthetics depress myocardial contractility significantly, but ventricular function and cardiac output, as in the awake state, are still modulated to some degree by the demands of peripheral tissues and by the integrated autonomic set-points for arterial pressure and central blood volume. Narcotics and other intravenous anesthetics have little effect on myocardial tissues, but they produce centrally mediated changes in the autonomic state and may directly alter the tone of peripheral vascular smooth muscle. Nevertheless, provided that relatively normal arterial pressures are maintained, metabolic and myogenic regional autoregulation maintains adequate perfusion of the myocardium and other specialized tissues in proportion to their respective metabolic needs.

In patients with coronary artery disease, vascular obstruction becomes the limiting factor in coronary blood flow. Under these circumstances, the adequacy of the balance between myocardial oxygen supply and demand largely reflects the workload imposed on the myocardium and the interval and pressures available for perfusion of this tissue. Therefore the anesthetic plan for the management of patients with coronary artery disease places special priority on adequate control of the overall hemodynamic environment, with special emphasis on factors that influence cardiac work and myocardial perfusion. The principles of anesthetic management for patients with valvular, myocardial, and other cardiac disorders reflect the specific factors, such as elevated vascular resistance or bradycardia, that permit continuing compensation for the pathophysiology associated with each condition. In some cases, therapeutic intervention is needed to correct disequilibrium and provide hemodynamics compatible with the maintenance of adequate cardiac output.

REFERENCES

1. Adams RJ, Schwartz A: Comparative mechanisms for contraction of cardiac and skeletal muscle. *Chest* 1980; 78(suppl):123–139.
2. Patterson S, Starling EH: On the mechanical factors which determine the output of the heart. *J Physiol* 1914; 48:357–379.
3. Braunwald E, Ross J Jr, Sonnenblick EH: Mechanism of contraction of the normal and failing heart. Part II. *N Engl J Med* 1967; 277:853–863.
4. Berne RM, Levy MN: *Cardiovascular Physiology*, ed 3. St. Louis, CV Mosby, 1977.
5. Gordon AM, Huxley AF, Julian FJ: The variation in isometric tension

with sarcomere length in vertebrate muscle fibres. *J Physiol* 1966; 184:170–192.

6. Fozzard HA: Heart: Excitation-contraction coupling. *Annu Rev Physiol* 1977; 39:201–220.

7. Borg TK, Caulfield JB: The collagen matrix of the heart. *Fed Proc* 1981; 40:2037–2041.

8. Robinson TF, Factor SM, Sonnenblick EH: The heart as a suction pump. *Sci Am* 1986; 254:83–91.

9. Allen DD, Kentish JC: The cellular basis of the length-tension relation in cardiac muscle. *J Mol Cell Cardiol* 1985; 17:821–840.

10. Langer GA: The intrinsic control of myocardial contraction—ionic factors. *N Engl J Med* 1971; 285:1065–1071.

11. Jewell BR: A re-examination of the influence of muscle length on myocardial performance. *Circ Res* 1987; 40:221–230.

12. Chapman RA: Control of cardiac contractility at the cellular level. *Am J Physiol* 1983; 245:H535–H552.

13. Reuter H: Exchange of calcium ions in the mammalian myocardium. *Circ Res* 1974; 34:599–605.

14. Mancini DM, LeJemtel TH, Factor S, et al: Central and peripheral components of cardiac failure. *Am J Med* 1986; 80(suppl 2B):2–13.

15. Braunwald E: Control of myocardial oxygen consumption. *Am J Cardiol* 1971; 27:416–432.

16. Sethna DH, Moffitt EA: An appreciation of the coronary circulation. *Anesth Analg* 1986; 65:294–305.

17. Parmley WW, Chuck L: Length-dependent changes in myocardial contractile state. *Am J Physiol* 1973; 224:1195–1199.

18. Roach MR: Biophysical analyses of blood vessel walls and blood flow. *Annu Rev Physiol* 1977; 39:51–71.

19. Sonnenblick EH, Strobeck JE: Derived indexes of ventricular and myocardial functions. *N Engl J Med* 1977; 296:978–982.

20. Braunwald E, Ross J Jr, Sonnenblick EH: Mechanisms of contraction of the normal and failing heart (Part III). *N Engl J Med* 1967; 277:910–920.

21. Rubin SA, Swan HJC: Implications of peripheral circulatory control: Implications of vasodilator therapy in heart failure. *Cardiovasc Clin* 1984; 14:19–29.

22. O'Rourke MF: Vascular impedance in studies of arterial and cardiac function. *Physiol Rev* 1982; 62:570–623.

23. Parmley WW, Tyberg JV, Glantz SA: Cardiac dynamics. *Annu Rev Physiol* 1977; 39:277–299.

24. Guyton AC: Regulation of cardiac output. *Anesthesiology* 1968; 20:314–326.

25. Braunwald E: Regulation of the circulation. *N Engl J Med* 1974; 290:1124–1129 (Part I); 1420–1425 (Part II).

26. Nicoll PA: Structure and function of minute vessels in autoregulation. *Circ Res* 1964; 15(suppl I):245–252.

27. Segal SS, Duling BR: Flow control among microvessels coordinated by intercellular conduction. *Science* 1987; 234:868–870.
28. Berne RM: Metabolic regulation of blood flow. *Circ Res* 1964; 15(suppl I):261–268.
29. Feigl EO: Coronary physiology. *Physiol Rev* 1983; 63:1–168.
30. Shepherd JT, Vanhoutte PM: Role of the venous system in circulatory control. *Mayo Clin Proc* 1978; 53:247–255.
31. Lurie AA: Anesthesia and the systemic venous circulation. *Anesthesiology* 1963; 24:368–395.
32. Bishop VS, Peterson DF, Horwitz LD: Factors influencing cardiac performance, in Guyton AC, Cowley AW (eds): *Cardiovascular Physiology II,* volume 9. Baltimore, University Park Press, 1976, pp 239–273.
33. Spencer MP, Greiss FC: Dynamics of ventricular ejection. *Circ Res* 1962; 10:274–279.
34. Watson WE, Seelye E, Smith AC: The action of thiopentone on the vascular distensibility of the hand. *Br J Anaesth* 1962; 34:19–23.
35. Price HL, Linde HW, Jones RE, et al: Sympathoadrenal responses to general anesthesia in man and their relation to hemodynamics. *Anesthesiology* 1959; 20:563–575.
36. Tweed WA, Minuck M, Mymin D: Circulatory responses to ketamine anesthesia. *Anesthesiology* 1972; 37:613–619.
37. Kawamura R, Stanley TH, English JB, et al: Cardiovascular responses to nitrous oxide exposure for two hours in man. *Anesth Analg* 1980; 59:93–99.
38. Waxman K, Shoemaker WC, Lippmann M: Cardiovascular effects of anesthetic induction with ketamine. *Anesth Analg* 1980; 59:355–358.
39. Stoelting RK, Gibbs PS: Hemodynamic effects of morphine and morphine-nitrous oxide in valvular heart disease and coronary artery disease. *Anesthesiology* 1973; 38:45–52.
40. Demas K, Wyner J, Muhm FG, et al: Anaesthesia for heart transplantation. *Br J Anaesth* 1986; 58:1357–1364.
41. Lowenstein E, Hallowell P, Levine FH, et al: Cardiovascular response to large doses of intravenous morphine in man. *N Engl J Med* 1969; 281:1389–1393.
42. Edde RR: Hemodynamic changes prior to and after sternotomy in patients anesthetized with high-dose fentanyl. *Anesthesiology* 1981; 55:444–446.
43. Hall GM: Fentanyl and the metabolic response to surgery (editorial). *Br J Anaesth* 1980; 52:561–562.
44. Zurick AM, Urzua J, Yared J-P, et al: Comparison of hemodynamic and hormonal effects of large single-dose fentanyl anesthesia and halothane/nitrous oxide anesthesia for coronary artery surgery. *Anesth Analg* 1982; 61:521–526.
45. Stanley TH, Webster LR: Anesthetic requirements and cardiovascular effects of fentanyl-oxygen and fentanyl-diazepam-oxygen anesthesia in man. *Anesth Analg* 1978; 57:411–416.

46. Moffitt EA, Sethna DH: The coronary circulation and myocardial oxygenation in coronary artery disease. *Anesth Analg* 1986; 65:395–410.
47. Zelis R. Mansour EJ, Capone RJ, et al: The cardiovascular effects of morphine. *J Clin Invest* 1974; 54:1247–1258.
48. Rosow CE: Sufentanil citrate: A new opioid analgesic for use in anesthesia. *Pharmacotherapy* 1984; 4:11–19.
49. Marty J, Nitenberg A, Blanchet F, et al: Effects of droperidol on left ventricular performances in humans. *Anesthesiology* 1982; 157:22–25.
50. Housmans PR, Murat I: Comparative effects of halothane, enflurane, and isoflurane at equipotent anesthetic concentrations on isolated ventricular myocardium of the ferret. I. Contractility. *Anesthesiology* 1988; 69:451–463.
51. Bahlman SH, Eger EI II, Halsey MJ, et al: The cardiovascular effects of halothane in man during spontaneous ventilation. *Anesthesiology* 1972; 36:494–502.
52. Eger EI II, Smith NT, Stoelting RL, et al: Cardiovascular effects of halothane in man. *Anesthesiology* 1970; 32:396–409.
53. Smith NT, Ingels NB, Daughters GT II, et al: Contribution of asynergic contraction to halothane-induced myocardial depression. *Anesth Analg* 1980; 59:178–185.
54. Smith NT, Eger EI II, Stoelting RK: The cardiovascular and sympathomimetic responses to the addition of nitrous oxide to halothane in man. *Anesthesiology* 1970; 32:410–421.
55. Mote PS, Pruett JK, Gramling ZW: Effects of halothane and enflurane on right ventricular performance in hearts of dogs anesthetized with pentobarbital sodium. *Anesthesiology* 1983; 58:53–60.
56. Rathod R, Jacobs HK, Kramer NE, et al: Echocardiographic assessment of ventricular performance following induction with two anesthetics. *Anesthesiology* 1978; 49:86–90.
57. Calverley RK, Smith NT, Prys-Roberts C, et al: Cardiovascular effects of enflurane anesthesia during controlled ventilation in man. *Anesth Analg* 1978; 57:619–628.
58. Calverley RK, Smith NT, Jones CW, et al: Ventilatory and cardiovascular effects of enflurane anesthesia during spontaneous ventilation in man. *Anesth Analg* 1978; 57:610–618.
59. Smith NT, Calverley RK, Prys-Roberts C, et al: Impact of nitrous oxide on the circulation during enflurane anesthesia in man. *Anesthesiology* 1978; 48:345–349.
60. Cromwell TH, Stevens WC, Eger EI II, et al: The cardiovascular effects of compound 469 (Forane) during spontaneous ventilation and CO_2 challenge in man. *Anesthesiology* 1971; 35:17–25.
61. Stevens WC, Cromwell TH, Halsey MJ, et al: The cardiovascular effects of a new inhalation anesthetic, Forane, in human volunteers at constant arterial carbon dioxide tension. *Anesthesiology* 1971; 35:8–16.
62. Bosnjak ZJ, Kampine JP: Effects of halothane, enflurane, and isoflurane on the SA node. *Anesthesiology* 1983; 58:314–321.

63. Atlee JL, Rusy BF: Atrioventricular conduction times and atrioventricular nodal conductivity during enflurane anesthesia in dogs. *Anesthesiology* 1977; 47:498–503.

64. Ghonheim MM, Uamada T: Etomidate: A clinical and electroencephalographic comparison with thiopental. *Anesth Analg* 1977; 56:479–485.

65. Dhadphale PR, Jackson APF, Alseri S: Comparison of anesthesia with diazepam and ketamine vs. morphine in patients undergoing heart-valve replacement. *Anesthesiology* 1970; 51:200–203.

66. Sonntag H: Actions of anesthetics on the coronary circulation in normal subjects and patients with ischemic heart disease. *Int Anesthesiol Clin* 1980; 18:111–135.

67. Nettles DC, Herrin TJ, Mullen JG: Ketamine induction in poor-risk patients. *Anesth Analg* 1973; 52:59–64.

68. Martyn JAJ, Snider MT, Szyfelbeing SK, et al: Right ventricular dysfunction in acute thermal injury. *Ann Surg* 1980; 191:330–335.

69. Merin RG: Is anesthesia beneficial for the ischemic heart? (editorial). *Anesthesiology* 1980; 53:439–440.

70. Merin RG, Verdouw PD, deJong JW: Dose-dependent depression of cardiac function and metabolism by halothane in swine. *Anesthesiology* 1977; 46:417–423.

71. Klocke FJ, Ellis AK, Orlick AE: Sympathetic influences on coronary perfusion and evolving concepts of driving pressure, resistance, and transmural flow regulation. *Anesthesiology* 1980; 52:1–5.

72. Reiz S, Ostman M: Regional coronary hemodynamics during isoflurane–nitrous oxide anesthesia in patients with ischemic heart disease. *Anesth Analg* 1985; 64:570–576.

73. Priebe H-J: Isoflurane and coronary hemodynamics. *Anesthesiology* 1989; 71:960–976.

74. Tatekawa S, Trabar KB, Hantler CB, et al: Effects of isoflurane on myocardial blood flow, function, and oxygen consumption in the presence of critical coronary stenosis in dogs. *Anesth Analg* 1987; 66:1073–1082.

75. Hoffman JIE: Determinants and prediction of transmural myocardial perfusion. *Circulation* 1978; 58:381–391.

76. Lell WA, Walker DR, Blackstone EH, et al: Evaluation of myocardial damage in patients undergoing coronary artery bypass procedures with halothane-N20 anesthesia and adjuvants. *Anesth Analg* 1977; 56:556–563.

77. Prys-Roberts C, Meloche R: Management of anesthesia in patients with hypertension or ischemic heart disease. *Int Anesthesiol Clin* 1979; 18:181–217.

78. Prys-Roberts C, Meloche R, Foex P: Studies of anaesthesia in relation to hypertension. I. Cardiovascular responses of treated and untreated patients. *Br J Anaesth* 1971; 43:122–137.

79. Moffitt EA, Sethna DH, Gray RJ, et al: Rate-pressure product correlates poorly with myocardial oxygen consumption during anesthesia in coronary patients. *Can Anaesth Soc J* 1984; 31:5–12.

80. Gobel FL, Nordstrom LA, Nelson RR, et al: The rate pressure product as

an index of myocardial oxygen consumption during exercise in patients with angina pectoris. *Circulation* 1978; 57:549–556.

81. Hoffman JIE, Buckberg GD: Pathophysiology of subendocardial ischemia. *Br Med J* 1975; 1:76–79.

82. Massagee JT, McIntyre RW, Kates RA, et al: Effects of preoperative calcium entry blocker therapy on alpha-adrenergic responsiveness in patients undergoing coronary revascularization. *Anesthesiology* 1987; 67:485–491.

83. Schulte-Sasse U, Tarnow J: Effects of short-term infusion of nifedipine or verapamil on systemic hemodynamics and left ventricular myocardial contractility in patients prior to coronary artery bypass surgery. *Anesthesiology* 1987; 67:492–497.

84. Thomas SJ, Lowenstein E: Anesthetic management of the patient with valvular heart disease. *Int Anesthesiol Clin* 1978; 17:67–96.

85. Frank S, Johnson A, Ross J Jr: Natural history of valvular aortic stenosis. *Br Heart J* 1973; 35:41–46.

86. Stone JG, Hoar PF, Calabro JR, et al: Afterload reduction and preload augmentation improve the anesthetic management of patients with cardiac failure and valvular regurgitation. *Anesth Analg* 1980; 59:737–742.

87. Arandi DT, Carleton RA: The deleterious role of tachycardia in mitral stenosis. *Circulation* 1967; 36:511–516.

88. Befeler B, Kamen AR, MacLoed MB: Coronary artery disease and left ventricular function in mitral stenosis. *Chest* 1970; 57:435–439.

89. Stone JG, Hoar PF, Faltas AN, et al: Nitroprusside and mitral stenosis. *Anesth Analg* 1980; 59:662–665.

90. Selzer A, Katayama F: Mitral regurgitation: Clinical patterns, pathophysiology, and natural history. *Medicine* 1972; 51:337–366.

91. Ross J Jr: Acute displacement of the diastolic pressure-volume curve of the left ventricle. *Circulation* 1979; 59:32–37.

92. Krantz EM, Viljoen JF, Schermer R, et al: Mitral valve prolapse. *Anesth Analg* 1980; 59:379–383.

93. Marks AR, Choong CY, Sanfilippo AJ, et al: Identification of high-risk and low-risk subgroups of patients with mitral valve prolapse. *N Engl J Med* 1989; 320:1031–1036.

94. Lanier E, Prough DS: Intraoperative diagnosis of hypertrophic obstructive cardiomyopathy. *Anesthesiology* 1984; 60:61–63.

95. Anderson KP, Stinson EB, Derby GC, et al: Vulnerability of patients with obstructive hypertrophic cardiomyopathy to ventricular arrhythmia during induction in the operating room. Analysis of 17 patients. *Am J Cardiol* 1983; 51:811–816.

96. Loubser P, Suh K, Cohen S: Adverse effects of spinal anesthesia in a patient with idiopathic hypertrophic subaortic stenosis. *Anesthesiology* 1984; 60:228–230.

97. Thompson RC, Liberthoson RR, Lowenstein E: Perioperative anesthetic risk of noncardiac surgery in hypertrophic obstructive cardiomyopathy. *JAMA* 1985; 254:2419–2421.

98. Mangano DT: Monitoring pulmonary arterial pressure in coronary-artery disease. *Anesthesiology* 1980; 53:364–370.

99. Rao TLK: Cardiac monitoring for the noncardiac surgical patient. *Semin Anesth* 1983; 2:241–250.

100. Geha DG, Davis NJ, Lappas DG: Persistent atrial arrhythmias associated with placement of a Swan-Ganz catheter. *Anesthesiology* 1973; 39:651–653.

101. Jobes DR, Schwartz AJ, Greenhow DE, et al: Safer jugular vein cannulation: Recognition of arterial puncture and the external jugular route. *Anesthesiology* 1983; 59:353–355.

102. Swan HJC, Ganz W, Forrester J, et al: Catheterization of the heart in man with use of a flow-directed balloon-tipped catheter. *N Engl J Med* 1970; 283:447–451.

103. Simon AB: Perioperative management of the pacemaker patient. *Anesthesiology* 1977; 46:127–131.

104. Zaidan JR: Pacemakers. *Anesthesiology* 1984; 60:319–334.

105. Sadowski AR, Moyers JR: Anesthetic management of the Wolff-Parkinson-White syndrome. *Anesthesiology* 1979; 51:553–556.

106. Otteni JC, Pottecher T, Bronner G, et al: Prolongation of the Q-T interval and sudden cardiac arrest following right radical neck dissection. *Anesthesiology* 1983; 59:358–361.

107. Galloway PA, Glass PSA: Anesthetic implications of prolonged QT interval syndromes. *Anesth Analg* 1985; 64:612–620.

108. Diaz JH, Friesen RH: Anesthetic management of congenital complete heart block in childhood. *Anesth Analg* 1979; 58:334–336.

7

Pulmonary Function During Anesthesia

The lungs are part of a multiorgan system complex that provides tissues with continual elimination of carbon dioxide and the delivery of oxygen. To maintain the capillary oxygen tensions compatible with sustained aerobic metabolism, lung tissues allow the transfer of several hundred milliliters of oxygen from alveolar air each minute, although maximal skeletal muscle activity can further increase the requirements for oxygen delivery 15-fold. The cardiovascular system, discussed in the previous chapter, provides the pumping function that circulates blood to and through the lungs, major vascular conduits, and tissue exchange beds. The physical carriage of oxygen and carbon dioxide from lungs to tissues is one of the functions of blood, described separately in Chapter 10.

The sections that follow review the fundamental characteristics of the lungs as a site for gas exchange, the function of the chest wall, diaphragm, and associated musculature as a ventilatory mechanism or "air pump," and the mechanical and chemical factors that maintain the appropriate matching of gas and blood flow within this organ system. Also discussed are the effects of anesthetics on ventilatory mechanics, on the matching of ventilation and pulmonary blood flow, and on the neurally integrated regulation of ventilatory effort. The assessment of lung dysfunction and the impact of these factors on the anesthetic plan both for healthy patients and for those patients with lung disease are summarized.

PULMONARY MECHANICS AND THE WORK OF BREATHING

Lung Volumes

Measurements of gas volumes within the lungs and the pressures at which they are achieved are used to derive parameters that describe the physical conditions under which air or other gas mixtures move into or out of the lungs. This discipline, pulmonary mechanics, does not describe the process of molecular gas exchange; rather, it is a quantitative description of the physical interactions between pressure and volume that can be used to assess the efficiency of the ventilatory process.

Lung volume at rest (functional residual capacity [FRC]) reflects the physical equilibrium between anatomic determinants of recoil within the lung itself and the opposing tendency of the chest walls to spring outward. In effect, FRC describes the natural resting position of the lungs in the absence of muscular contraction or imposed movement. The concept of FRC is of great importance in understanding the changes in lung function that occur during anesthesia because it reflects the net interaction of those factors that influence the state of the lungs and the surrounding soft tissues. Normally about 3 L, FRC is reduced by about 25% upon assumption of the supine position. It represents approximately one half of total lung capacity (TLC) (Fig 7–1).

Total lung capacity itself is traditionally subdivided into component volumes representing the contributions of maximal inspiration (inspiratory reserve volume [IRV]), exhalation (expiratory reserve volume [ERV]), and the residual, nonexchangeable volume of gas remaining in the lungs even after a maximal expiratory effort (residual volume [RV]). Two thirds of the energy expended by the respiratory diaphragm and accessory respiratory muscles in the process of inflating the lung beyond FRC is stored in the form of elastic recoil and subsequently returned during the exhalation phase of the ventilatory cycle.[1] This energy is then expressed in the form of pressures transmitted to the airways, producing bulk movement of gas volume within the tracheobronchial tree.

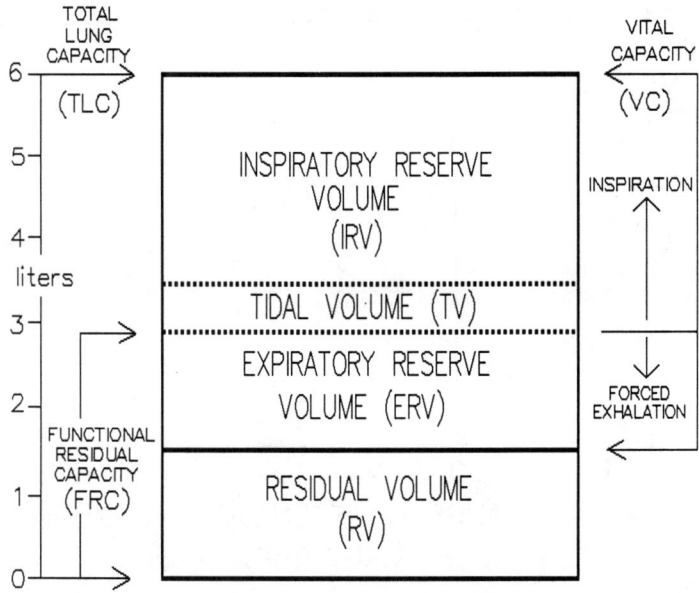

FIG 7–1.
Approximate distribution of intrathoracic gas volume among the components of total lung capacity *(TLC)* in normal adults. The sum of residual volume *(RV)* and vital capacity *(VC)* determines *TLC* and reflects "nonexchangeable" and "exchangeable" gas volumes, respectively. Functional residual capacity *(FRC)* is lung volume at rest in the absence of respiratory muscle activity.

Compliance and Elastance

When gas flow ceases, the net change in volume and the gradient or difference in alveolar distending pressure required to achieve that volume is used to quantitate elastic recoil by means of measurements of compliance, or its reciprocal value, elastance. The springlike qualities of elastic structures such as the lung or the thorax dictate that the tension developed during changes in volume is directly proportional to the extent of their physical displacement or stretch. For an ideal spring, the relationship between change in length and tension is linear (Hooke's law); for the respiratory system as a whole the relationship is ideal only over a limited range of lung volumes greater than FRC (Fig 7–2). The slope of this relationship between pressure and volume defines compliance, and its value when lung volume is equal to FRC is termed "specific" compliance.

The elastic structural elements of the lung are the major source of its recoil, but alveolar surface tension also contributes to lung elastance, and thus is one determinant of measured lung, or *"pulmo-*

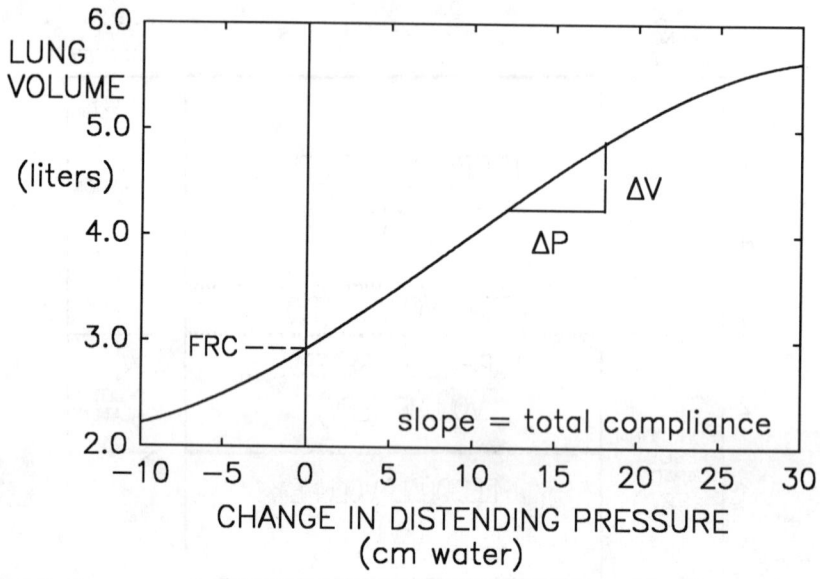

FIG 7–2.
Relationship between changes in total lung volume (ΔV) and net distending pressure (ΔP) (alveolar minus intrapleural pressure). The slope of the relationship defines total pulmonary compliance and reflects the mechanical properties both of lung tissues and the surrounding thoracic structures. Net distending pressures are shown here *relative* to the pressure at FRC, which is therefore zero by definition.

nary" compliance.[2] Measurements of total *respiratory* compliance are determined by the elastic properties of both the lung (pulmonary compliance) and of the chest wall and other nonpulmonary elements as if they were springlike components connected in a parallel arrangement. The use of the term *elastance* instead of *compliance* allows these components to be added algebraically, simplifying the mathematic analysis as well as conveying more directly the anatomic basis from which they are derived.[1]

Lung volume is a major determinant of total respiratory compliance. During quiet tidal breathing, the work of breathing is determined by both the volume of inspired gas and the pressure gradient that must be generated to achieve that volume. With low flow velocities and minimal airway resistance, almost all ventilatory work is "elastic" work derived directly from compliance. Inspiration is initiated by the contraction of the diaphragm and the intercostal muscles. Exhalation, in contrast, is passive: the elastic elements of the chest wall that were stretched during inspiration return lung volume back to FRC without additional expenditure of energy.

Resistance and Conductance

As ventilatory rate and tidal volume increase, however, higher rates of gas flow velocity within the tracheobronchial tree generate turbulence and friction. Consequently, energy beyond that required simply to stretch elastic elements is consumed by frictional loss in direct proportion to peak airflow velocity. The increased ventilatory demands of heavy exercise can generate a 100-fold increase in the work of breathing, more than one half of which is needed to meet "resistive" energy losses that are consumed and not returned during the process of exhalation.

In contrast to compliance, resistance is a flow-dependent parameter computed from the ratio of net airway driving pressure to volume of gas flow. Total *respiratory* resistance is the sum of *pulmonary*, or lung resistance, and chest wall resistance.[3] Lung resistance itself is further subdivided to distinguish between airway resistance and resistance

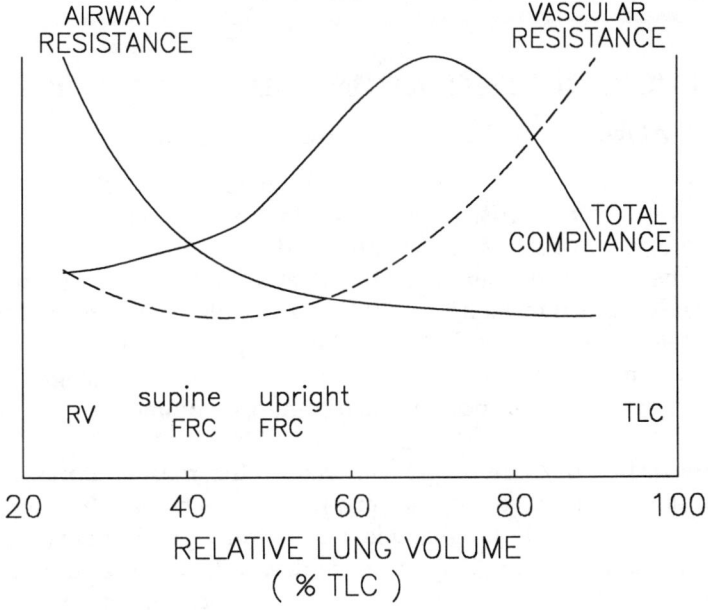

FIG 7–3.
Relative change in pulmonary mechanics and vascular resistance associated with variations in lung volume. When tidal breathing in the upright position carries lung volume to values just above *FRC*, intrathoracic resistance to the movement of pulmonary gases and blood flow is minimal, and total respiratory compliance is near its optimal value. Airway resistance rises sharply with loss of lung volume, and compliance falls to minimum values under these circumstances.

due to viscous or internal tissue movement, which is usually insignificant. Like compliance, respiratory resistance, and airway resistance in particular, is determined in large part by lung volume (Fig 7–3). The diameter of small airways is modulated by the tethering effect of the elastic fibers that surround them; for any given volumetric respiratory gas flow rate, air flow velocity must be inversely proportional to the summed cross-sectional area of the conducting airways.[4]

During quiet breathing, the majority of resistive loss occurs in the nasal passages and other tissues of the upper airway. As air flow velocity increases, however, resistance in the lower conducting airways of the tracheobronchial tree assumes progressively greater importance. Additional nonrecoverable energy expenditures are also incurred under these circumstances by the progressively greater physical distortions of the lung and chest wall soft tissues that inevitably occur with vigorous ventilatory efforts.[3] Conductance, the reciprocal of resistance, provides an alternative conceptual framework for analysis of the flow-dependent factors that determine the work of breathing.[4]

MATCHING OF VENTILATION AND BLOOD FLOW

Pleural, Alveolar, and Pulmonary Artery Pressures

Since molecular gas exchange in the lungs ultimately occurs by a process of passive diffusion, efficient pulmonary function requires that the appropriate volumes of gas and blood be maintained in close proximity. The simple "balloon in a bell jar" classroom model for lung inflation belies the extraordinarily subtle and complex mechanisms that actually determine the distribution of inhaled gas volumes. Nor do conventional mechanical models provide an accurate analogy for the mechanisms that influence the distribution of pulmonary blood flow within those tissues.

The respiratory diaphragm is certainly the most important active component required for normal inspiratory mechanics. Shortening of diaphragmatic muscle fibers evoked by normal phrenic nerve activity causes the domes of the diaphragm to descend by 1 to 2 cm with each tidal breath; a 6- to 7-cm excursion can be produced during vigorous active hyperventilation. The resultant caudal displacement of abdominal viscera is facilitated by simultaneous reflexive reciprocal inhibition of the musculature of the abdominal wall.

However, lung volume increases not only along the cephalad-caudad direction, but also across the dorsal-ventral thoracic axis. The active contraction of the external intercostal muscles elevates the lower chest wall, making thoracic expansion a three-dimensional process: the action of the chest wall and the diaphragm combines to provide a true respiratory "bellows." The contribution of intercostal muscle activity to normal, quiet inspiration is variable, but the functional reserve of this mechanism is sufficiently great that it can substitute adequately even for bilateral diaphragmatic paralysis.[5]

The preferential expansion of the diaphragmatic end of the thoracic cylinder during the coordinated contraction of the diaphragm and intercostal muscles is particularly well suited to both the elastic properties of the lungs and to the forces that distribute pulmonary blood flow. With upright posture, the lung, in effect, "hangs" from the apical pleural surface of the chest wall, coupled to the inner surface of the chest wall by the subatmospheric pressures that exist in the pleural space. Like a suction cup on a glass surface, negative pressures are generated by both the inward recoil of the elastic lung parenchyma and by the effect of gravity on its mass, since both forces are opposed by the tendency of the chest wall to expand outward. Measurement of pleural pressures at different points of the chest wall, therefore, reveals a gravity-dependent gradient: pressures at the apices are usually about 5 cm H_2O more negative than those at the lung bases of upright subjects.

Upper airway and alveolar pressures are in direct continuity through the tracheobronchial tree. By definition, therefore, they are equal throughout the lung under the no-airflow conditions at which FRC must be measured. When the lung is at rest, net "transmural" or alveolar distending pressures (alveolar minus pleural pressures) must therefore follow a gravitational gradient, greatest in uppermost areas of the lung and at minimal values at the lung bases near the diaphragmatic surface. Consequently, the air spaces of upper or "independent" lung fields can be considered to be relatively overdistended even at FRC. "Dependent" areas closer to the lung bases undergo slight compression of their volume by their own weight and the weight of the pulmonary blood volume that they contain; they rest, in effect, on a diaphragmatic "shelf."

The variable degree to which lung expansion occurs because of these gravitational forces also imposes unique mechanical properties upon each lung region. Regional lung compliance is low in the apices: elastic tissues there are already under tension because of large distending transmural pressure gradients. Further apical volume increases would require large additional increases in alveolar distending pressures and therefore would produce a further reduction in regional lung compliance in these areas. In contrast, compliance is relatively

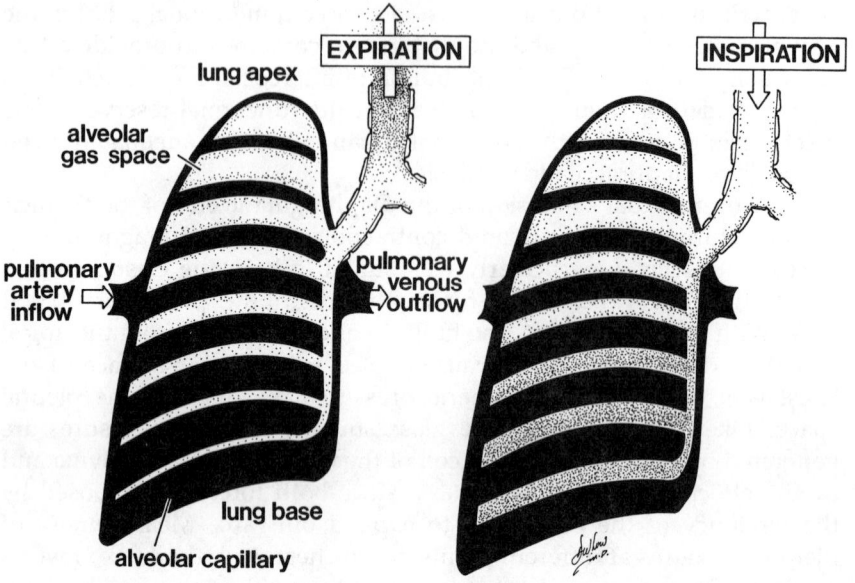

FIG 7–4.
Conceptual depiction of the distribution of intrapulmonary gas and blood along gravitational gradients in the upright posture. Apical alveolar gas spaces, even at end-expiration, are relatively overdistended, noncompliant, and poorly perfused. Although relatively underexpanded and overperfused at FRC, during inspiration the lung bases are moved by the diaphragmatic descent of each tidal breath into the range of regional lung volume at which they exhibit maximum compliance. Consequently the bulk of each tidal breath *(stippled areas)* is preferentially distributed downward to those areas that also receive the preponderance of pulmonary blood flow *(black areas)*, accomplishing the matching of ventilation and perfusion distribution.

high in the lower third of the lungs: lung fields in dependent areas are incompletely distended at FRC; increases in volume there can be accommodated with minimal initial increases in the tension produced by elastic recoil, and thus with very small increases in transmural pressure.

The active caudad motion of the diaphragm and outward elevation of the chest wall produced by intercostal muscle action release dependent lung fields from the external compression imposed by the weight of the heart and other intrathoracic structures, and by the chest wall itself. Thus in dependent lung fields, regional respiratory compliance is high, and may further increase during inspiration. As a consequence, inspired tidal gas volume is preferentially distributed to dependent lung fields (Fig 7–4). In contrast, alveolar airspaces in apical areas are relatively overdistended even at rest, and they receive very little further expansion, and thus only minimal alveolar ventilation, with inspiration during normal tidal breathing.[6]

By creating a gradient for regional lung compliance, gravity not only determines the distribution of inspired gas volumes but also partitions and distributes pulmonary blood volume and blood flow directly. In normal subjects, regional lung perfusion is decreased in direct proportion to the vertical displacement of the lung field above heart level. The pressures within the pulmonary artery are sufficiently low that there is a virtual hydrostatic failure of alveolar perfusion in the most independent lung zones in upright subjects.[1]

There is no "siphon" effect to maintain net driving pressures across the pulmonary circulation analogous to the one that occurs in the cerebral circulation because the pulmonary capillaries have little intrinsic structural stiffness, and, unlike their cerebral counterparts, they are not surrounded by a rigid container. The behavior of the pulmonary alveolar vasculature is, in fact, that of a Starling resistor: a parallel array of collapsible vascular segments through which blood flow occurs only when intraluminal hydrostatic pressures exceed the external compressive forces imposed by the surrounding alveolar gas spaces.[7]

Intra-alveolar gas pressures vary with the ventilatory cycle, but they remain positive during at least some part of exhalation in a spontaneous breathing pattern, and for virtually all of the cycle during controlled mechanical ventilation. In subapical areas, vascular pressures may be high enough to permit intermittent or variable "waterfall" blood flow during most of spontaneous, or at least part of positive pressure, mechanical ventilation. In the most dependent areas, alveolar capillary blood pressures are capable of generating continuous blood flow at rates determined simply by the net driving pressure across the capillary itself. These compliant vascular channels in dependent lung segments also serve as a reservoir for pulmonary blood volume, buffering transient discrepancies between left and right ventricular stroke volumes.[8]

Alveolar Architecture

Gravitational effects can also alter the distribution of pulmonary blood flow indirectly by modifying vascular resistance in the lung. Simplistic functional models depict the pulmonary capillary as a tube of circular cross-section traveling near or through a gas-filled alveolar space. Data derived from both anatomic studies and physiologic modeling of the pulmonary circulation indicate, however, that alveolar capillaries do not actually resemble this traditional concept. Rather, they are thin-walled, platelike vascular sheets enclosing alveolar airspaces.[9] This conformation not only makes alveolar capillaries exquisitely sensitive to external compression by the pressures imposed by the surrounding alveolar gas, but also makes pulmonary capillary cross-sectional area and the hydraulic resistance to pulmonary blood flow dependent on the degree of lung inflation existing in that lung region.

Measurements of pulmonary vascular resistance (PVR), in fact, confirm that it is lowest at FRC (Fig 7–3) and may be increased significantly by changes in either the overall lung volume or the local forces affecting regional lung volumes. As lung volume approaches TLC, increasing distention of alveolar airspaces brings closer together opposing pulmonary capillary walls, and thereby selectively closes those segments of the pulmonary vascular tree in the most independent areas.[10] When lung volume is reduced to values below FRC, PVR also increases, probably because there is kinking of large, cylindric precapillary pulmonary vascular structures.[11]

Ventilation-Perfusion Profiles

Classic analysis of the distribution of ventilation and perfusion throughout the lung described a model with three distinct zones of lung parenchyma characterized as underperfused, intermittently perfused, or continuously perfused.[12] It is far more likely, however, that regional variations in the extent to which lung tissues receive pulmonary blood flow occur not in three distinct areas, but rather along a continuous gravitational gradient, with some local effects of superimposed, nongravitational factors.

In any case, what appears to be a gravitationally induced maldistribution of pulmonary blood flow is, in fact, an appropriate diversion or partitioning of pulmonary blood flow to alveoli, which, for reasons described previously herein, also receive the majority of the gas volumes associated with each inspired breath. Since the change in net transmural or alveolar distending pressures is equal throughout the lung, there is a preferential distribution of incoming tidal gas to dependent lung zones as inspiratory muscle activity moves these areas into their range of maximal compliance. Simultaneously, these predominantly dependent areas maintain good ventilation-perfusion (V/Q) matching because they also receive the majority of cardiac output; PVR in these areas is low, and their capillaries are continuously patent. The process of regional lung expansion dictated by the gravitational gradient for net transmural pressures at FRC also minimizes PVR in those areas in which lung volume is relatively compressed.

Active Mechanisms

Although the overall distribution of ventilation and blood flow is therefore determined largely by the mechanical qualities of the lung–chest wall unit and by gravitational pressure gradients, active contraction of the smooth muscle within the bronchi and the vasculature of the lung appears to provide an additional mechanism for the matching of ventilation and perfusion. Hypoxic pulmonary vasoconstriction (HPV) is a locally mediated response that improves overall V/Q matching[13] by diverting pulmonary blood flow away from unventilated or underventilated regions in which alveolar or pulmonary vascular oxygen tensions are low.[14] Another, but probably less important, mechanism by which V/Q matching established by mechanical factors is further "fine tuned" is hypocapnic bronchoconstriction, a phenomenon that reduces small airway caliber, and thus increases airway resistance, in poorly perfused lung zones.[15]

Nonrespiratory Functions

The nonrespiratory functions of the lung are important but neither as well studied nor as widely appreciated as those related to gas exchange. The pulmonary vascular bed provides a compliant fluid reservoir, or "buffer," between the right and left ventricles. Transient surges of venous return as large as 200 mL can be accommodated while producing only minimal changes in diastolic pressure and cardiac chamber volume. The lung parenchyma is also a metabolically active tissue that synthesizes surfactant, local vasoactive mediators such as histamine, and also produces or facilitates the activation of hormonal substances such as angiotensin, which have effects on nonpulmonary circulatory beds. The lung also provides for the absorption of particulates, albumin and other proteins, inorganic salts, urea, and many drugs, including curare.[16]

The absorption of vasoactive substances from pulmonary arterial blood is a highly selective but poorly understood phenomenon that appears to clear or deactivate many of the exogenous and endogenous substances that are continually released from other tissue beds. This organ also serves a more obvious function: it is a mechanical filter, removing fibrin, other products of hemostasis, and various forms of intravascular debris before they can enter the arterial circulation and cause potentially disastrous embolization of other organs. The ability of pulmonary mast cells to produce heparin also suggests that this organ may be an important determinant of the overall control of blood coagulability.[17]

CONTROL OF VENTILATION

Central Components

The control of the timing and the depth of spontaneous ventilatory patterns is accomplished by a complex of neuronal and chemical feedback loops. Some of the essential components of this system, however, remain poorly defined. Respiratory drive, as evidenced by the contraction of respiratory muscles, is automatic, rhythmic, and continuously maintained despite wide variations in the general level of consciousness. These motor impulses appear to originate in medullary neuron clusters. Both dorsal and ventral respiratory cell body groups have been identified.[18]

In contrast to the classic view that the dorsal and ventral respiratory groups (DRG and VRG, respectively) function as reciprocally inhibiting rhythm generators, it now appears that the origins of respiratory rhythmicity reside solely in the DRG. The VRG probably acts as a processing station to project respiratory drive to both the diaphragm and the accessory muscles of respiration, although the spinal cord may also play an essential role in the overall integration of respiratory muscle activity (Fig 7–5).

The classic pneumotaxic center (PNC) and apneustic center (APC) of the pons and upper medulla appear to receive and process a continuous flow of afferent information from the chemoreceptors and mechanoreceptors associated with respiration. These brain centers limit the duration and the extent of lung inflation but appear to possess little intrinsic rhythmicity. Voluntary ventilatory patterns and the ventilatory responses to anxiety or other altered emotional states require the additional participation of cerebral cortical areas, probably by way of pontine centers.

Increased respiratory muscle activity and even hyperventilation with decreased alveolar carbon dioxide tensions can also occur as a result of acute pain, or by stimulation of cutaneous temperature receptors. These mechanisms have been widely used in medical practice to stimulate ventilation in newborn infants, in sedated subjects, and in other patients with respiratory depression for a variety of reasons. Passive movement of the limbs and vibrations of various body tissues may also produce a reflex increase in respiratory rate or tidal volume.

Interneurons of the spinal cord modulate phrenic nerve excitation and diaphragmatic muscle activity. They also provide the cyclic and coordinated inhibition of the abdominal muscles that is seen during inspiration, as well as the reflexive relaxation of most accessory and aux-

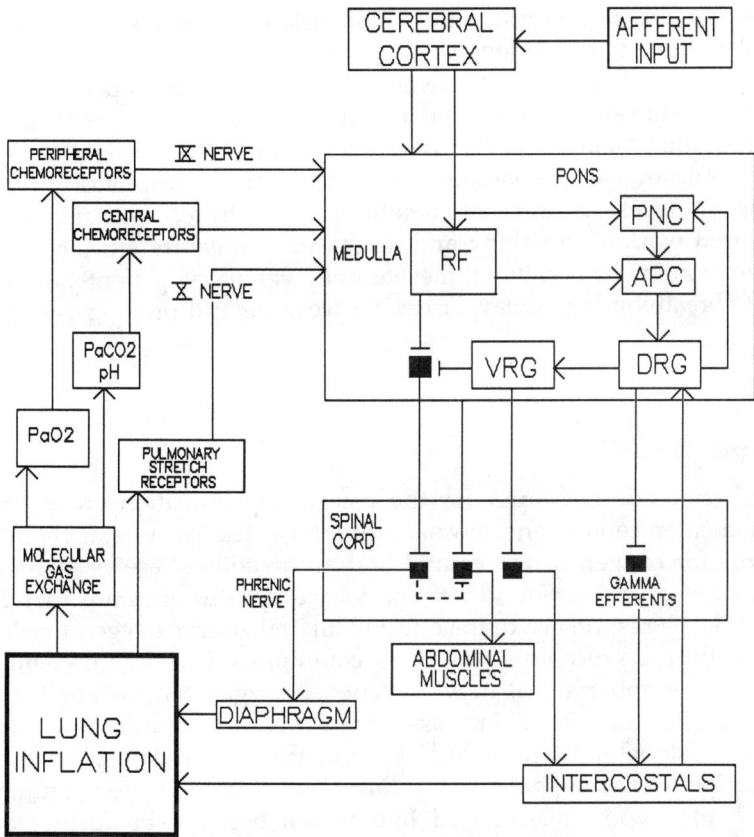

FIG 7–5.
Schematic depiction of the complex interconnection of afferent, efferent, and central components of ventilatory control. Input comes not only from mechanoreceptors and chemoreceptors but also from higher centers mediating sensory and psychologic activity. Major integrative centers exist in the pneumotaxic center *(PNC),* apneustic center *(APC),* reticular formation *(RF),* and the dorsal and ventral respiratory neuron groups *(DRG, VRG)* of the medulla and the pons. In addition, there are also little-understood integrative centers within the medulla and spinal cord that synchronize reciprocal inhibition of the muscles of the abdominal wall *(dashed lines).*

iliary inspiratory muscles during exhalation. The intercostal muscles, however, appear to be under direct medullary control.[18] Reflex relaxation of abdominal and paravertebral musculature during slow, quiet breathing facilitates abdominal examination and lumbar puncture, a clinically evident phenomenon frequently utilized to facilitate these maneuvers.

Contractions of the intercostal muscles during inspiration elevate the lower ribs and improve the volumetric effectiveness of diaphragmatic excursion by stiffening the upper anterior chest wall. "Paradoxical" inward chest wall movements may be seen in patients with residual paralysis of intercostal muscles at the end of an anesthetic incorporating neuromuscular blockade. Loss of the strength or the synchronization of the various components of the respiratory muscle group produces discoordinate breathing, a syndrome characterized by increased work of breathing and decreased ventilatory efficiency. Not uncommon in chronically ill, mechanically ventilated patients, discoordinate breathing may delay successful weaning and prolong ventilator dependence.[19]

Receptor Input

Specific afferent input for the control of ventilation comes from both chemoreceptors and mechanoreceptors. The peripheral chemoreceptors for oxygen in the carotid and aortic bodies receive extremely high rates of blood flow; their specialized cytochromes are therefore immediately responsive to the effect of altered arterial oxygen tensions. Although these receptors produce a continuous discharge transmitted by the glossopharyngeal nerve whenever oxygen tensions are below 500 mm Hg, their input increases ventilation significantly only when tensions fall below 60 mm Hg.[18] The increase in ventilatory drive produced by arterial hypoxemia is a linear function of oxygen saturation (Fig 7–6). Hypoxemia-induced hyperventilation can be further augmented by coexisting acidosis, or by hypercarbia.[20]

Other essential chemoreceptors that participate in the normal control of spontaneous ventilation and ventilatory drive are located centrally, on the ventral medullary surface of the brain stem in direct proximity to cerebrospinal fluid. Unlike the almost instantaneous sensitivity of peripheral chemoreceptors, these specialized areas exhibit delayed responses, and only after there have been changes in arterial carbon dioxide tension. Central responses appear to be stimulated directly by cerebrospinal fluid carbon dioxide or pH.

Central receptors are insensitive to changes in arterial or cerebrospinal fluid oxygen tension, although their activity is suppressed in a nonspecific manner by local tissue hypoxia. In the absence of peripheral chemoreceptor input, ventilation is proportional to cerebrospinal fluid pH, which may be metabolically adjusted during the complex process of adaptation to chronic acid-base imbalance, or as part of the process of acclimation to high altitudes.

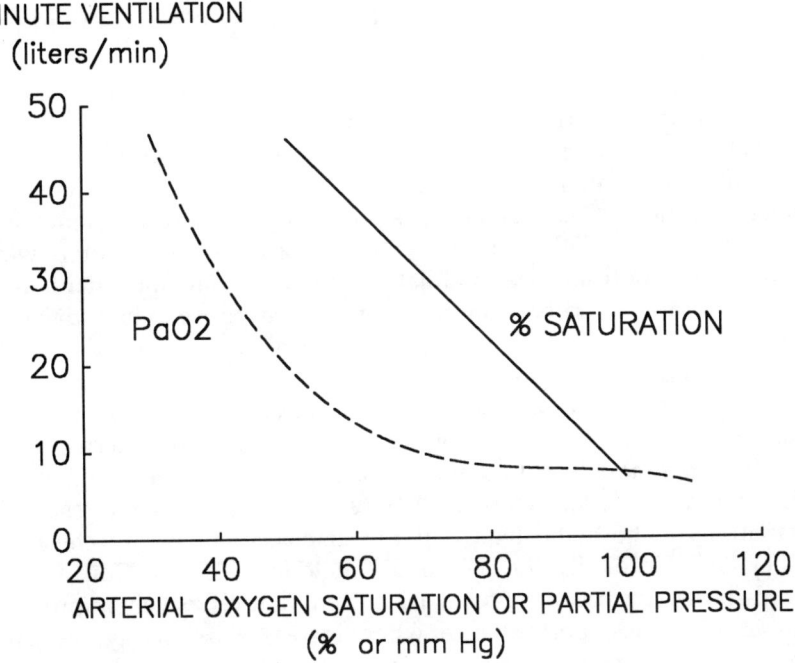

MINUTE VENTILATION
(liters/min)

ARTERIAL OXYGEN SATURATION OR PARTIAL PRESSURE
(% or mm Hg)

FIG 7–6.
Reductions of arterial oxygen saturation stimulate increases in minute ventilation in a direct and linear fashion. The complex shape of the oxygen-hemoglobin dissociation curve produces a curvilinear relationship for the ventilatory response to hypoxia if it is defined in terms of arterial oxygen tension.

Integration of Ventilatory Control

The integration of peripheral and central chemoreceptor input occurs in a complex and nonadditive manner within medullary centers (Fig 7–5). In normal unanesthetized subjects, central and peripheral chemoreceptor input ultimately modulates the amplitude and the frequency of ventilatory efforts, but is not required for the initiation of diaphragmatic movement. Spontaneous ventilation is, in fact, maintained despite the presence of central hypocarbia during voluntary hyperventilation. A rhythmic, spontaneous ventilatory pattern is also usually apparent during emergence from anesthesia even before there is a full return of consciousness in patients who have been passively hyperventilated to arterial carbon dioxide levels less than 20 mm Hg.[21]

The spontaneous and rhythmic discharge of medullary and spinal cord respiratory neurons, therefore, appears to be an intrinsic property of the neuronal tissues and pathways involved in control of ventilation. However, the rate and pattern of neuronal discharge and carbon dioxide responsiveness are clearly modified by both the pontine pneumotaxic center and by higher neural structures exerting their influence on the reticular formation. Carbon dioxide modifies ventilatory patterns but does not itself initiate spontaneous respiratory efforts.

Afferent input from lung and chest wall mechanoreceptors conducted to the APC also determines the timing of the components of the respiratory cycle. Other input from specialized stretch receptors within bronchial smooth muscle modulates respiratory rate and tidal volume, providing an inspiratory "shutoff" signal in response to lung distention and subsequent airway distortion. The classic Hering-Breuer reflex, which can produce complete interruption of inspiratory effort, requires tidal volumes of 1 L or more, and is usually not a functionally important element of spontaneous or controlled ventilation patterns.[18]

The gamma-efferent spindle muscle systems of intercostal muscles function as important chest wall "stretch receptors." They respond to variations in both the load and the displacement of the chest wall. They may provide the essential anatomic element for a spinal cord–based, servocontrol feedback system that reflexively improves inspiratory muscle performance when increases in airway resistance, common during general anesthesia, magnify the work of breathing.[22]

Other components of the diffuse system that provides control of ventilation are found within the respiratory epithelium of the nose, pharynx, larynx, and trachea. They contain poorly defined areas that respond to chemical or to particulate irritation by initiating a sneeze, cough, or, in some cases, prolonged apnea. Stimulation of these receptors by pungent anesthetic vapors, in fact, frequently disrupts inhalational anesthetic induction. Better-defined, fast-adapting irritant receptors found in the epithelium of the tracheobronchial tree can abbreviate the duration of exhalation and may even cause histamine-mediated bronchospasm on a local basis. This may explain the acute increases in airway resistance that follow the aspiration of gastric acid.

Finally, there are the specialized structures involved in the regulation of pulmonary blood volume, "type J" (juxtacapillary) receptors found in close proximity to the pulmonary capillaries. Normally quiescent, these receptors provide input that travels along vagal pathways to produce subjective sensations of dyspnea, as well as shallow tachypnea and bradycardia, when stimulated by increases in lung water, lung tissue inflammation, or congestion of the pulmonary circulation by volume overload or heart failure.

Evaluation of Lung Function

The primary function of the lung is gas exchange. Oxygen and carbon dioxide diffuse passively along the partial pressure gradients established by blood flow and gas movement on either side of an anatomic barrier composed primarily of alveolar epithelium and pulmonary capillary endothelium. This barrier is sufficiently thin that reduced diffusing capacity due to "alveolar-capillary block" is rarely a cause of impaired gas exchange, and is largely a diagnosis of exclusion.[23] However, this term has been applied to a clinical syndrome of dyspnea and impaired oxygenation that occurs in patients with interstitial pulmonary fibrosis, alveolar proteinosis, asbestosis, scleroderma, or pulmonary edema. Although the symptoms experienced by these patients could be due to the actual separation of capillary endothelium from alveolar epithelial layers within the lung parenchyma, they can be adequately explained on the basis of V/Q mismatching alone.

Normally, 50 to 70 m^2 of alveolar surface area are available for the diffusion of respiratory gases. The pulmonary capillaries that surround alveolar gas spaces are layered between epithelial sheets perforated by respiratory bronchioles and alveolar ducts. In addition, connective tissue struts, or "posts," provide structural continuity, transforming the gross anatomic increases in lung volume that occur with each inspiration into increased alveolar dimensions. Anatomic loss of alveolar surface area can limit pulmonary gas exchange if the normal alveolar microarchitecture is destroyed pathologically. The obliteration of alveolar walls by caustic chemical vapors or by the progressive deterioration associated with emphysema inevitably merges adjacent small alveolar areas into larger units that have a reduced total surface area relative to the volumes of gas that they contain.

$P(A-a)o_2$

Most commonly, however, the efficiency of gas exchange within the lung is impaired not by anatomic destruction, but by the functional loss of surfaces available for gas diffusion. The most frequent cause of an increased gradient between alveolar and arterial oxygen tensions $(P[A-a]o_2)$ is the mismatching of pulmonary ventilation and blood flow.[24]

$P(A-a)o_2$ is a sensitive indicator of the efficiency of gas exchange because the physicochemical characteristics of hemoglobin impose a ceiling for oxygen content in end-capillary alveolar blood. Consequently even the optimal functioning of many alveolar gas exchange units cannot compensate for other units in which end-capillary blood is less than fully saturated with oxygen because of V/Q mismatching. Although assessment of oxygenation by measurement of the degree to which hemoglobin is saturated with oxygen is essential for the calculation of oxygen transport and analysis of the delivery of oxygen to peripheral tissues,[25] it has little value as a monitor of gas exchange per se, unless pulmonary dysfunction is severe. The diffusion of oxygen from alveolar gas occurs along partial pressure gradients, and the discrepancy between gas tensions in gas and blood, not the amount of oxygen carried in arterial blood, reflects most accurately any impairment of this process.

The complex shape of the oxygen-hemoglobin dissociation curve (see Chapter 10) is such that the relationship between oxygen tension and the saturation of hemoglobin is virtually indifferent to changes in oxygen tension above 150 mm Hg, even though changes in arterial oxygen pressure (Pao_2) at this or higher levels may indicate significant impairment of the efficiency of gas exchange in patients receiving supplemental oxygen therapy. For all practical purposes, therefore, oxygen content is independent of oxygen partial pressure in patients once arterial blood is fully saturated with oxygen. Measurements of the saturation of arterial blood can confirm the general adequacy of oxygenation, however, when measurements of Pao_2 are either impractical or impossible. In contrast, measurement of $P(A-a)o_2$, normally 10 mm Hg or less, has become the most important overall indicator of the effectiveness and the efficiency of pulmonary gas exchange, and it usually provides the definitive, objective basis for initiating and adjusting therapeutic interventions.

Analysis of V/Q Matching

Despite remarkably precise matching in the normal lung, many of the 300 million alveolar gas exchange units receive less than the optimal proportions of blood flow and tidal gas volumes. The overall average volumetric ratio of alveolar ventilation to cardiac output is about 0.8. This figure does not, however, convey the extensive regional variations in V/Q matching that normally occur, nor can it describe localized deviations from this value in pathologic states. However, techniques that can measure multiple inert gases simultaneously can be used to generate V/Q "profiles" describing both the mode and the distribution of V/Q ratios as a continuum from the lowest to the highest values.[26]

In normal subjects both ventilation and perfusion are restricted to alveolar units with V/Q ratios at or just below approximately 1.0 (Fig 7–7). Consequently there is virtually no true shunt (perfused but unventilated alveoli, V/Q ratio of 0) and no true alveolar dead space (ventilated but unperfused gas exchange units, infinite V/Q ratio) under these circumstances. The small but finite $P(A-a)o_2$ seen in normal subjects largely reflects the 1% or 2% of cardiac output that avoids participation in the pulmonary gas exchange process as it traverses extrapulmonary anatomic "shunt" channels in the bronchial and coronary circulations.

Venous Admixture

When disease, aging, or external processes interfere with V/Q matching, however, the profile spreads across a far wider base of ratios. Efficiency of gas exchange declines under these circumstances,

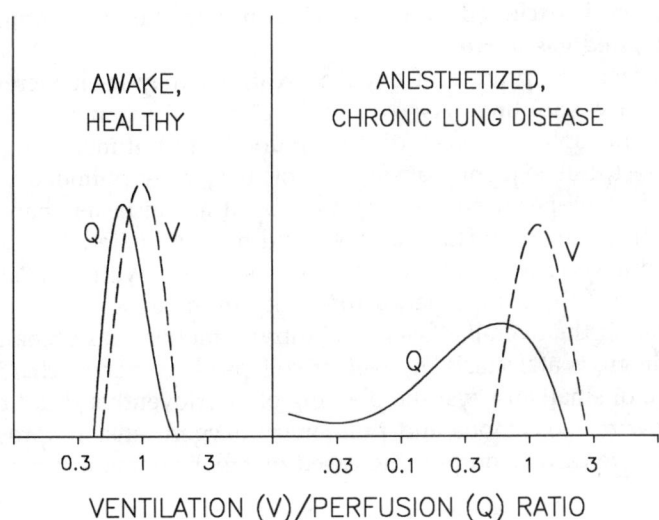

FIG 7–7.
Distribution profiles for pulmonary ventilation *(V)* and blood flow *(Q)*, when tightly matched in normal subjects *(left panel)* and when markedly disrupted, as during general anesthesia in patients with lung disease *(right panel)*. Severe disease may generate some degree of true shunting (V/Q ratio equals 0), but rarely results in measurable true alveolar dead space (infinite V/Q ratio) in the absence of pulmonary vascular embolization.

and thus net $P(A-a)O_2$ increases. The total fraction of cardiac output that would have to be excluded entirely from the gas exchange in order to produce the measured discrepancy between arterial and alveolar oxygen tensions is termed *venous admixture*. This term includes the consequences of both intrapulmonary and extrapulmonary "physiologic" shunting, where blood is either diverted away from alveolar airspaces, and thus does not perfuse lung tissue at all, and also includes the inefficiencies of oxygenation that occur because there are areas with low V/Q ratios in which ventilation occurs but at rates inadequate for locally available pulmonary blood flow.

The contributions of the components that determine venous admixture can be estimated by imposed oxygen breathing. At a high inspired fraction of oxygen (FIO_2), there is a partial pressure gradient and a molecular supply of oxygen sufficient to provide oxygenation of pulmonary capillary blood to near-optimal levels, even when ventilation is conducted through lung zones with alveoli characterized by low V/Q ratios. A large $P(A-a)O_2$ value produced by diffuse V/Q mismatching will be reduced significantly at an FIO_2 value of 1.0. If the $P(A-a)O_2$ is due to true, or "physiologic," shunt, however, increases in FIO_2 will not improve arterial oxygenation because blood flow in these areas, by definition, is excluded from contact with, and therefore indifferent to, the inspired gas mixture.

In fact, the process of oxygen breathing may itself increase intrapulmonary shunting. As oxygen displaces nitrogen in alveolar gas spaces, the splinting effect of this predominant but inert component of air is lost. Subsequently absorption of oxygen by pulmonary capillary blood in well-perfused areas may occur at a rate faster than it is provided through conducting airways, and may ultimately lead to the collapse of alveoli with very low V/Q ratios. Along with this "absorption atelectasis," there are other factors that can increase venous admixture and impair the overall efficiency of intrapulmonary gas exchange. They include gross atelectasis or alveolar collapse by other mechanisms, the closure of small airways, the opening of arteriovenous shunt channels, and low mixed venous and pulmonary oxygen tensions produced by inadequate cardiac output, increased metabolic demand for oxygen, or anemia.[23]

Alveolar Ventilation and Dead Space

Arterial carbon dioxide tensions, in general, reflect total or minute ventilation ($\dot{V}E$), but they are related more precisely to net alveolar ventilation. It is this factor that actually limits the excretion of carbon dioxide from the lungs. The difference between total and alveolar ventilation represents wasted or "dead space" ventilation, the volume of inspired and exhaled gas that does not participate in gas exchange at an alveolar level. *Total* or "physiologic" dead space includes both *anatomic* dead space, the unavoidable gas volume of the conducting, nonexchanging elements of the tracheobronchial tree and upper airway, and *alveolar* dead space, the volume of ventilation conducted to alveolar gas exchange units that are not perfused.

Like alveolar shunt, alveolar dead space is one extreme of the spectrum of V/Q ratios, and probably does not exist to a significant degree in normal lungs. Anatomic dead space due to to-and-fro bulk gas movement within the nasopharynx and the oropharynx, and through the lower conducting airways of the tracheobronchial tree, accounts for virtually all of the wasted fraction of a normal tidal volume. Total dead space can be expressed either volumetrically, approximately 150 mL of a normal tidal breath at rest, or as a fraction of tidal volume (V_D/V_T), normally about 0.3.

Total dead space is a conceptual analogue of venous admixture applied to the analysis of carbon dioxide exchange. It is a measure of wasted ventilation, just as venous admixture is a measure of wasted pulmonary blood flow. However, whereas arterial oxygen tensions at any F_{IO_2} value reflect primarily the efficiency of molecular gas exchange, arterial carbon dioxide tensions are inversely proportional to the adequacy of the ventilatory process. Because of the ease with which carbon dioxide passes through alveolar tissues, its arterial tension is related to the volumetric, nonmolecular efficiency of bulk gas movement within the lung, rather than to the fine structure of the pulmonary tissues themselves.

Arterial carbon dioxide tensions are also relatively insensitive to variations in the efficiency of molecular gas exchange in most spontaneously breathing patients unless lung disease is profound. Under most conditions reduced excretion of carbon dioxide from lung regions with high V/Q ratios is readily offset by increases in total or alveolar ventilation. Because ventilatory adequacy is defined relative to metabolic rate and the production of carbon dioxide, the criteria for ventilatory failure may be changed dramatically by metabolic state, temperature, or other nonpulmonary factors, even when simple ventilatory parameters or the process of pulmonary gas exchange itself remains unaltered.

End-Tidal Carbon Dioxide

Dilution of carbon dioxide–containing alveolar gas by carbon dioxide–free dead space gas produces an inevitable discrepancy between the tension of carbon dioxide in arterial blood and that in collected exhaled gases. An alternative approach, end-tidal gas sampling, ignores the early phase of exhalation and therefore reduces the effects of anatomic dead space. It allows estimation of alveolar carbon dioxide tensions and can be used to determine whether there have been relative changes in the volume of alveolar dead space or the production of carbon dioxide. The difference between arterial and end-tidal carbon dioxide is conceptually analogous to $P(A-a)o_2$: it increases with greater severity of lung disease or progressively severe impairment of V/Q matching because a greater proportion of gas exchange units function at high, nonoptimal V/Q ratios.

Inadequate cardiac output can also be a limiting factor in the delivery of carbon dioxide to lung tissues. The almost inevitable association of low cardiac output and pulmonary artery hypotension also exaggerates preexisting V/Q mismatching by generating more extensive zones that are well ventilated but poorly perfused. Localized pulmonary vascular obstruction by thrombus, gas bubbles, or other emboli will also produce large areas of unperfused lung tissue. If they continue to be ventilated, there is an immediate and dramatic reduction of end-tidal carbon dioxide and an increase in arterial carbon dioxide. This increased gradient between arterial and end-tidal values indicates the impaired efficiency of carbon dioxide excretion.

Carbon Dioxide Responsiveness

Under normal conditions arterial oxygen tension does not determine directly the characteristics of ventilation. In fact, Pao_2 varies widely, determined primarily by Fio_2. The amount of oxygen carried in arterial blood, however, is relatively constant, normalized by the shape of the oxygen-hemoglobin dissociation relationship. Ventilatory responses to variations in oxygenation do occur at pathologic extremes of desaturation, or under conditions of gross hyperoxia as a manifestation of oxygen toxicity.[27]

In contrast, arterial carbon dioxide tension is constantly and tightly regulated: increases in $\dot{V}E$ may be 2 L/mm Hg of arterial carbon dioxide pressure ($Paco_2$), or even greater. Consequently, spontaneous increases in total alveolar ventilation frequently mask the impaired efficiency of carbon dioxide excretion associated with the V/Q mismatching produced by mild to moderate lung disease. Carbon dioxide retention occurs very late in the natural history of these events. With terminal disease, other organ systems have already begun compensatory activities such as increased hemoglobin to optimize oxygen-carrying capacity, or enhanced production and retention of bicarbonate by renal mechanisms to normalize the acid-base status disruptions associated with chronic respiratory acidosis.

Lung Volumes, Spirometry, and Flow-Volume Loops

Measurements of the mechanical properties of the lungs and the chest wall and the assessment of the work required for pulmonary ventilation can provide a rational basis for diagnosis and, in some cases, a guide for therapeutic intervention. Static lung volumes are obtained with spirometry, plethysmography, or gas dilution techniques. Lung volumes containing two or more component subvolumes are "capacities." Vital capacity (VC) is the volume of respiratory gas inspired by a subject during a maximal effort, beginning from a forced end-expiratory state and ending at full inspired volume. VC contains the inspiratory and expiratory reserve volumes (IRV and ERV) as well as tidal volume (TV; Fig 7–1). The intrathoracic volume of gas remaining after a forced expiration is designated residual volume (RV). The sum of RV and VC equals total lung capacity (TLC).

Oxygen breathing after a forced exhalation can be used to measure the lung volume "above," or greater than, RV, at which residual nitrogen from previous inhalations of air begins to contribute to the exhaled gas volume. This lung volume appears to reflect that point at which there may be closure of small airways during a normal ventilatory cycle.[28] To facilitate direct comparison with FRC and other measurements of absolute, rather than relative, lung volumes, closing volume (CV) is usually added to. RV, yielding the term *closing capacity* (CC).

Spirometry also provides timed volumetric studies that can be of greater value than static measurements alone in the assessment of diseases in which there is obstruction or restriction of exhaled gas flow. Timing the course of a forced vital capacity (FVC) allows precise determination of the volume exhaled within the first second ($FEV_{1.0}$); both restrictive and obstructive lung disease can reduce $FEV_{1.0}$ to abnormally low values. Consequently this information may be more useful for diagnostic purposes if expressed as a fraction of total expired gas flow ($FEV_{1.0}/FVC$). Unlike obstructive disease, restrictive processes reduce both $FEV_{1.0}$ and FVC, and therefore yield low $FEV_{1.0}$ values with a normal $FEV_{1.0}/FVC$ ratio.

Significant pulmonary obstructive processes, however, characteristically depress $FEV_{1.0}$ while FVC itself is well maintained. Thus a ratio of $FEV_{1.0}/FVC$ of less than 65% is frequently used to indicate the presence of an obstructive pulmonary process. A sustained ventilatory challenge can also be used to establish maximal breathing capacity (MBC, now termed maximal voluntary ventilation, or MVV). This assessment adds to intrinsic pulmonary factors the cardiovascular and muscular requirements associated with the work of breathing itself. Indices of expired flow velocity, such as maximum midexpiratory flow rate (MMEFR), vary directly with airway caliber; they may be less dependent on the degree of patient effort than those pulmonary function tests requiring sustained ventilatory work.

Continuous measurements of relative lung volumes and approximation of lung inflation pressures with use of an esophageal balloon to estimate pleural pressures can be employed to generate oscilloscopic flow-volume and flow-pressure loops that describe the dynamic changes in pulmonary compliance occurring throughout the spontaneous ventilatory cycle. The area inside the flow-pressure loop is proportional to the resistive, nonelastic component of respiratory work, which can be twice as high in patients with obstructive lung disease as in patients with normal lungs taking breaths of the same size. Flow-volume loops permit easy identification of obstruction to exhaled gas flow. The proximity of airflow obstruction to the extremes of lung volume associated with a ventilatory cycle can be used to determine whether the obstruction exists at large or at small airways, or even at extrathoracic sites.

Time, expense, and the degree of patient cooperation and tolerance required by spirometry in its various forms limit the application of this technique as a routine diagnostic test. Alternate approaches, including transient external airway obstruction and the measurement of oscillatory airway pressures, have also been explored as useful diagnostic tools. The specificity and the reproducibility of these approaches appear adequately established, but questions remain as to whether they are sufficiently sensitive to allow diagnosis of obstructive or restrictive lung disease at stages earlier than can be obtained from the clinical history, the patient's activity level, or such simple analyses of maximum expiratory air flow as the "match test."[29]

Nevertheless, clinical spirometry and calculation of $FEV_{1.0}/FVC$ ratio and MMEF appear to be both valid and appropriate for objective assessment of pulmonary function when patients are scheduled for thoracic or upper abdominal surgery, or when they have signs, symptoms, or history of intrinsic or extrinsic lung disease. They may also be indicated in subjects who are morbidly obese or elderly. Spirometric tests of pulmonary function permit objective confirmation of tentative diagnoses already made on clinical grounds, and they may quantify the severity of the disease process. Arterial blood gases can confirm the severity of advanced pulmonary disease and they may be useful in establishing the goals of preoperative preparation, or the need for supplemental oxygen therapy perioperatively.[29, 30]

For patients with lung disease who require pulmonary resection, more extensive evaluation of regional lung blood flow and ventilation can be obtained with use of pulmonary angiography or radioisotope scans that display regional V/Q matching profiles.[31] Although a general relationship between preoperative pulmonary dysfunction and postoperative pulmonary morbidity and mortality is widely assumed and accepted, no single measurement has been shown to have consistent predictive value. However, severe limitations of expiratory flow and significant abnormalities of arterial blood gases do appear to be associated with a high frequency of postoperative pulmonary complications.[32] If it has produced a reduction of both integrated cardiopulmonary and skeletal muscle functional reserve, a severe chronic pulmonary disease process that limits maximal voluntary ventilation or total body oxygen consumption is most frequently associated with postoperative pulmonary catastrophe in patients scheduled for thoracotomy.[33]

PULMONARY FUNCTION DURING ANESTHESIA

The effects of anesthesia on pulmonary function are determined primarily by the mechanical consequences of positional change and by altered respiratory muscle activity and tone.[34] The anesthetic agents themselves alter the pattern of spontaneous ventilation, neuronal responsiveness to chemical stimuli such as oxygen and carbon dioxide, and appear to impair the intrinsic pulmonary vascular mechanisms that normally maintain optimal V/Q matching. Of lesser but still significant concern are the changes in lung function that reflect anesthetic-induced circulatory effects and the mechanical consequences of the positive airway pressure required for mechanical or manually controlled ventilation. Other coincident factors that appear to be significant in altering pulmonary function perioperatively are the site of surgery, the alteration of inspired gas mixtures or the use of selective "one-lung" ventilation, the degree, location, and duration of postoperative pain and its treatment, and, finally, the interaction between preexisting lung disease and the details of perioperative management.

The invention of practical electrode systems for the measurement of oxygen tensions in blood three decades ago permitted confirmation and extensive analysis of early observations that anesthetized patients almost invariably have impaired efficiency of oxygenation.[35] The conclusion that $P(A-a)o_2$ was increased by the process of anesthesia itself or by the effects of the drugs with which anesthesia is produced was easily reached and confirmed. The mechanism has been far more difficult to establish,[36] however, since assumptions that impaired oxygenation during anesthesia simply reflected inadequate ventilation, inappropriate choice of Fio_2, or diffuse "miliary" or microatelectasis were not supported by continuing investigation.[24]

Changes in Lung Volumes and Mechanics

It is now well established that the fundamental physical change associated with the process of anesthesia is a reduced volume of gas within the lungs, evident primarily as a fall in FRC. After the induction of general anesthesia, FRC falls to values 15% to 20% below those normally associated with the assumption of the supine position.[37] Loss of lung volume appears to occur almost immediately after anesthetic induction and does not occur progressively with prolonged anesthesia,[38, 39] although FRC can be subsequently compromised even further by placement of surgical packs, retractors, and other devices used to improve exposure during abdominal surgery.[40] These changes in lung volume are also independent of the mode of ventilation and are not altered significantly by the use of neuromuscular blocking drugs.[41] A similar reduction in FRC is also seen after regional anesthesia that extends cephalad to at least a midthoracic level.[42]

The decline in FRC that occurs after anesthetic induction, about 750 mL, has a profound effect on pulmonary mechanics. The slight decrease in chest wall tension at the new point of equilibrium is inadequate to offset the reduced lung compliance associated with smaller lung volumes, so total respiratory compliance is reduced. At lung volumes below normal FRC, airway caliber also decreases. Frictional resistance to airflow therefore increases, especially at the higher gas flow velocities usually associated with mechanically controlled ventilation.

If the fall in FRC brings lung volume to values at or less than closing capacity, there may be actual closure of small airways, and resultant air trapping.[43] Small airway closure during anesthesia, however, would appear to be more important in determining regional gas flow patterns than it is in dictating the changes in lung mechanics and volume that normally occur as a consequence of the induction of anesthesia.[34]

At lower long volumes, reduced total airway cross-sectional area not only makes resistance to gas flow extremely sensitive to any further variations in bronchomotor tone, but also dictates that the velocity of gas movement, and therefore the likelihood of turbulence in the airways, is increased. In effect, both the elastic and the resistive components of work of ventilation are increased significantly by the alteration of pulmonary mechanics occurring during anesthesia because of reduced lung volume, even when abnormalities of the ventilatory pattern are excluded.

Spontaneous Breathing

As was known a century ago, however, the gross pattern of respiratory muscle activity and its timing also change dramatically after anesthetic induction or other forms of drug-induced loss of consciousness.[2] The contribution of the intercostal muscles to each tidal breath diminishes progressively with increasing depth of anesthesia (see Chapter 2). Ultimately intercostal activity ceases, and breathing becomes a solely diaphragmatic event at surgical levels of anesthesia.[39]

In the unanesthetized individual, tidal exhalation occurs by the passive return of energy that has been stored elastically during inspiration. During anesthesia, however, exhalation is active because of the additional energy required for abdominal muscular contraction. The abdominal wall musculature may also fail to relax completely during subsequent inspiratory efforts, providing an element of active resistance to diaphragmatic movement during tidal breathing in anesthetized subjects, and further elevating the work of breathing under these circumstances.

The diaphragm also functions differently during anesthesia. Although still the primary motivator for initiation of inspiration, it no longer maintains the resting tension during exhalation seen in the unanesthetized subject. Lightly anesthetized individuals, therefore, have abrupt, "choppy" respiratory efforts. Episodic diaphragmatic contractions opposed by sustained abdominal muscle contractions may also produce a "rocking" or paradoxic inward motion of the upper thorax if intercostal activity has not yet returned.

The mechanism by which FRC is reduced during anesthesia is therefore probably quite complex (Fig 7–8). Diaphragmatic and intercostal muscle tone, synchronization, and activation, as well as the reciprocal phasic inhibition of other respiratory muscles throughout the respiratory cycle, normally optimize the mechanical efficiency of inspiration and minimize the intrusion of the abdominal viscera into the thoracic cavity. This complex, integrated process is progressively impaired and then abolished by deeper levels of general anesthesia.

The resting position of the diaphragm is always more cephalad

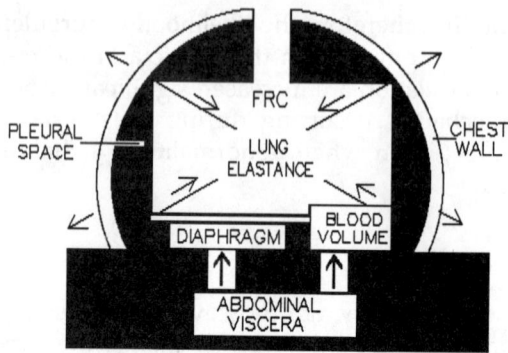

FIG 7–8.
Conceptual relationship of the forces that determine lung volume at rest *(FRC)* during anesthesia in the supine position. Loss of *FRC* during anesthesia may reflect cephalad displacement of the diaphragm, perhaps facilitated by the pressure of the abdominal viscera. Outward traction by the chest wall is reduced because of intercostal paralysis or a reduced contribution by surface-active agents in alveolar fluid, increasing lung elastance and reducing *FRC*. There is also some evidence for encroachment on intrathoracic gas volume by translocation of venous blood volume from abdominal to thoracic areas.

during anesthesia than it is during the awake state.[44] In supine subjects the inspiratory excursions of the diaphragm are restricted dorsally by the weight of the abdominal contents, and tidal volumes delivered passively during mechanical controlled ventilation are distributed almost entirely to the more independent, and therefore less well-perfused, ventral or anterior lung zones.[41]

During spontaneous breathing and light anesthesia, absence of active intercostal activity limits chest expansion in the anteroposterior direction and reduces the size of each tidal breath.[45] FRC in anesthetized subjects may be further reduced during spontaneous ventilation by an influx of venous blood volume from peripheral to central sites,[2] or even by increased surface tension in alveolar gas exchange units.[46] Whatever the exact contribution of each of these factors, the mechanical properties of the lungs and of the thorax with which they are intimately associated are fundamentally altered by the anesthetic state. Neither large tidal volumes, "sighs," nor superimposition or positive end-expiratory pressure (PEEP) appears to prevent the fall in FRC that occurs during general anesthesia.[24, 41]

Disruption of V/Q Matching

In addition to alteration of pulmonary mechanics, efficiency of gas exchange is compromised during anesthesia. The change in the mechanical and elastic properties of the lung, diaphragm, and chest wall disrupt the fragile and subtle interactions between regional lung compliance and pulmonary vascular resistance that normally maintain precise V/Q matching.

The preferential distribution of tidal gas flow to those lung fields receiving the majority of pulmonary capillary blood is lost during anesthesia when the diaphragmatic areas become compressed by the cephalad displacement of the diaphragm. Consequently the peridiaphragmatic lung areas have increased airway resistance and demonstrate reduced lung compliance. Apical and anterior or ventral lung fields, however, become more compliant and therefore receive greater fractions of each tidal breath during anesthesia, even though the perfusion of these areas remains inadequate because of the persistent gravitational effects that largely determine the distribution of pulmonary blood flow in both awake and anesthetized subjects.

The efficiency with which hypoxic pulmonary vasoconstriction (HPV) can provide additional adjustment of V/Q matching may also be impaired or abolished directly by the actions of potent inhalational agents,[47] or by the high F_{IO_2} values commonly used during general anesthesia.[14] Most importantly, however, induction of anesthesia disrupts the normal, gravitationally determined matching of ventilation and perfusion, alters regional and vascular resistance to gas flow within the tracheobronchial tree, eliminates the bellows-like movement of the lower thorax normally mediated by synchronized intercostal muscle contractions, and interferes with both the tonic and the phasic qualities of diaphragmatic tone and motion.

In the normal lung these changes nevertheless rarely produce significant alveolar shunt or dead space. Total venous admixture usually increases from 1% to about 10%, but the subsequent increase in $P(A-a)o_2$ is largely a reflection of impaired V/Q matching over what is still a relatively narrow and tightly controlled range of V/Q ratios.[24] The same process of V/Q mismatching, however, causes V_D/V_T to increase from 0.3 to about 0.5 as the V/Q profile acquires a greater spread to either side of the optimal value of about 0.8 (Fig 7–7). The alveolar effects of positive pressure ventilation may also contribute to this alteration of the shape of the V/Q profile.[48]

When profound impairment of V/Q matching or extensive alveolar shunting and dead space do occur, however, they may produce gross arterial hypoxemia. This degree of V/Q mismatching usually suggests extensive preexisting lung disease, complete suppression of HPV by inhalational anesthetics, or inadequate cardiac output and associated systemic and pulmonary arterial hypotension.[23] A severe breakdown of V/Q matching can also occur as a consequence of acute parenchymal lung disease after the aspiration of gastric acid,[49] fluid overload, airway barotrauma, diffuse lung tissue injury,[50] or, in rarer cases, a manifestation of the toxic effects of oxygen.[51]

Positioning and One-Lung Techniques

Pulmonary gas exchange may be mechanically disrupted if the surgical procedure requires lateral positioning or the use of selective one-lung ventilation. Lateral positioning increases the length of the vertical gravitational axis. External compression of the dependent lung by the weight of the thorax and mediastinal structures also produces a severe reduction of regional FRC, decreasing compliance and increasing pulmonary vascular and airway resistance. Consequently the effects of thoracotomy and one-lung ventilation on pulmonary gas exchange are complex and variable. In general, patients with healthy lungs tolerate both the lateral position and the imposition of one-lung ventilation well, despite some degree of V/Q mismatching. Patients with intrinsic lung disease may experience moderate to profound hypoxemia, however, even when high FIO_2 values are present.[6]

A fall in arterial oxygen tension to levels of 50 mm Hg or less during one-lung anesthesia despite high FIO_2 occurs when pulmonary dysfunction is coincident with a simultaneous decrease in mixed venous oxygen content due to inadequate delivery of oxygen to peripheral tissues.[52] The application of PEEP under these circumstances produces unpredictable results because the precise mechanism for V/Q mismatching varies with the nature and the extent of the underlying pathology. Predictability of response to PEEP is further compromised by variations in the adequacy of cardiac output and the prevailing mechanical factors that distort the thorax and alter venous return.[53] PEEP therapy therefore remains empirical: contemporary standards suggest initial application of low levels of PEEP to the dependent (ventilated) lung, followed by trials of constant positive airway pressure (CPAP) to the nonventilated lung and, if necessary, a subsequent increase in the levels of PEEP to the dependent lung until maximal or adequate oxygenation is achieved.[54]

VENTILATION DURING ANESTHESIA

The maintenance of spontaneous respiration during inhalational anesthesia is accompanied by an increase in respiratory rate and reduced time available for exhalation. Trichloroethylene and diethyl ether were particularly potent stimuli for tachypnea during anesthesia in previous eras, but in current practice halothane produces a similar pattern. Respiratory rate increases in proportion to increasing depth of anesthesia, a phenomenon that partially offsets the reductions in tidal volume that occur because normal intercostal muscle activity is lost.[45]

Consequently, $\dot{V}E$ may remain near preinduction values, but the efficiency of the ventilatory pattern is decreased. Tachypnea, in effect, multiplies the impact of anatomic dead space and invariably results in reduced net alveolar ventilation, with a subsequent rise in arterial carbon dioxide tensions.[55] No similar compensatory effect on respiratory rate occurs with enflurane or isoflurane: both of these halogenated ethers depress both $\dot{V}E$ and alveolar ventilation profoundly,[56] unless the anesthetic agents are carried in a gas mixture that includes significant fractions of nitrous oxide and the patients are subject to some degree of surgical stimulation.[57]

Carbon Dioxide Responsiveness

Spontaneous respiration during inhalational anesthesia is also characterized by decreased responsiveness to the chemical factors that modulate ventilatory drive.[58] The loss of responsiveness to carbon dioxide produced by all the inhalational anesthetic agents can be quantified precisely by the carbon dioxide–ventilatory response relationship in which both the sensitivity of ventilatory responsiveness and the minimum value of arterial carbon dioxide required to produce an increase in $\dot{V}E$ can be assessed.

For clinical purposes, halothane, enflurane, and isoflurane can be considered to produce significant, and roughly equivalent, dose-related reductions in the sensitivity of ventilatory response to endogenous carbon dioxide.[56, 59] This respiratory depression is conveyed by the reduction of the slope of the relationship, which appears to be largely a function of anesthetic depth (Fig 7–9).

The carbon dioxide–ventilatory response relationship during inhalational anesthesia is also notable for the presence of an X-intercept 5 to 10 mm Hg below the equilibrium point maintained during unstimulated, spontaneous ventilation.[60] This apneic or respiratory "threshold"[61] reflects the consequences of the functional deafferentation of medullary respiratory centers that inevitably accompanies a state of general anesthesia. Rarely seen in unsedated subjects,[21] the apneic threshold is the minimal arterial or end-tidal carbon dioxide tension required for continuing ventilatory efforts when patients are isolated by the anesthetic

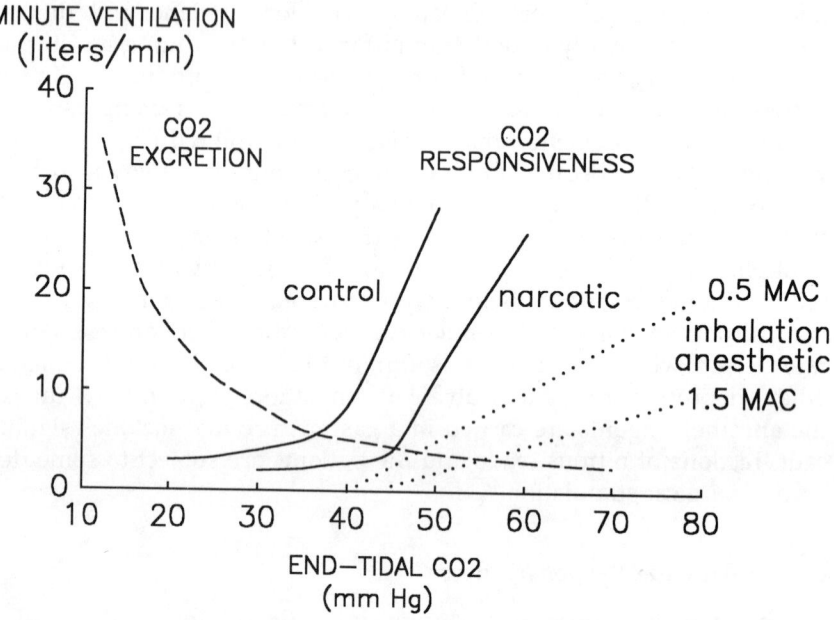

FIG 7–9.
Spontaneous ventilatory responses to imposed changes in carbon dioxide in unanesthetized awake and in lightly narcotized subjects *(solid lines)* and during light and surgical
levels of inhalational anesthesia *(dotted lines)*. The relationship between mechanically
controlled ventilation and the carbon dioxide levels produced by that degree of alveolar
ventilation produces a carbon dioxide excretion hyperbola *(dashed line)*. The points at
which the various ventilatory response curves cross this hyperbola represent the typical
ventilatory equilibrium "set-point" reached during spontaneous breathing under those conditions, in the absence of other forms of respiratory stimulation. Response curves for
awake and lightly narcotized subjects do not cross the X-axis, and therefore have no apneic threshold, because ventilation under these circumstances is initiated by factors other
than carbon dioxide.

state from the normal forms of sensory input and reticular formation
activity that usually modulate and initiate ventilatory patterns. Apneic
threshold is a process-specific, and not a drug-specific, phenomenon.
It occurs even with the use of anesthetic agents such as diethyl ether,
which itself is a direct respiratory stimulant capable of generating sustained hypocarbia during spontaneous hyperventilation.

Small doses of parenteral narcotics can produce an isolated rightward shift of the carbon dioxide–ventilatory response relationship: a
higher equilibrium point for carbon dioxide tension is established, although the intrinsic sensitivity of carbon dioxide responsiveness may
remain unchanged. With dosage increased to amounts commonly used

perioperatively, however, narcotics almost invariably produce sufficient generalized sedation and medullary depression that the slope of the relationship ultimately becomes depressed in a fashion similar to that described for anesthesia with inhalational agents or, to a lesser extent, during natural sleep.[62]

Response to Hypoxia

Even more dramatic than the anesthesia-related decline in carbon dioxide responsiveness and appearance of an apneic threshold is the depression of ventilatory responses to isocarbic hypoxemia, attenuated or abolished by virtually all of the narcotics and inhalational anesthetics in current use.[63, 64] Residual anesthetic-induced depression implies, virtually by definition, an increased risk of postoperative hypoxemia.

Rigidity

A ventilatory phenomenon that may be unique to narcotics is their ability to precipitate acute skeletal muscle rigidity so severe that spontaneous or even passive pulmonary ventilation may be impossible.[65] Ventilation may also be compromised by glottic rigidity and obstruction of the upper airway.[66] Narcotic-induced rigidity appears to be caused by the direct stimulation of *mu* receptors of the basal ganglia; it shows many of the characteristics of parkinsonism, as well as those of related, drug-induced extrapyramidal syndromes.[67]

This narcotic side effect has also been reported with morphine,[68] as well as after administration of the newer synthetic opioids, fentanyl and alfentanil. It can be reversed specifically with narcotic antagonists,[65] or prevented by paralysis of skeletal muscle with neuromuscular blocking drugs[69] in anticipation of administration of narcotics.

Airway Resistance

Inhalational anesthetics have been characterized as having bronchodilator properties, but this may be difficult to demonstrate in vivo, since airway resistance is already at its minimal value at FRC.[70] The reduction of FRC associated with general anesthesia, however, decreases airway tethering and enhances the bronchoconstrictor effect of any further loss of lung volume or increase in bronchomotor tone.[71]

The primary criterion for the selection of anesthetic agents for patients with reactive airways, therefore, should be their ability to ablate reflex-mediated bronchoconstriction in response to tracheal intubation or surgical stimulation.[70, 72] In fact, halothane, enflurane, and isoflurane all blunt bronchospasm clinically to an extent far more dramatic than would be expected from their effects on isolated strips of tracheal smooth muscle.[73] A similar antibronchospastic property has been reported for ketamine and for nebulized atropine,[74] which suggests that cholinergic reflex pathways may be important in the genesis of intraoperative bronchospasm.[75]

Other Effects

Very little is known about the effects of anesthetics on those aspects of lung function that do not relate directly to ventilation or gas exchange. Impairment of alveolar macrophage and mucociliary activity within the tracheobronchial tree by anesthetic agents could increase susceptibility to perioperative infection. Halothane and enflurane do, indeed, reduce ciliary activity in a dose-dependent manner even when inspired gas mixtures are warmed and humidified.[76] Halothane may also depress the effectiveness of alveolar macrophages, even at concentrations less than those that decrease ciliary activity.[77] Prolonged exposure to dry anesthetic gases of any type causes obvious destruction of tracheobronchial epithelial cells.[78]

POSTOPERATIVE PULMONARY DYSFUNCTION

Functional reserve for pulmonary gas exchange is sufficiently great in most patients that extraction of oxygen from inspired gases and excretion of carbon dioxide are grossly adequate throughout the perioperative course. More rigorous measurement of subclinical indices suggests, however, a virtually universal impairment of these functions after anesthesia and surgery.

The cause of postoperative pulmonary dysfunction is multifactorial. Mechanical impairment is commonplace: failure to adequately antagonize neuromuscular blockade produces residual weakness of the accessory muscles of respiration, or, less commonly, overt and complete diaphragmatic paralysis. Lesser degrees of skeletal muscle weakness can still produce bulbar muscle weakness and upper airway obstruction, increasing the work of breathing and limiting tidal volume extrinsically. Nor does adequate muscle strength guarantee effective pulmonary ventilation: poorly synchronized or discoordinate activation breathing may increase the work of breathing sufficiently that it ultimately leads to postoperative ventilatory failure.[19]

Topical diaphragmatic hypothermia is common in open chest procedures or after cardiopulmonary bypass and the use of iced cardioplegic solutions. The effects of these factors are sufficiently profound to produce gross functional impairment of respiratory muscle activity. In addition, mechanical dysfunction and injury to the lung itself during thoracic surgery may increase lung water and not only compromise gas exchange but also increase the work required for adequate ventilation. Other extrinsic factors, such as abdominal binders or elastic chest bandages, may constrict thoracic mechanics and contribute directly to postoperative pulmonary dysfunction.

Persistent V/Q Mismatch

The most common cause of impaired postoperative efficiency of gas exchange, however, is a persistent mismatch of ventilation and perfusion due to failure to return to preoperative lung volumes. After upper abdominal surgery, in particular, vital capacity is significantly reduced for 24 to 48 hours.[79] This may reflect the general level of somnolence associated with residual anesthetic effects and the use of narcotics to treat postoperative pain, but an equally important factor appears to be reflex abdominal wall muscle spasm. These changes in the behavior of the primary and accessory muscles of ventilation preclude the prompt resumption of the vigorous inspiratory efforts needed to restore FRC to preoperative values.

Voluntary "splinting," a failure to breathe deeply because of incisional pain, appears to be a less-important factor than was once believed, since neural blockade of sensory pathways with use of epidural or local anesthetic agents after abdominal surgery effectively eliminates the perception of incisional pain, yet does not restore vital capacity.[42, 80] Positive airway pressure before tracheal extubation is similarly ineffective.[81] Return of normal diaphragmatic mechanics and restoration of effective and synchronized respiratory muscle activity postoperatively, however, may be accelerated by sustained and active voluntary deep breathing in patients who have previously experienced a full return of neuromuscular and neurologic function. Incentive spirometry alone may not be effective in accomplishing adequate utilization of diaphragmatic excursion.[82]

Postoperative ventilatory dysfunction and impaired V/Q matching sometimes reflect nonpulmonary events. Even trauma outside of the chest can produce a syndrome of "shock lung," or adult respiratory distress syndrome (ARDS), characterized by an increase in pulmonary vascular resistance, decreased lung compliance, and a loss of FRC.[83] Toxin-induced changes in pulmonary capillary permeability or sustained increases in sympathoadrenal activity[84] may also change the quality of the lung parenchyma and contribute to increases in $P(A-a)O_2$.[85] The metabolic requirements of tissues responding to massive trauma may simultaneously increase oxygen extraction from capillary blood, producing arterial hypoxemia by magnifying the effects of normal venous admixture, even without the presence of significant pulmonary injury.[86] Impaired efficiency of gas exchange also occurs after increases in lung water due to intravenous fluid overload or left ventricular congestive heart failure.

Ventilatory Depression

Almost one third of a surgical patient population consisting of healthy adults and children will experience transient arterial hypoxemia during transport to the postanesthetic recovery facility if allowed to breathe air unsupplemented with additional oxygen.[87] Most commonly, relative hypoventilation after emergence from anesthesia reflects anesthetic- or narcotic-induced central depression of ventilatory responsiveness. Both arterial and alveolar carbon dioxide tensions are increased because there is a persistent flattening and "rightward" shift of the relationship between carbon dioxide and ventilatory response, generating a new point of ventilatory equilibrium.[88] Conversely, depressed $\dot{V}E$ may be an appropriate response of fully restored central ventilatory mechanisms if sustained intraoperative hyperventilation has lowered total body stores of carbon dioxide sufficiently to produce prolonged arterial hypocapnia.[89]

Whatever the precise mechanism for acute postoperative hypoventilation, supplementation of inspired oxygen postoperatively usually provides a volumetric supply of oxygen adequate to meet aerobic metabolic requirements elevated by shivering or by the cardiovascular stimulation associated with acute pain. Arterial oxygen tensions may, however, be markedly depressed for brief periods of time if alveolar oxygen is displaced by the large amounts of nitrous oxide exhaled in the first few minutes after the discontinuation of an anesthetic gas mixture containing this agent especially if patient is not provided a high inspired fraction of oxygen.[90] However, the contribution of "diffusion anoxia" to postoperative hypoxemia in anesthetic practice appears to be significant only for patients with coincident hypoventilation, or those with a substantial degree of V/Q mismatching because of intrinsic lung disease.[91]

ANESTHETIC IMPLICATIONS OF LUNG DISEASE

Unlike hemodynamic variables, pulmonary mechanics and the matching of lung ventilation and blood flow are relatively independent of the specific pharmacology of anesthetic agents. Consequently, the guidelines for anesthetic management of patients with chronic lung disease are much less specific than those described in Chapter 6 for patients with coronary or valvular heart disease. In addition, although there are on-line monitoring techniques for pulmonary mechanics[92] and for respiratory function, they are neither as widely employed nor as well understood as the cardiovascular pressure and flow displays routinely utilized for the management of patients with heart disease. In general, the anesthetic plan compensates for preexisting pulmonary disease, but does little to control or correct underlying abnormalities.

Perioperative risk is reduced when the pulmonary function of patients with chronic lung disease is improved as much as possible before surgery.[93, 94] Acute bronchospastic disorders require bronchodilator therapy and adequate hydration, and bronchitic patients need suppression of active infection and the adequate clearance of tracheobronchial secretions. All patients with impaired vital capacities appear to benefit from incentive spirometry or other maneuvers that will increase inspiratory reserve volume and expedite the full return of FRC postoperatively.[30]

The lung–chest wall unit and the complex neural mechanisms that initiate, modulate, and control ventilation itself are fragile. Once damaged, the remarkable efficiency of gas exchange seen in normal individuals can rarely be reestablished, even with vigorous therapy. Consequently the incidence and severity of postoperative pulmonary complications remain largely a function of the presence and the extent of preexisting pulmonary disease.[32, 95] Postoperative pulmonary morbidity and mortality are usually not determined by the details of anesthetic management, but rather reflect a preexisting disease process and the extent and site of the surgical procedure.

Nevertheless, some fundamental principles of respiratory physiology and pathophysiology can be incorporated effectively into the anesthetic plan designed for patients with chronic obstructive, restrictive, or parenchymal lung disorders. Ultimately, impairment of gas exchange during surgery is due to the exaggerated spread of V/Q distribution profiles in patients with intrinsic lung disease.[49] In patients with chronic obstructive lung disease (COLD), therefore, impaired oxygenation responds to increased inspired oxygen tension because it reflects relative, rather than complete, underventilation of large numbers of alveolar gas exchange units. Thus the anesthetic plan should include flexibility in adjusting FIO_2. This, in turn, encourages the administration of inhalational rather than narcotic-based anesthesia, since the intravenous techniques may be difficult to manage successfully without the simultaneous use of nitrous oxide in concentrations of 60% or more.

The fact that the potent anesthetic agents can be delivered in a gas mixture free of nitrous oxide is especially important when nitrous oxide is contraindicated by the presence of a pneumothorax, or when anesthesia is planned for patients at high risk of spontaneous pneumothorax, such as in individuals with bullous emphysema. Alternate forms of controlled ventilation, such as high-frequency oscillation (HFO), may also be of particular value under these circumstances.[96]

High-dose intravenous narcotic techniques that do not require nitrous oxide for adequate sedation and amnesia may also be useful in these applications, especially for severely compromised cardiac patients; the high plasma levels of narcotics may produce sustained[97] or episodic[98] sedation and depression of carbon dioxide responsiveness postoperatively, however. This may preclude early extubation and ambulation of patients with COLD. Pharmacologic antagonism of narcotic-induced respiratory depression and infusions of nonspecific central respiratory stimulants such as doxapram[99] have also been employed under these circumstances, but they can produce hemodynamic side effects[100] and result in inadequate postoperative analgesia.[101]

Bronchospastic Disorders

Halothane is a frequent choice for the anesthetic management of patients with COLD characterized by reactive airways.[102] Clinical experience suggests, however, that there may be little difference in outcome when any of the potent halogenated inhalational anesthetics are used.[103, 104] In adequate inspired concentrations, they all appear to confer sufficient protection against intraoperative bronchospasm,[105] appears to be primarily a reflex response to the mechanical irritation produced by tracheal intubation.[106] Specific β-adrenergic or anticholinergic[74, 75] bronchodilators or the preoperative use of mast cell stabilizers can also be incorporated into the perioperative plan for management of these patients. These agents may also be administered in aerosolized form intraoperatively in anticipation of periods of intense tracheobronchial stimulation.[107]

Other Forms of COLD

Patients with emphysema or other forms of COLD not associated with bronchospasm or increased airway reactivity will not benefit from the use of bronchodilator agents in preparation for surgery. Similarly, there is no reason to expect that suppression of increased bronchomotor activity by inhalational anesthetics will make a significant contribution to anesthetic management. In fact, inhalational anesthetic agents are of value in these circumstances primarily because they provide flexibility of inspired oxygen tensions. Unfortunately they may also suppress both hypoxic pulmonary vasoconstriction and hypocapnic bronchoconstriction, compensatory mechanisms that support adequate V/Q matching in patients with impaired efficiency of gas exchange.

Patients with emphysema may experience further mismatching of ventilation and pulmonary blood flow if they become hypotensive, or if the myocardial-depressant properties of anesthetic agents produce marked reductions in cardiac output. In both situations, there is a further increase in the fraction of alveolar gas exchange units that are inadequately perfused. Positive pressure ventilation and PEEP, in particular, may not be well tolerated because increased alveolar pressures further inflate already distended lung zones, and total dead space fraction is even further increased.[49] In addition, the reduced lung elastance in patients with emphysema transmits a greater fraction of positive airway pressures to the mediastinal contents, reducing venous return and cardiac output, and once again compromising alveolar gas exchange.

In patients with grossly impaired V/Q matching, the maintenance of normal carbon dioxide tensions may require significant increases in $\dot{V}E$. Increasing tidal volume may also, however, generate increased alveolar dead space and excessively high airway pressures. Increases in respiratory rate reduce the time available for exhalation, and may predispose to air trapping in patients requiring a prolonged expiratory phase. Alternate strategies for ventilation, such as the use of a "jet" ventilator technique, may be required for patients with severe COLD, especially when parenchymal lung diseases restrict lung expansion.

The respiratory musculature has considerable ability to compensate automatically and effectively for the modest increase in resistive loads that occur inevitably during spontaneous respiration in anesthetized patients.[108] Nevertheless the ventilatory workload imposed on massively obese patients in the supine position can actually precipitate abrupt and lethal ventilatory failure.[109]

Chronic infiltrative and fibrotic lung diseases and extrinsic restrictive conditions such as kyphoscoliosis are associated with loss of lung volume, reduced pulmonary compliance, and a requirement for energy expenditure during spontaneous breathing under anesthesia that may be unattainable.[110] Acute changes in the physical characteristics of lung tissue due to pulmonary edema, adult respiratory distress syndrome (ARDS), and aspiration pneumonitis appear to respond well to the application of PEEP and the use of gas mixtures with high F_{IO_2}. Oxygenation improves as venous admixture is reduced and some redistribution of lung water is facilitated, but there is an almost inevitable increase in alveolar dead space[49] that may require a compensatory increase in $\dot{V}_E$.

Regardless of the exact nature of the pulmonary pathology encountered, the choice of anesthetic agent itself clearly is less important than the degree to which fundamental principles of perioperative management are observed. Although a regional anesthetic is frequently requested as a logical choice for patients who are pulmonary "cripples," spinal and epidural anesthesia permit continuous functioning of all accessory and auxiliary ventilatory mechanisms only during peripheral surgery where the level of sensory and motor blockade is relatively low. In addition, the mechanical consequences of surgical intervention into the upper abdomen remain the primary intraoperative factor in determining the incidence and severity of postoperative pulmonary morbidity, regardless of the anesthetic technique employed.[111]

Arterial blood gases remain normal during surgery in most patients having upper abdominal procedures under regional anesthesia, yet these patients subsequently demonstrate loss of lung volume and a degree of compromise in vital capacity equivalent to their counterparts receiving general anesthesia.[112] For the same type of surgery, outcome even for patients with severe COLD appears to be independent of the selection of general, as opposed to regional, anesthesia.[113] Where the surgery or underlying acute pulmonary disease process predicts a high risk of postoperative ventilatory compromise, general anesthesia may, in fact, be preferable because it facilitates early and complete control of both ventilatory pattern and inspired oxygen concentration.

SUMMARY

The interdependence of pulmonary structure and function has been firmly established. The remarkable efficiency of pulmonary gas exchange reflects an extraordinarily complex and intimate relationship between the lung tissues themselves, the chest wall, and intrathoracic vascular and tracheobronchial structures. Active local and neurally mediated reflex mechanisms compensate for gravitational and mechanical factors, "fine-tuning" regional pulmonary perfusion and airway caliber and adjusting the performance of the muscles required for efficient ventilation on a breath-by-breath basis.

The increase in the gradient between alveolar and arterial oxygen that occurs during general anesthesia reflects a process-specific but not a drug-specific alteration in the mechanical properties of the chest wall, an event associated with subsequent loss of intrathoracic gas volume. Both pulmonary mechanics and blood flow are exquisitely sensitive to changes in lung volume, and some active responses, such as hypoxic pulmonary vasoconstriction, may be depressed directly by the action of the potent inhalational anesthetics.

Studies of pulmonary and ventilatory function in anesthetized subjects also suggest that there is a consistent depression of the ventilatory response to endogenous carbon dioxide and to hypoxemia. The nervous system dysfunction characteristic of general anesthesia also produces a diffuse, dose-related disruption of the usual synchrony between the thoracic and abdominal muscular components of the ventilatory apparatus.

An optimal anesthetic plan for patients with lung disease includes meticulous preoperative treatment of reversible pulmonary changes and symptoms, and sufficient flexibility of technique to allow increases in F_{IO_2} or the augmentation of $\dot{V}_E$ as needed. All of the halogenated inhalational anesthetics appear to be sufficiently potent to minimize the reflexive increases in airway resistance that follow tracheal intubation or other forms of stimulation if these drugs are used in adequate inspired concentrations. Patients with bronchospastic disease may, however, require additional adrenergic or anticholinergic measures. The cardiovascular consequences of the anesthetic technique employed are also important for patients with lung disease: pulmonary artery pressures high enough to ensure perfusion of all lung fields are essential if optimal ventilation-perfusion matching is to be maintained.

REFERENCES

1. Slonim NB, Hamilton LH: *Respiratory Physiology,* ed 5. St Louis, CV Mosby, 1987.
2. Marsh HM, Southorn PA, Rehder K: Anesthesia, sedation and the chest wall. *Int Anesthesiol Clin* 1984; 22:1–12.
3. Ferris BG, Mead J, Opie LH: Partitioning of respiratory flow resistance in man. *J Appl Physiol* 1964; 19:653–658.
4. Briscoe WA, DuBois AB: The relationship between airway resistance, airway conductance and lung volume in subjects of different age and body size. *J Clin Invest* 1958; 37:1279–1285.
5. Campbell EJM: An electromyographic examination of the role of the intercostal muscles in breathing in man. *J Physiol* 1955; 129:12–26.
6. Kaneko K, Milic-Emili J, Dolovich MB, et al: Regional distribution of ventilation and perfusion as a function of body position. *J Appl Physiol* 1966; 21:767–777.
7. Fung YC, Sobin SS: Elasticity of the pulmonary alveolar sheet. *Circ Res* 1972; 30:451–469.
8. Demling RH: The lung as a reservoir for fluid. *Int Anesthesiol Clin* 1977; 15:107–123.
9. Staub NC: The interdependence of pulmonary structure and function. *Anesthesiology* 1963; 24:831–854.
10. Whittenberger JL, MacGregor M, Berglund E, et al: Influence of state of inflation of the lung on pulmonary vascular resistance. *J Appl Physiol* 1960; 15:878–882.
11. Benumof JL: Mechanism of decreased blood flow to atelectatic lung. *J Appl Physiol* 1979; 46:1047–1048.
12. West JB, Dollery CT, Naimark A: Distribution of blood flow in isolated lung; relation to vascular and alveolar pressures. *J Appl Physiol* 1964; 19:713–724.
13. Prefault CH, Engel LA: Vertical distribution of perfusion and inspired gas in supine man. *Respir Physiol* 1981; 43:209–219.
14. Isawa T, Teshima T, Hirano T, et al: Regulation of regional perfusion distribution in the lungs. *Am Rev Respir Dis* 1978; 118:55–63.
15. Coon RL, Kampine JP: Hypocapnic bronchoconstriction and inhalation anesthetics. *Anesthesiology* 1975; 43:635–641.
16. Bakhle YS, Vane JR: Pharmacokinetic function of the pulmonary circulation. *Physiol Rev* 1974; 54:1007–1045.
17. Warren BA: Fibrinolytic properties of vascular endothelium. *Br J Exp Pathol* 1963; 44:365–372.
18. Berger AJ, Mitchell RA, Severinghaus JW: Regulation of respiration (3 parts). *N Engl J Med* 1977; 297:92–97, 138–143, 194–201.
19. Pontoppidan H, Geffin B, Lowenstein E: Acute respiratory failure in the adult. *N Engl J Med* 1972; 287:690–698.
20. Severinghaus JW: Proposed standard determination of ventilatory responses to hypoxia and hypercapnia in man. *Chest* 1976; 70(suppl):129–131.

21. Markello R, Cutter JA, King BD: Hyperventilation studies during nitrous oxide–narcotic–relaxant anesthesia. *Anesthesiology* 1963; 24:225–230.
22. Nunn JF, Ezi-Ashi TI: The respiratory effects of resistance to breathing in anesthetized man. *Anesthesiology* 1961; 22:174–185.
23. Marshall BE, Wyche MQ Jr: Hypoxemia during and after anesthesia. *Anesthesiology* 1972; 37:178–209.
24. Dueck R: Gas exchange. *Int Anesthesiol Clin* 1984; 22:13–28.
25. Finch CA, Lenfant C: Oxygen transports in man. *N Engl J Med* 1972; 286:407–415.
26. West JB, Dollery CT: Distribution of blood flow and ventilation-perfusion ratio in the lung, measured with radioactive carbon dioxide. *J Appl Physiol* 1960; 15:405–410.
27. Winter PM, Smith G: The toxicity of oxygen. *Anesthesiology* 1972; 37:210–241.
28. Craig DB, Wahba WM, Don HF, et al: "Closing volume" and its relationship to gas exchange in seated and supine positions. *J Appl Physiol* 1971; 31:717–721.
29. Bolton JWR, Weiman DS, Haynes JL, et al: Stair climbing as an indicator of pulmonary function. *Chest* 1987; 92:783–788.
30. Rigg JRA, Jones NL: Clinical assessment of respiratory function. *Br J Anaesth* 1978; 50:3–13.
31. Baier H: Assessment of unilateral lung function. *Anesthesiology* 1980; 52:240–247.
32. Mittman C: Assessment of operative risk in thoracic surgery. *Am Rev Respir Dis* 1961; 84:197–207.
33. Eugene J, Brown SE, Light RW, et al: Maximum oxygen consumption: A physiologic guide to pulmonary resection. *Surg Forum* 1982; 33:260–262.
34. Rehder K, Sessler AD, Marsh HM: General anesthesia and the lung. *Am Rev Respir Dis* 1975; 11:541–563.
35. Nunn JF, Payne JP: Hypoxaemia after general anaesthesia. *Lancet* 1962; 2:631–632.
36. Nunn JF, Bergman NA, Coleman AJ: Factors influencing the arterial oxygen tension during anesthesia with artificial ventilation. *Br J Anaesth* 1965; 37:898–914.
37. Don HR, Wahba M, Cuadrado L: The effects of anesthesia and 100 percent oxygen on the functional residual capacity of the lungs. *Anesthesiology* 1970; 32:521–529.
38. Panday J, Nunn JF: Failure to demonstrate progressive falls of arterial Po_2 during anaesthesia. *Anaesthesia* 1968; 23:38–46.
39. Don H: The mechanical properties of the respiratory system during anesthesia. *Int Anesthesiol Clin* 1977; 15:113–136.
40. Wyche MQ, Teichner RL, Kallos T, et al: Effects of continuous positive-pressure breathing on functional residual capacity and arterial oxygenation during intra-abdominal operations. *Anesthesiology* 1973; 38:68–74.
41. Froese AB, Bryan AC: Effects of anesthesia and paralysis on diaphragmatic mechanics in man. *Anesthesiology* 1974; 41:242–255.

42. Wahba WM, Don HF, Craig DB: Post-operative epidural anesthesia: Effects on lung volumes. *Can Anaesth Soc J* 1975; 22:519–527.
43. Don HF, Wahba WM, Craig DB: Airways closure, gas trapping, and the functional residual capacity during anesthesia. *Anesthesiology* 1972; 36:533–539.
44. Muller N, Volgyesi G, Becker L, et al: Diaphragmatic muscle tone. *J Appl Physiol* 1979; 47:279–284.
45. Jones JG, Faithfull D, Jordan C, et al: Rib cage movement during halothane anaesthesia in man. *Br J Anaesth* 1979; 51:399–407.
46. Scheidt M, Hyatt RE, Rehder K: Effects of rib cage or abdominal restriction on lung mechanics. *J Appl Physiol* 1981; 51:1115–1121.
47. Sykes MK, Seed RF, Kafer ER, et al: The effect of inhalational anaesthetics on hypoxic pulmonary vasoconstriction and pulmonary vascular resistance in the perfused lungs of the dog and cat. *Br J Anaesth* 1972; 44:776–788.
48. Conway CM: Haemodynamic effects of pulmonary ventilation. *Br J Anaesth* 1975; 47:761–766.
49. West JB: Ventilation-perfusion relationships. *Am Rev Respir Dis* 1977; 116:919–931.
50. Modig J: Adult respiratory distress syndrome; pathogenesis and treatment. *Acta Chir Scand* 1986; 152:241–249.
51. Sackner MA, Landa J, Hirsch J, et al: Pulmonary effects of oxygen breathing. *Ann Intern Med* 1975; 82:40–43.
52. Mithoefer JC, Ramirez C, Cook W: The effect of mixed venous oxygenation on arterial blood in chronic obstructive pulmonary disease. *Am Rev Respir Dis* 1978; 117:259–264.
53. Alfery DD, Benumoff JF, Trousdale FR: Improving oxygenation during one-lung ventilation in dogs: The effects of positive end-expiratory pressure and blood flow restriction to the nonventilated. *Anesthesiology* 1981; 55:381–385.
54. Benumof JL: One-lung ventilation: Which lung should be PEEPed? *Anesthesiology* 1982; 56:161–162.
55. Askrog VF, Pender JW, Smith TC: Changes in respiratory dead space during halothane, cyclopropane, and nitrous oxide anesthesia. *Anesthesiology* 1964; 25:342–352.
56. Fourcade HE, Stevens WC, Larson P Jr, et al: The ventilatory effects of Forane, a new inhaled anesthetic. *Anesthesiology* 1971; 35:26–31.
57. Eger EI II, Dolan WM, Stevens WC, et al: Surgical stimulation antagonizes the respiratory depression produced by Forane. *Anesthesiology* 1972; 36:544–549.
58. Drummond GB: Factors influencing the control of breathing. *Int Anesthesiol Clin* 1984; 22:59–74.
59. Knill RL, Manninen PH, Clement JL: Ventilation and chemoreflexes during enflurane sedation and anaesthesia in man. *Can Anaesth Soc J* 1979; 26:353–360.
60. Hickey RF, Fourcade HE, Eger EI II, et al: The effects of ether,

halothane, and Forane on apneic thresholds in man. *Anesthesiology* 1971; 35:32–37.

61. Hanks EC, Ngai SH, Fink BR: Respiratory threshold for carbon dioxide in anesthetized man. *Anesthesiology* 1961; 22:393–397.

62. Forrest WH Jr, Bellville JW: The effect of sleep plus morphine on the respiratory response to carbon dioxide. *Anesthesiology* 1964; 25:137–141.

63. Cullen DJ: The effects of halothane on respiratory and cardiovascular responses to hypoxia in dogs: A dose-response study. *Anesthesiology* 1970; 33:487–496.

64. Knill RL, Kieraszwicz HT, Dodgson BG, et al: Chemical regulation of ventilation during isoflurane sedation and anaesthesia in humans. *Can Anaesth Soc J* 1983; 30:607–614.

65. Holderness MC, Chase PE, Dripps RD: A narcotic analgesic and a butyrophenone with nitrous oxide for general anesthesia. *Anesthesiology* 1963; 24:336–340.

66. Scamman FL: Fentanyl-02-N20 rigidity and pulmonary compliance. *Anesth Analg* 1983; 62:332–334.

67. Benthuysen JL, Smith NT, Sanford TJ, et al: Physiology of alfentanil-induced rigidity. *Anesthesiology* 1986; 64:440–446.

68. Freund FG, Martin W, Wong KC, et al: Abdominal rigidity induced by morphine and nitrous oxide. *Anesthesiology* 1973; 38:358–362.

69. Hill AB, Nahrwold ML, DeRosayro AM, et al: Prevention of rigidity during fentanyl-oxygen induction of anesthesia. *Anesthesiology* 1981; 55:452–454.

70. Hirshman CA, Edelstein G, Peetz S, et al: Mechanism of action of inhalational anesthesia on airways. *Anesthesiology* 1982; 56:107–111.

71. Lehane JR: The effect of anesthesia on airway caliber. *Int Anesthesiol Clin* 1984; 22:29–43.

72. Vettermann J, Beck KC, Lindahl SGE, et al: Actions of enflurane, isoflurane, vecuronium, atracurium, and pancuronium on pulmonary resistance in dogs. *Anesthesiology* 1988; 69:688–695.

73. Fletcher SW, Flacke W, Alper MH: The actions of general anesthetics on tracheal smooth muscle. *Anesthesiology* 1968; 29:517–522.

74. Gross NJ, Bankwala Z: Effects of anticholinergic bronchodilator on arterial blood gases of hypoxemic patients with chronic obstructive pulmonary disease: A comparison with a beta-adrenergic agent. *Am Rev Respir Dis* 1987; 136:1091–1094.

75. Ingram RH, McFadden ER Jr: Localization and mechanisms of airway responses. *N Engl J Med* 1977; 297:596–600.

76. Lee KS, Park SS: Effect of halothane, enflurane, and nitrous oxide on tracheal ciliary activity in vitro. *Anesth Analg* 1980; 59:426–430.

77. Manawadu BR, LaForce FM: Impairment of pulmonary antibacterial defense mechanisms by halothane anesthesia. *Chest* 1979; 75(suppl):242–243.

78. Chalon J, Loew DAY, Malebranche J: Effects of dry anesthetic gases on tracheobronchial ciliated epithelium. *Anesthesiology* 1972; 37:338–343.

79. Stein M, Koota GM, Simon M, et al: Pulmonary evaluation of surgical patients. *JAMA* 1962; 181:765–770.
80. Jakobson S, Ivarsson J: Effects of intercostal nerve blocks (etidocaine 0.5%) on chest wall mechanics in cholecystectomized patients. *Acta Anaesthesiol Scand* 1977; 21:497–503.
81. Quan SF, Falltrick RT, Schlobohm RM: Extubation from ambient or expiratory positive airway pressure in adults. *Anesthesiology* 1981; 55:53–56.
82. Chuter TAM, Weissman C, Starker PM, et al: Effect of incentive spirometry on diaphragmatic function after surgery. *Surgery* 1989; 105:488–493.
83. Bergofsky EH: Pulmonary insufficiency after nonthoracic trauma: Shock lung. *Am J Med Sci* 1974; 264:92–101.
84. De Oliveira GG, Antonio MP: Role of the central nervous system in the adult respiratory distress syndrome. *Crit Care Med* 1987; 15:844–849.
85. Blaisdell FW: Pathophysiology of the respiratory distress syndrome. *Arch Surg* 1974; 108:44–49.
86. Kelman GR, Nunn JF, Prys-Roberts C: The influence of cardiac output on arterial oxygenation: A theoretical study. *Br J Anaesth* 1967; 39:450–457.
87. Pullerits J, Burrows FA, Roy WL: Arterial desaturation in healthy children during transfer to the recovery room. *Can J Anaesth* 1987; 34:470–473.
88. Edelist G, Osorio A: Postanesthetic initiation of spontaneous ventilation after passive hyperventilation. *Anesthesiology* 1969; 31:222–227.
89. Salvatore AJ, Sullivan SF, Papper EM: Postoperative hypoventilation and hypoxemia in man after hyperventilation. *N Engl J Med* 1969; 280:467–470.
90. Fink BR: Diffusion anoxia. *Anesthesiology* 1955; 16:511–519.
91. Frumin MJ, Edelist G: Diffusion anoxia: A critical reappraisal. *Anesthesiology* 1969; 31:243–249.
92. Wilson RS: Monitoring the lung: Mechanics and volume. *Anesthesiology* 1976; 45:135–145.
93. Stein M, Cassara EL: Preoperative pulmonary evaluation and therapy for surgery patients. *JAMA* 1970; 211:787–790.
94. Gracey DR, Divertie MB, Didier EP: Preoperative pulmonary preparation in patients with chronic obstructive pulmonary disease. *Chest* 1979; 76:123–129.
95. Latimer RG, Dickman M, Day WC: Ventilatory patterns and pulmonary complications after upper abdominal surgery determined by preoperative and postoperative computerized spirometry and blood. *Am J Surg* 1971; 122:622–632.
96. Butler WJ, Bohn DJ, Bryan AC, et al: Ventilation by high-frequency oscillation in humans. *Anesth Analg* 1980; 59:577–584.
97. Cartwright P, Prys-Roberts C, Gill K, et al: Ventilatory depression related to plasma fentanyl concentrations during and after anesthesia in humans. *Anesth Analg* 1983; 62:966–974.

98. Adams AP, Pybus DA: Delayed respiratory depression after use of fentanyl during anesthesia. *Br Med J* 1978; 1:1612.
99. Gupta PK, Dundee JW: The effect of an infusion of doxapram on morphine analgesia. *Anaesthesia* 1974; 29:40–43.
100. Jaffe RS, Moldenhauer CC, Hug CC, et al: Nalbuphine antagonism of fentanyl-induced ventilatory depression: A randomized trial. *Anesthesiology* 1988; 68:254–260.
101. Romagnoli A, Keats AS: Ceiling effect for respiratory depression by nalbuphine. *Clin Pharmacol Ther* 1980; 27:478–485.
102. Echeverria M, Gelb AW, Wexler HR, et al: Enflurane and halothane in status asthmaticus. *Chest* 1986; 89:152–154.
103. Rodriguez R, Gold MI: Enflurane as primary anesthetic agent for patients with chronic obstructive pulmonary disease. *Anesth Analg* 1976; 55:806–809.
104. Gold MI, Schwam SJ, Goldberg M: Chronic obstructive pulmonary disease and respiratory complications. *Anesth Analg* 1983; 62:975–981.
105. Hirshman CA, Bergman NA: Halothane and enflurane protect against bronchospasm in an asthma dog model. *Anesth Analg* 1978; 57:629–633.
106. Gal TJ: Pulmonary mechanics in normal subjects following endotracheal intubation. *Anesthesiology* 1980; 52:27–35.
107. Gold MI: Anesthesia and bronchoconstrictive disease. *Adv Anesth* 1988; 5:203–236.
108. Moote CA, Knill RL, Clement JL: Ventilatory compensation for continuous inspiratory resistive and elastic loads during halothane anesthesia in humans. *Anesthesiology* 1986; 64:582–589.
109. Tsueda K, Debrand M, Zeok SS, et al: Obesity supine death syndrome: Reports of two morbidly obese patients. *Anesth Analg* 1979; 58:345–347.
110. Kafer ER: Respiratory and cardiovascular functions in scoliosis and the principles of anesthetic management. *Anesthesiology* 1980; 52:339–351.
111. Boutros AR, Weisel M: Comparison of the effects of three anesthetic techniques on patients with severe pulmonary obstructive disease. *Can Anaesth Soc J* 1971; 18:286–292.
112. Askrog VF, Smith TC, Eckenhoff JE: Changes in pulmonary ventilation during spinal anesthesia. *Surg Gynecol Obstet* 1964; 119:563–567.
113. Ravin MB: Comparison of spinal and general anesthesia for lower abdominal surgery in patients with chronic obstructive pulmonary disease. *Anesthesiology* 1971; 35:319–322.

8

Hepatic, Metabolic, and Splanchnic Function

The liver is ideally sited in the circulation to carry out its manifold functions of exchange, enzymatic modification, and synthesis. A unique system of dual perfusion delivers both fully oxygenated blood and blood rich in nutrients absorbed from the gastrointestinal tract. Unlike the changes seen in the cardiovascular and pulmonary systems, altered hepatic function during anesthesia is not due to mechanical restrictions nor to anatomic disruptions. Thus the effects of anesthesia are not easily explained by physical analogy or by input-output analysis. In addition, the autonomic control loops for hepatic metabolism are not neural pathways, but are enzymatic and hormonal mechanisms; they are far less discrete and certainly less well understood than those that maintain cardiopulmonary homeostasis.

Nevertheless, formulation of a rational anesthetic plan requires an understanding of the integrated nature of hepatic metabolism and splanchnic blood flow. Familiarity with the effects of anesthetics on hepatic and on splanchnic visceral function also permits the identification of priorities for management of patients with hepatic, gastrointestinal, and metabolic diseases.

HEPATIC AND METABOLIC FUNCTION

As described in Chapter 7, the elastic structure of lung tissue facilitates the continuous matching of pulmonary ventilation and blood flow that maintains efficient gas exchange. Similarly, the effectiveness with which hepatocytes extract and exchange metabolic substrates from liver blood flow results largely from their unique platelike cellular microarchitecture. Unlike other tissues, there is no structurally continuous capillary network. Instead, the hepatic microcirculation and exchange bed consists of blood-filled sinusoidal cavities in which a thin, porous layer of endothelial cells represents the only barrier between blood and liver tissue.

The liver, in effect, functions as a dense and metabolically active sponge, with immense surface area of almost infinite molecular permeability. Salts, carbohydrates, lipids, and even protein molecules move freely and efficiently between the intrahepatic blood volume and the hepatocytes of the liver parenchyma. Larger elements, such as inorganic particles, cellular debris, and bacteria, are actively cleared by the phagocytic action of the endothelial Kupffer cells.

Liver Blood Flow

Representing about one quarter of cardiac output, liver blood flow is determined largely, but not entirely, by available arterial perfusion pressures. The hepatic artery normally provides only about 25% of total hepatic blood flow, although it delivers two thirds of the oxygen consumed by this organ. Most hepatic perfusion is conducted to the liver sinusoids through the portal venous system. Arteriolar smooth muscle cells distributed along the hepatic artery participate in a modest degree of local, active adjustment of vascular resistance. Hepatic artery vascular resistance falls significantly in response to declines in intrahepatic blood volume or reductions of sinusoidal pressure.

A "reciprocal" relationship between hepatic artery and portal vein blood flow[1] can be demonstrated by clamping the portal vein: there is an immediate increase in hepatic artery blood flow, even when systemic arterial pressure is unchanged, although its relatively small contribution to total liver blood flow limits the effectiveness of these autoregulatory changes. Consequently, obstruction of the portal vein is almost invariably associated with decreased delivery of oxygen, increased oxygen extraction, and reduced hepatic venous and tissue oxygen tensions. Complete reciprocity is also rarely achieved when hepatic artery flow is selectively compromised: portal vein blood flow is limited by the low hydrostatic driving pressures in this system, and by the effects of additional sites of vascular resistance in the splanchnic tissue exchange beds through which it must first pass.

Glucose Homeostasis

Carbohydrates are the only metabolic energy source utilized by all tissues. In addition, glucose is the preferred substrate for the nervous system, since this organ is unable to meet its minimum energy requirements using noncarbohydrate aerobic or anaerobic biochemical pathways. Hepatic tissues not only provide the metabolic machinery for the conversion of a wide variety of substances into glucose, but they also function as a depot for glucose storage in the form of its phosphate polymer, glycogen (Fig 8–1). The "glucostatic" function of the liver, however, involves far more than the conversion of glucose to glycogen (glyconeogenesis) and its reconversion back to glucose (glycogenolysis). In fact, these pathways are only the most obvious elements of a complex system that provides the hormonal stimulation and feedback control for all aspects of carbohydrate metabolism.

Blood glucose levels primarily reflect the timing and the magnitude of insulin and glucagon release from the pancreas, but cortisol, growth hormone, catecholamines, and vasopressin (antidiuretic hormone) stimulate lipolysis and proteolysis, generating ketones and glycerol. These alternate energy sources can be consumed by skeletal and heart muscle tissues, freeing carbohydrates for specific consumption by those tissues that do not have these metabolic alternatives. Hepatic glycogen stores represent a relatively limited carbohydrate reserve. Twelve to 24 hours of fasting or restricted carbohydrate intake exhausts this resource and initiates the complex sequence of metabolic processes that maintain blood glucose levels by the active degradation (catabolism) of fat, protein, and other compounds.

Hormonally facilitated intrahepatic generation of glucose (gluconeogenesis) from amino acids and from the lactate produced by skeletal muscle and other metabolically active tissues under anaerobic conditions ultimately reestablishes glucose homeostasis. Body lipid and protein stores are therefore not inert, but participate in the constant transformation and exchange of molecular substrates, which provides the basis for glucose homeostasis. Rather than serve merely as an emergency source of metabolic fuel during acute carbohydrate shortages, peripheral tissues containing lipid and protein molecules are continuing components of a dynamic process of constant metabolic activity modulated by endocrine and hepatocellular mechanisms.[2]

Molecular Synthesis

The interconversion of metabolic substrates and the degradation of high-energy phosphates take place primarily at mitochondrial sites

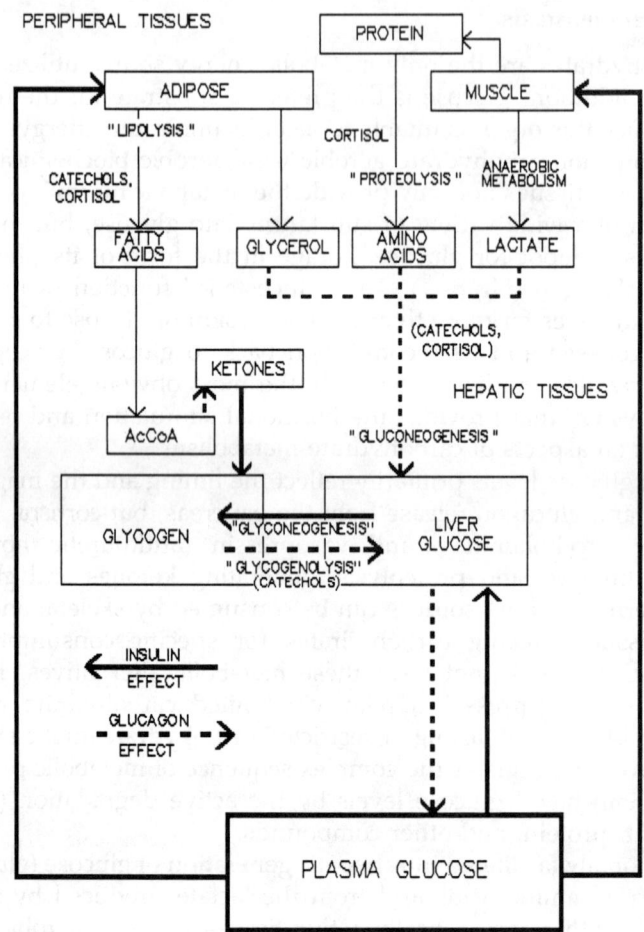

FIG 8–1.
Carbohydrate homeostasis achieved by the interaction of the synthetic (anabolic) actions of insulin *(heavy solid arrows)* and the opposing catabolic actions of glucagon *(dashed arrows).* Major effects of cortisol and catecholamines are also indicated; parentheses indicate actions in concert with insulin or with glucagon.

within liver cells. Generation of proteins and most forms of synthetic (anabolic) metabolism is accomplished on the intracellular membrane surfaces of the endoplasmic reticulum. Albumin and virtually all other plasma proteins except gamma globulin are of hepatic origin, as are all coagulation factors except for factor VIII. Although its physiologic role remains unknown, plasma or "pseudo"-cholinesterase is also synthesized intrahepatically.

Other synthetic functions of the hepatocyte include generation of fatty acids from carbohydrates, cholesterol metabolism, and synthesis of the specialized lipoproteins in plasma that are required for fatty acid and cholesterol transport to peripheral tissues. Hepatocytes also recycle hemoglobin from damaged erythrocytes, converting albumin-bound bilirubin into a more water-soluble form suitable for biliary excretion by a process of conjugation with glucuronic acid. Once excreted, conjugated bilirubin undergoes further conversion within the intestinal lumen to urobilinogen and urobilin. Urobilinogen is subsequently reabsorbed into the portal circulation to complete an enterohepatic cycle.[3] These bile salts facilitate absorption of both ingested lipid and the lipid-soluble vitamins A, E, and, in particular, K, which is essential for the normal synthesis of procoagulant factors II, VII, IX, and X.

Biodegradation

Normal liver function encompasses not only the synthesis of new molecules but also the destruction or deactivation of endogenous and exogenous chemical compounds carried in portal venous blood. Ammonia generated by the breakdown of amino acids or produced by gastrointestinal bacteria is extracted from the portal circulation and detoxified hepatically by conversion to urea. Because it is water soluble, urea is excreted efficiently into the urine.

Hepatocytes also deactivate the facilitators of primary fibrinolysis. Aldosterone and vasopressin are cleared from portal venous blood by hepatic tissues; similarly, hepatocytes are responsible for the biodegradation of histamine, serotonin, prostaglandins, and other substances that are synthesized in the gastrointestinal tract, its associated vascular and neural structures, or released from endocrine neoplasms that occur in this area. The metabolic capacity and the unique location of the liver, like those of the lung, provide an effective metabolic filtering system. In effect, hepatic capacity for biodegradation isolates the rest of the body from the effects of the localized release of potent substances generated in the metabolically active tissues perfused by the splanchnic circulation.

Pathways of Biotransformation

The enzyme systems that catalyze the biotransformation of both endogenous and exogenous ("xenobiotic") biologically active substances can be physically separated from other hepatocellular systems by a process of tissue homogenation and ultracentrifugation. They are commonly referred to as "microsomal" enzymes because they remain intimately associated with disrupted endoplasmic reticulum: the membrane fragments form nonanatomic "microsomes" during this in vitro purification process.

Functionally, hepatic microsomal systems are nonspecific and are described as being mixed oxidase enzyme systems because oxidation in some form, primarily hydroxylation, characterizes nonconjugative (type I) hepatic drug biotransformation (Fig 8–2). Hepatocytes, in fact, contain ample assortments of enzymes for oxidative dealkylation, deamination, demethylation, and desulfuration. Oxidative dehalogenation is also an important pathway for the metabolism of the anesthetic agents methoxyflurane, enflurane, and halothane. A pigment, cytochrome P-450, appears to be a key element in these and other en-

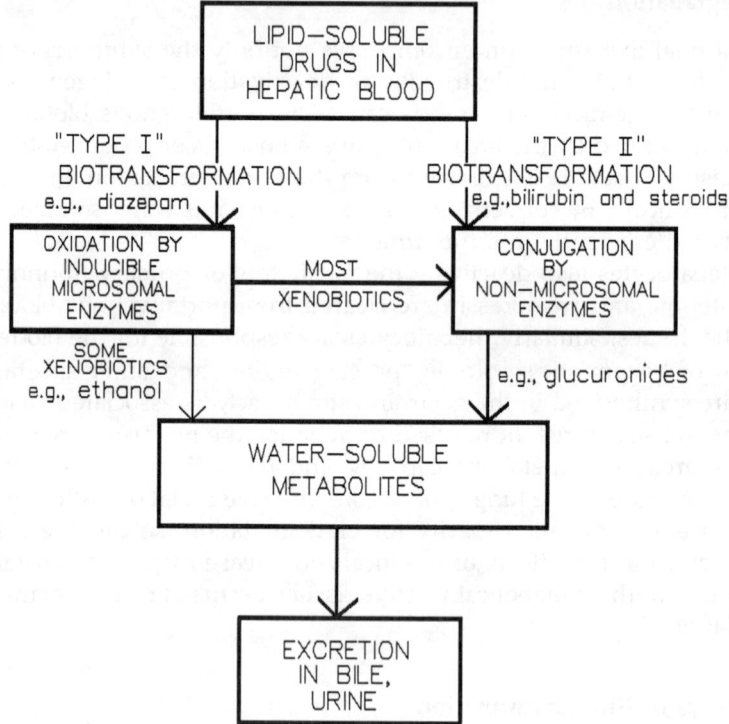

FIG 8–2.
Major pathways for hepatic biotransformation of endogenous and pharmacologic (xenobiotic) substances. Ultimately, hepatic biotransformation converts the parent molecules to forms both less active and more soluble in water for easy elimination into bile and urine.

zyme systems that, in the process of oxidizing drug molecules, generate water and nicotinamide adenine dinucleotide phosphate.[4]

Type II hepatic pathways include those resulting in the conjugation of molecules with glucuronides or the acetylation, sulfation, and other processes of inactivation that represent the addition to, rather than the destruction of, the original chemical structure. These enzymatic pathways are nonmicrosomal. For the most part, they are responsible for the normal hepatic biotransformation of endogenous substances, including steroidal hormones. Most xenobiotics undergo sequential biotransformation, with both initial oxidative deactivation and subsequent conjugation. This process increases water solubility and facilitates excretion, but requires the utilization of both type I and type II pathways. Alcohols are oxidized and then excreted directly without conjugation.

The enzymatic activity of type I systems is rapidly enhanced or "induced" by exposure to any of a large number of compounds, including phenobarbital and phenytoin, and by exposure to some anesthetics.[4, 5] Type II pathways are more substrate-specific and thus are not readily inducible. In general, maximal type I enzymatic capacity is dependent on the degree of chronic enzyme induction that has occurred. For type II pathways, maximal metabolic activity is directly proportional to the mass of well-perfused, normally functioning hepatic tissue available. Both pathways function to reduce the biologic activity of the molecules on which they act, and to increase their solubility in water, facilitating the termination of their clinical effect, at least in part, by a process of urinary or biliary excretion.

ASSESSMENT OF LIVER FUNCTION

Hepatocellular Disease

Various assessment systems have been used to categorize acute liver dysfunction. All acknowledge that there is a fundamental distinction between disease due to a primary process of intrinsic hepatocellular damage and disorders due to mechanical obstruction of biliary tract outflow or similar extrinsic processes.[6] Acute parenchymal liver disease most often occurs as infectious viral hepatitis (type A), serum viral hepatitis (type B), or one of a variety of less well-understood forms of acute, subacute, or other (type C) hepatitis. In addition, hepatic inflammation and destruction may occur as the consequence of the direct toxic effects of alcohol, hydrocarbons, or other chemicals, or may follow hypoxia or generalized sepsis. It may also be associated with intrinsic cardiac disease, or with pregnancy.

Whatever the etiologic factor, hepatocellular injury produces significant and occasionally massive elevations in the serum concentrations of the transaminase enzymes, aspartate aminotransferase or alanine aminotransferase (AST or ALT), or of lactic dehydrogenase (LDH), especially the LDH-5 isoenzyme fraction. These changes mark clearly the onset of acute hepatitis. They also may provide an indication of the extent of hepatocellular injury, but they do not provide quantitative information regarding the remaining level of hepatic function or functional reserve, and therefore should not be considered to be "liver function tests."

Although there are genetically determined abnormalities of hepatocellular function that can be considered as chronic parenchymal liver diseases, this entity most often presents clinically as chronic hepatitis, a persistent inflammatory process. Cause is frequently unknown. If progressive, however, chronic hepatitis may ultimately produce sufficient parenchymal destruction and subsequent fibrosis of hepatic tissues that the sequelae are indistinguishable from cirrhosis due to chronic alcoholism or other forms of chemical hepatotoxicity. Cirrhosis, therefore, merely describes the anatomic and physical consequences of massive inflammation, parenchymal destruction, and fibrotic replacement within the liver, regardless of cause. The degree of fibrous replacement required to produce hypertension in the portal circulation is sufficiently great that it usually is accompanied by clinically obvious hepatic dysfunction, or even hepatic failure.

Jaundice and Biliary Tract Obstruction

Biliary obstruction either within the liver or at extrahepatic sites can produce jaundice and malaise. Intrahepatic cholestasis due to inflammation or to drug effects produces acute elevation of conjugated bilirubin. In addition, there is usually some evidence of hepatocellular injury, frequently in the form of elevated transaminase enzyme concentrations. If the obstruction of the biliary tract is extrahepatic or posthepatic, however, the increase in conjugated bilirubin is accompanied by significant serum concentrations of alkaline phosphatase, an enzyme released from injured biliary tract epithelial cells. Jaundice associated with normal serum enzyme levels therefore suggests a "prehepatic" mechanism: the ability of the liver to process bilirubin is being overwhelmed as, for example, by abrupt and massive amounts of free hemoglobin, such as occurs after generalized hemolysis of red blood cells or the resorption of a large hematoma.

Indices of Liver Function

Analysis of hepatocellular and biliary tract enzymes and bilirubin levels provides important diagnostic data but little quantitative information regarding liver function itself. Bromsulphalein retention and other similar challenges to hepatic drug clearance can, however, provide estimates of hepatic functional reserve, although they reflect both intrinsic hepatocellular capacity and liver blood flow, itself subject to extrinsic factors such as cardiac output and sympathoadrenal state.

Measurements of the proteins synthesized within the liver may provide the most direct assessment of hepatocellular capacity. Hypoalbuminemia (less than 3 to 5 g/100 mL) is seen consistently in patients with overt liver failure. Albumin synthesis by hepatic tissues, stimulated directly by the expansion of extracellular fluid volume, may be limited significantly by reduced hepatocellular capacity, although it is also compromised by impaired nutritional status.[7] A decline in the serum concentrations of albumin reduces plasma oncotic pressures and causes a net dislocation of intravascular water into tissues, disrupting both pulmonary and cerebral function.[8] Contraction of intravascular volume then stimulates activation of the renin-aldosterone system, producing retention of sodium and additional reabsorption of water by renal tubular mechanisms (Chapter 9).

The coagulopathy associated with liver failure also reflects decreased hepatic protein synthesis. Once the functional mass of hepatic tissue is reduced to one third or less of its normal value, clotting factor deficiencies are reflected directly as a prolongation of both prothrombin and partial thromboplastin times. Coagulopathy is a relatively late sign of evolving hepatic dysfunction, although the turnover rate of clotting factors is sufficiently rapid to make these tests useful in following the course of acute hepatic failure.[6]

ANESTHETICS AND HEPATIC FUNCTION

Hyperglycemia

Reversible depression of biochemical function occurs in virtually all organ systems during exposure to anesthetic agents. The metabolic processes that take place in the hepatic parenchyma are assumed to be influenced less dramatically by anesthesia than are hepatic circulation and oxygenation, although there are virtually no techniques available to monitor hepatocellular metabolism during anesthesia.

Glucose homeostasis is, in fact, transiently disrupted during routine general anesthesia. Hyperglycemia is usually mild and not associated with ketosis, however, suggesting that insulin production and release are still sufficient for adequate utilization of carbohydrates, at least in nondiabetic subjects. Direct suppression of pancreatic insulin release by halothane is, nevertheless, demonstrable in vitro.[9] Intrahepatic conversion of lactate to glucose is also impaired by inhalational anesthetics in a dose-related fashion.[10] The ubiquitous nature of hyperglycemia during general anesthesia suggests that this mild metabolic dysfunction reflects a nonspecific, stress-related state of catecholamine-induced glycogenolysis. In fact, the sympathoadrenal blockade produced by high epidural anesthesia prevents catecholamine release and also minimizes disruption of perioperative glucose homeostasis.[11]

Enterohepatic Cycles

The enterohepatic circulation of water-solubilized drugs from the intestinal lumen into portal venous blood and on to the liver parenchyma functions normally during anesthesia, at least for conjugated bile products and many drugs. Hours after intravenous administration in high dosage, fentanyl may produce sudden and severe respiratory depression even after spontaneous return of awareness and normal carbon dioxide responsiveness.[12] This phenomenon of recurrent respiratory depression is attributable directly to the appearance of a delayed rise in plasma concentrations of fentanyl after secondary intestinal reabsorption of this drug following its secretion from the gastric mucosa or the biliary tract.[13] Similar enterohepatic "recycling" may occur with other narcotics if they are used as part of a high-dose intravenous technique that generates a large, initial enteric pool of active drug, or if the primary metabolites retain residual narcotic potency.

Postanesthetic Dysfunction

Measurements of change in serum levels of hepatocellular enzymes suggest that a small fraction of the surgical population who do not have evidence of preoperative liver disease nevertheless demonstrate subclinical parenchymal liver injury after anesthesia and surgery. Unsuspected hepatic dysfunction from exacerbated residual viral hepatitis may explain this phenomenon, which occurs in one of every 2,000 patients; the mechanism is not known, but appears to be independent of the choice of anesthetic agents.[14] Since patients undergoing surgical procedures on or in close proximity to the liver itself have a significantly higher incidence of postoperative enzyme elevation than those having peripheral surgery, there may be a physical, rather than a purely pharmacologic, explanation.[15] The effect of anesthesia on postoperative hepatic synthetic function as judged by albumin synthesis or production of coagulation factors is currently not known.

Hepatic Toxicity

Hepatic toxicity, unlike transient anesthetic disruption of hepatic and metabolic function, implies irreversible destruction of liver tissues. Carbon tetrachloride provides the classic model for hepatotoxicity, producing hepatic damage that is dose related, consistent in microscopic appearance, and easily reproduced in animal experiments. The evidence implicating other halogenated hydrocarbons, such as chloroform and trichloroethylene, is somewhat less compelling, but still impressive.

Among the inhalational anesthetics currently in use, halothane alone possesses the chemical structure of a halogenated hydrocarbon. It is also the only agent for which hepatotoxicity remains a significant issue[16] three decades after its introduction into clinical use. Halothane-associated hepatic injury produces no pathologically unique pattern of damage and therefore remains a tissue diagnosis of exclusion. Nevertheless, the incidence of otherwise-unexplained massive hepatic necrosis is sufficiently great (1 or 2 per 10,000 halothane anesthetics) and its outcome severe enough (more than 50% mortality) to warrant continuing investigation of the mechanism by which this, or other anesthetics, can cause hepatocellular injury.[17, 18]

Mechanisms of Halothane-related Injury

There appears to be little controversy that hepatic injury after exposure to halothane reflects, in some way, the biochemical transformation of this anesthetic within the liver by metabolic pathways. About one quarter of a clinical dose of halothane undergoes oxidative (type I) dehalogenation, a process that generates inorganic chloride, bromide, and trifluoracetate.[19] Some of the metabolites have the potential to produce adverse effects if present in very high concentrations, but there appears to be little direct hepatotoxicity due to these substances under clinical conditions. Consequently, there has been great interest in other possible pathways for the metabolism of this drug.

The formation of unstable, "reactive intermediate" molecules with unpaired electrons could produce direct injury to hepatocellular membrane structures during reductive metabolism, a phenomenon that might occur during hepatic hypoxia. Unfortunately, these free-radical species exist only transiently, and thus are not measurable directly. In addition, animal models used to demonstrate a relationship between halothane, hypoxia, and hepatic injury require a coincident state of microsomal enzyme induction.[20] Since reductive pathways are thought to be noninducible, current concepts of biotransformation do not provide a single coherent metabolic explanation for hepatic injury after halothane exposure.[21]

Further complicating the assessment of the role of biotransformation of halothane in human hepatotoxicity are the clinical circumstances of its occurrence. There is a statistical association between occupational[22, 23] or repeated anesthetic exposure[24] to halothane and the subsequent appearance of hepatic injury. The frequency with which halothane-related hepatic injury is associated with eosinophilia also suggests an immune mechanism involving prior exposure and sensitization.[25] Observations of lymphocyte stimulation by halothane exposure[26] support this hypothesis. There is also recent evidence that specific antibodies are formed against halothane-damaged hepatocytes in children,[27] once thought to be free of the risk of hepatic injury after halothane exposure.

These biochemical and clinical findings can be reconciled by postulating two separate mechanisms for halothane-related hepatic injury: (1) the formation of free-radicals that destroy hepatic tissues when generated by noninducible reductive pathways under conditions of hepatic hypoxia or ischemia or (2) an inducible immune-mediated form of hepatitis in which a haptene capable of eliciting an antibody response is generated by sequential oxidative and conjugative halothane metabolism and then attaches to hepatic tissues directly. The first pathway would apply to the hypoxic "animal model" for halothane hepatitis. The second pathway would be consistent with reports of enflurane hepatitis[28] and cross-sensitivity to halogenated anesthetic agents.[29]

Obesity, characterized metabolically by increased microsomal enzyme activity, enlarged hepatic mass, increased liver blood flow, and enhanced rates of anesthetic biotransformation,[30] could be predicted to be a contributory risk factor for either mechanism.[31] Ultimately, "halothane hepatitis" may be redefined not as a unique entity but rather as a group of anesthetic-related hepatic sequelae that share massive centrilobular hepatic necrosis as a common, final pathologic lesion.[32]

Intraoperative Hepatic Blood Flow

The mechanisms by which anesthetics alter splanchnic and hepatic blood flow are less speculative than those used to explain postanesthetic hepatic injury. Total splanchnic blood flow falls about 25% from awake levels during virtually all types of anesthesia, both regional and general, and appears to be independent of the agent selected.[33] For spinal and epidural techniques, the decline in splanchnic perfusion reflects the fall in mean arterial pressure that usually follows the pharmacologic sympathectomy produced by autonomic blockade, subsequent vasodilation, and reduced venous return.

The vasculature of the splanchnic viscera demonstrates little intrinsic autoregulation.[34] When narcotic-based or other "light" anesthetic approaches that maintain or increase sympathoadrenal tone are used, neurally mediated vasoconstriction and the elevation of plasma catecholamines by surgical stress increase splanchnic resistance significantly, which may compromise splanchnic perfusion despite adequate arterial perfusion pressures.[35, 36] Without local compensatory mechanisms, therefore, the splanchnic viscera appear to be at risk of ischemia whenever there is either a centrally integrated enhancement of sympathoadrenal tone[37] or generalized arterial hypotension. Local effects of vasoactive polypeptides may also be significant.[38]

Liver blood flow during anesthesia, therefore, is almost invariably reduced because it is largely dependent on splanchnic perfusion and portal blood flow. Unlike the splanchnic vasculature, however, the hepatic artery reliably demonstrates locally mediated autoregulation. Reduction in hepatic artery vascular resistance by intrinsic mechanisms limits participation in generalized arterial vasoconstriction and minimizes the effects of systemic arterial hypotension. A richly peptidergic neural network around the hepatic artery has, in fact, been identified microscopically.[39]

The reduction in total liver blood flow that occurs during anesthesia is large enough to lower hepatic tissue oxygen tensions. There does not appear to be a routine dependence on anaerobic metabolism, however, since lactate production does not increase.[40] Agent-specific anesthesia-induced spasm of the hepatic artery has been reported during halothane[41] and methoxyflurane[42] anesthesia. Under the general conditions of decreased overall hepatic blood flow that occur during anesthesia, these agents might produce a critical additional degree of hepatic ischemia that could play a role in subsequent hepatic injury produced by reductive pathways of biotransformation.

ANESTHESIA AND GASTROINTESTINAL FUNCTION

The mechanical aspects of gastrointestinal activity are profoundly disrupted by stress, disease, anxiety, direct surgical manipulation, and perioperative pain. Loss of peristalsis produces visceral atony and distention. Routine perioperative protocols, which include withholding of oral intake and the placement of nasogastric tubes or other similar devices to provide drainage of enteric and biliary secretions, anticipate these events. The return of gastrointestinal motility after intraperitoneal surgery commonly requires several days of convalescence, during which time the carbohydrates needed for metabolic balance and glucose homeostasis are provided intravenously. The degree to which the anesthetic state itself, or the agents with which it is produced, contribute to this generalized gastrointestinal dysfunction remains incompletely understood.

Stress

The neuroendocrine response to surgical stress and altered autonomic balance may explain much of the gastrointestinal disruption experienced by patients perioperatively. Sustained preoperative anxiety and sympathoadrenal activity depress gastric emptying and intestinal peristalsis: in contrast, anxiolytic therapy with benzodiazepines actually enhances gastric emptying and reduces the acidity of gastric secretions.[43] Acute increases in sympathetic activity during "light" anesthesia for abdominal surgery can produce not only changes in blood pressure and heart rate but also atony and intestinal distention: increases in the volume of the intestinal viscera due to loss of intrinsic visceral smooth muscle tone may cause protrusion from the open abdominal cavity.

Conversely, abrupt sympathectomy during spinal anesthesia or the use of physostigmine or other agents that enhance parasympathetic activity may produce a dramatic reduction of abdominal girth. There may also be sufficient impairment of sphincter tone that patients with marginal control can become incontinent. When compared with the use of parenteral narcotics for pain, postoperative sensory and sympathetic blockade with epidural local anesthetics reduces dramatically the time required for return of visceral activity and effective intestinal peristalsis.[44]

Narcotics

The potency with which narcotics depress gastrointestinal motility is the basis for both their therapeutic value in the treatment of enteritis and their ability to aggravate postoperative atony and constipation.[45] The role of these drugs in precipitating postoperative nausea and vomiting is less clear.

Pain itself, rather than analgesic therapy, may be the primary cause of these undesirable events in some patients.[46] In fact, in the early postoperative period, morphine appears to produce more potent acute analgesia, and less emesis, than does meperidine.[47] It may be associated with a higher incidence of vomiting later in the course of recovery, however, especially after ambulation.[48] Women appear to be affected by nausea and vomiting more frequently than do men. The importance of obesity as a factor predisposing to nausea and vomiting remains, however, in question.[49, 50] Nitrous oxide was once believed to be an important factor,[51] but it probably does not have significant effects on the incidence of nausea and vomiting.[47]

Aspiration of Gastric Contents

Narcotics certainly delay gastric emptying, increasing both the volume of retained gastric acid and the probability that food ingested preoperatively will remain in the stomach to be regurgitated during the induction of anesthesia. Originally described as Mendelson's syndrome in obstetric patients,[52] the aspiration of gastric contents into the tracheobronchial tree with subsequent generation of fulminant pneumonitis was ultimately acknowledged to be a major source of morbidity and mortality for all patients.[53]

Within 30 seconds of aspiration, gastric acid produces diffuse epithelial injury, bronchospasm, disruption of alveolar surfactant, and hemorrhage from pulmonary capillaries.[54] Alveolar gas spaces fill with protein-containing fluid, reducing significantly the number of functioning gas exchange units and producing a rapid fall in arterial oxygen tension. Direct irritation of the tracheobronchial tree by aspirated acid also produces an immediate, reactive bronchospasm. When the material aspirated is greater in volume than 25 mL or is extremely acid (pH

below 2.5), these two factors determine the eventual extent and severity of the injury, in effect, a chemical burn of the lung parenchyma.
Food or other particulate matter increases the likelihood of mechanical
obstruction of small airways and may produce local irritation and inflammation, with subsequent infection and abscess formation.

Intragastric Pressure

Initial observations of elevated intragastric pressure (IGP) during
the administration of succinylcholine were interpreted as evidence that
the use of this drug would further increase the risk of aspiration after
loss of consciousness during anesthetic induction.[55] Vigorous skeletal
muscle fasciculations produced by succinylcholine can, in fact, produce
significant elevations of IGP by a process of external compression of
gastric contents.[56]

However, the changes in IGP due to succinylcholine are sporadic,
small in magnitude, and accompanied by a simultaneous increase in
the gastroesophageal sphincter tone that usually maintains an effective
barrier to gastric reflux.[57] Transient enhancement of visceral sphincter
tone is an indication of the ability of succinylcholine to mimic acetylcholine at these sites, just as it does at many other sites that utilize cholinergic transmission. Consequently, sphincter tone at the gastroesophageal junction is reduced by atropine, but elevated by metoclopramide
or by other drugs that have centrally mediated cholinergic effects.[58]

The general effect of loss of consciousness itself on intra-abdominal
dynamics is to reduce IGP. Reduction of the resting tone of the respiratory diaphragm at end-expiration permits cephalad movement of the
viscera,[59] expanding intra-abdominal volume and reducing IGP at the
expense of pulmonary functional residual capacity (Chapter 7). Active
contractions of the abdominal wall musculature during the expiratory
phase of spontaneous ventilation during general anesthesia may, however, produce external compression of gastric contents. During surgical
levels of anesthesia with neuromuscular blockade and controlled ventilation, the tension of the abdominal wall and, presumably, IGP, both
fall to an extent determined by the degree of paralysis established as
part of the anesthetic plan (Fig 8–3).

IGP elevated by coughing, movement, or straining, in the absence
of accompanying improvement in gastroesophageal sphincter tone,
may nevertheless predispose to the regurgitation of gastric contents
during prolonged induction or emergence from anesthesia. Risk is additionally increased if there is transient hypoxemia, which further stimulates the vigor of respiratory muscle activity under these circum-

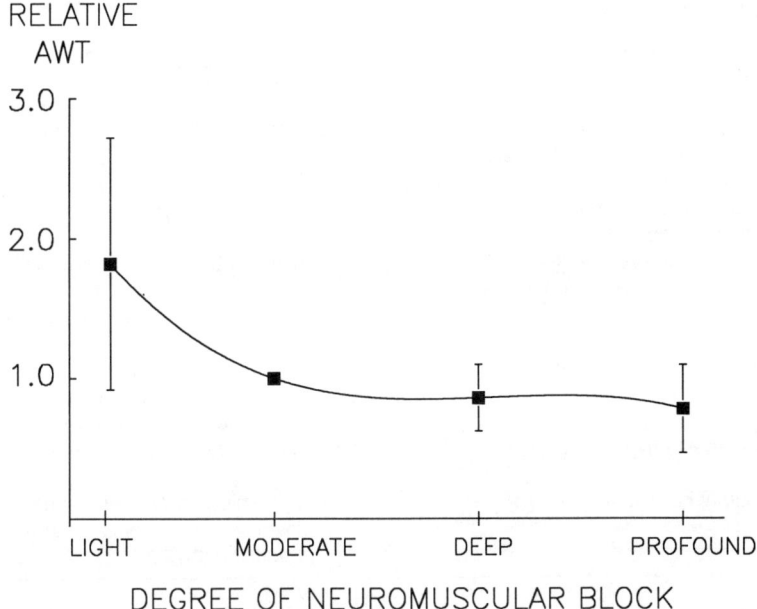

FIG 8-3.

Relative abdominal wall tension *(AWT)* as measured by instrumented surgical retractors during progressively more profound degrees of neuromuscular blockade. "Light" neuro-muscular blockade is defined as 80% or less twitch height depression from unparalyzed control values, "moderate" as 80% to 95% depression of evoked response, "deep" as 95% to 99% depression, and "profound" as the total abolition of evoked twitch response to stimulation of the ulnar nerve (author's data). *Bars* indicate standard deviation.

stances. Any prolonged period of drug-induced depression of consciousness without tracheal intubation, therefore, increases the likelihood of aspiration of gastric contents.[60,61] Even intravenous sedation with spontaneous breathing of nitrous oxide, a practice widely employed in office and outpatient settings for diagnostic or limited surgical procedures, can produce "silent" aspiration.

ANESTHETIC IMPLICATIONS OF LIVER DISEASE

Hepatic Failure

Hepatic failure is invariably associated with a wide spectrum of perioperative patient management problems (Table 8-1). Coagulopathy is due to reduced hepatocellular protein synthesis and to the inadequate absorption of the vitamin K required as a cofactor. Impaired hepatic

TABLE 8–1.

Clinical Consequences and Pathophysiology of Hepatic Failure and Cirrhosis

Clinical Abnormality	Pathophysiology
Elevated serum levels of transmission enzymes (AST, ALT) and lactate dehydrogenase isoenzyme-5 (LDH-5); hypoalbuminemia; prolongation of prothrombin time	Hepatocellular dysfunction or injury
Elevated serum levels of alkaline phosphatase; hyperbilirubinemia	Biliary tract obstruction, cholelithiasis
Hyponatremia	Water reabsorption in excess of sodium retention
Prolonged drug effects, increased Bromsulphalein retention	Decreased hepatic blood flow, loss of hepatic tissue, renal failure
Ascites	Portal hypertension, hypoalbuminemia
Relative arterial hypoxemia	Intrapulmonary shunting, increased lung water
High-output cardiac failure	Low systemic vascular resistance, pulmonary and systemic shunts, cardiomyopathy

clearance of the activators of fibrinolysis normally present in portal venous blood may also stimulate accelerated destruction of fibrin formed in the process of clotting.[62] The accumulation of ammonia, mercaptans, or other metabolic waste products normally detoxified by the liver frequently produces encephalopathy and cerebral edema.

Hypoalbuminemia reduces plasma oncotic pressure, further increasing brain tissue water in patients with cerebral edema. Sequestration of lung water ultimately compromises pulmonary gas exchange. These manifestations of general metabolic toxicity may also be accompanied by renal failure, for reasons that are not well understood, producing a preterminal hepatorenal syndrome.[63] Hypoglycemia and hyponatremia are part of this generalized disruption of metabolic balance common in patients with liver failure.

The pathophysiology of acute liver failure cannot be reversed. Physiologic functions are supported with metabolic replacement therapy, but pharmacologic measures serve only to stabilize the patient's condition in anticipation of spontaneous improvement of hepatocellular function or liver transplantation. If other surgery is required, decreased hepatic blood flow may produce potentially catastrophic deterioration in patients with severe or active preexisting hepatic disease. Once considered to be a desperation measure in patients with acute hepatitis or end-stage liver failure,[63, 64] surgery under these circumstances nevertheless remains associated with a mortality rate of at least 5%.[65] Resection of esophageal varices and portal decompression procedures are, however, commonly attempted in patients with severe but chronic hepatic disease.[66, 67]

Pharmacology

Even for patients with profound hepatic disease, there can be an objective, pharmacologic basis for the selection of an anesthetic plan. The clinical strategy is largely one that avoids the use of anesthetic agents and adjuvants subject to prolonged effects. The dynamics of inhalational anesthesia remain largely unchanged, but the pharmacology of intravenous agents may be significantly altered. The rates of plasma clearance for diazepam and for other intravenous drugs with relatively incomplete removal from splanchnic blood (low hepatic extraction ratios) are markedly reduced, since hepatocellular activity itself, rather than hepatic blood flow, largely determines their rates of biotransformation.[68, 69]

For drugs that are predominantly water soluble, the increases in the aqueous fraction of body weight reflecting sodium and water retention in patients with liver failure may enlarge their volumes of distribution (Fig 8–4), further extending the duration of their clinical effects.[70] The effects of a typical intubating dose of succinylcholine may also be significantly prolonged if hepatic functional capacity is reduced by more than 50%, a degree of liver failure associated with reduced activity of plasma cholinesterase.[71]

The altered disposition of drugs characterized by high hepatic extraction ratios is more variable, and therefore less predictable, than that seen with drugs having low ratios. The clearance of highly extracted drugs, such as lidocaine, verapamil, propranolol, meperidine, morphine, and pentazocine, is limited by cardiac output and hepatic blood flow, not by hepatocellular function or enzymatic activity.[69] Therefore decreased hepatic clearance of these drugs can be expected only when intrahepatic fibrosis, scarring, and destruction of the liver parenchyma produce increased intrahepatic vascular resistance, portal hypertension, and decreased hepatic blood flow. Chronic ethanol or drug abuse may eventually produce end-stage chronic liver disease and cirrhosis, but in earlier stages increased xenobiotic exposure also enhances the specific activity of hepatic microsomal enzyme systems.

Nevertheless, augmented hepatocellular capacity may not be protective against anesthetic-related side effects in patients with chronic liver disease. The risk of anesthetic overdosage or dose-related drug

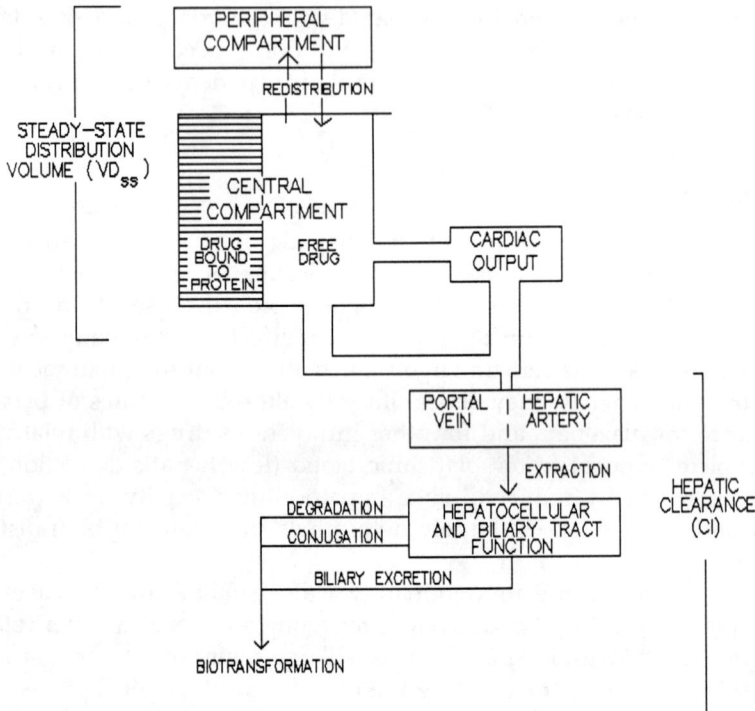

FIG 8–4.
Schematic representation of factors important for drug clearance by hepatic mechanisms. After intravenous injection, drug concentrations in plasma fall rapidly because of redistribution of "free" (not bound to plasma protein) drug molecules from the central to various peripheral distribution compartments, a process that ultimately determines the steady-state distribution volume *(VD_{ss})*. Simultaneously, cardiac output and vascular determinants of portal vein and hepatic artery blood flow deliver drug to hepatocytes, where extraction of free drug occurs by various metabolic processes. Hepatic clearance *(Cl)* of drugs with high extraction ratios is limited only by hepatic blood flow; hepatocellular mass and the extent of microsomal enzymatic induction determine the maximum rate of hepatic clearance for drugs with low extraction ratios. Drug elimination half-time *(T_{1/2β})* is prolonged when there are increases in VD_{ss}, the total volume to be cleared of drug, or by decreases in *Cl*, the rate at which plasma free of drug is generated. Clearance may also be delayed by increases in protein binding or accelerated by enhanced bioavailability of drug molecules.

toxicity after intravenous administration is enhanced for all drugs extensively bound to plasma protein. Hypoalbuminemia produces a dramatic increase in bioavailability: much higher concentrations of free drug may occur than are seen in normal patients.[72] In fact, by enhancing the availability of hepatically "clearable" (unbound) drug molecules, increased bioavailability may actually mask decreased intrinsic rates of hepatic drug clearance imposed by hepatocellular attrition. Renal dysfunction due to liver failure may also limit the clearance of drugs that require urinary elimination.[73]

Although no comparable alterations of pharmacokinetics occur when inhalational anesthetics are used for patients who have end-stage hepatic dysfunction, their anesthetic dose requirement may be extremely variable. In patients with liver failure, anesthetic pharmacodynamics are largely a function of the degree to which the metabolic dysfunction imposed by hepatic disease has compromised nervous system functional reserve. Chronic alcoholism actually appears to increase anesthetic requirements.[74-76] The acute depressant effects of hepatically induced cerebral edema and coma, however, clearly reduce the dosage or inspired concentrations required to produce a state of anesthesia.

Other Aspects of Management

The anesthetic implications of chronic liver failure also include the nonhepatic consequences of cirrhosis and related circulatory disturbances. Portal hypertension appears to open or to enlarge collateral splenic and esophageal vascular channels, creating the risk of spontaneous hemorrhage. Endocrine or metabolic factors may generate extensive arteriovenous splanchnic shunts and produce a state of generalized mesenteric vasodilation. Intrapulmonary right-to-left shunt channels and a loss of functional residual capacity due to the expansion of intra-abdominal volume by ascites may also contribute to significant impairment of pulmonary gas exchange. All these consequences influence the postoperative course to an extent greater than can be predicted solely from an assessment of "liver function tests."[77]

The experience gained by managing patients for orthotopic liver transplantation has provided a clinical model for the cardiovascular pathophysiology of end-stage liver failure.[78] It has revealed the extent to which this disease not only disrupts metabolic functions but also compromises circulatory homeostasis. In patients who maintain adequate myocardial function, the fall in systemic and pulmonary vascular resistance associated with the opening of shunts between the arterial and venous circulation produces a hyperdynamic cardiovascular system. Arterial blood pressure is low and the liver itself remains small, fibrotic, and underperfused, but cardiac output is chronically elevated.[79] Constant seepage of albumin from the liver surface into the abdominal cavity to form ascitic fluid further complicates the usual evaluation of perioperative intravascular volume shifts and overall fluid balance.

Accurate assessment of the circulating volume of patients with liver failure therefore usually requires invasive monitoring for measurement of ventricular preload to ensure optimal cardiac output. Arterial hypotension also compromises renal blood flow, exposing these patients to a high risk of renal ischemia if there is anesthetic-induced myocardial depression or failure to maintain adequate circulating blood volume perioperatively. Low plasma oncotic pressure and relative arterial hypotension may also produce an increase in aldosterone secretion and renal tubular sodium retention.[80] Hypokalemia may produce cardiac dysrhythmias if exacerbated by inadvertent hyperventilation during general anesthesia.

Liver Transplantation

The choice of anesthetic agents for liver transplantation remains an arbitrary one, since there are inadequate data to support the value of a specific anesthetic protocol. The donor liver is initially cold and not fully oxygenated, yet appears to resume some in vivo metabolic activity almost immediately.[81] Consequently, most anesthesiologists avoid the use of halothane under these circumstances, since it may predispose to the activation of reductive hepatic metabolic pathways and the formation of hepatotoxic free-radicals.

With a donor liver in place, there may be almost immediate arterial hypertension as systemic vascular resistance rapidly increases from subnormal toward normal values, suggesting the importance of circulating vasoactive agents in the etiology of the cardiovascular stigmata of chronic liver disease. Extensive diuresis and stabilization of blood pressure are generally established during the first few postoperative days, although supplemental calcium may be required to avoid myocardial depression due to low ionized calcium concentrations.[82] Depressed metabolism of the large amounts of citrate infused with blood products may also impair coagulation perioperatively.

Biliary Tract Disease

Patients with biliary tract disease, cholelithiasis in particular, are prone to spasm at the sphincter of Oddi. Biliary tract spasm not only is a source of severe perioperative pain but also may interfere with surgical exploration of the bile ducts and may compromise the diagnostic value of intraoperative cholangiography. Parenteral narcotics can precipitate sphincter spasm; they increase pressures within the common duct and obstruct biliary flow.[83] In equipotent dosages, all narcotic agonists produce biliary tract dysfunction with comparable incidence and severity. The effectiveness of naloxone in reversing narcotic-induced spasm supports the concept that this phenomenon is mediated by specific opiate receptors.[84]

Porphyria

Even a single intravenous dose of thiopental or other barbiturates can increase hepatic enzymatic activity of aminolevulinic acid synthase.[85] In patients with acute intermittent hepatic porphyria, this may generate excess porphyrin, a potent neurotoxin that causes seizures, coma, and paralysis.[86] Although a relatively rare genetic disease, acute intermittent porphyria may exist in a latent form, and no prior history of anesthetic intolerance may be noted at the time of surgery. However, its acute exacerbation after the xenobiotic induction of cytochrome P-450 enzymes can trigger a series of metabolic events with a mortality rate as high as 25%. Vigorous intravenous glucose therapy may be helpful in aborting the acute attack, but the use of ketamine or other nonbarbiturate induction agents is the preferred approach when patients at initial presentation do have a personal or family history consistent with the signs or symptoms of this metabolic disorder.[87]

ANESTHETIC IMPLICATIONS OF METABOLIC AND GASTROINTESTINAL DYSFUNCTION

Diabetes Mellitus

Diabetes mellitus is the most commonly encountered endocrinopathy. Characterized by fasting hyperglycemia and an intolerance of glucose challenge, it is also a diffuse metabolic disease that produces degeneration of the microcirculation in the kidney, retina, and many other tissues. It is associated with a severe and progressive peripheral neuropathy produced by mechanisms that are still unknown. A diagnosis of type I, juvenile-onset or insulin-dependent, diabetes mellitus implies the absence of functional endogenous insulin. The catabolic effects of glucagon are, therefore, not only unopposed by insulin but are further enhanced perioperatively by the cortisol and catecholamines released in response to surgical stress. Consequently, these patients are at risk of lipolysis, the release of fatty acids, and ketone production. Ketoacidosis may also occur if administration of exogenous insulin is interrupted or inadequate, even for a short period of time.

In contrast, type II, adult-onset or non-insulin-dependent diabetes mellitus, can be considered to be a state of relative resistance to the effects of endogenous insulin. This phenomenon is probably mediated by changes in the receptor population normally responsive to this hormone. The differences in the functional consequences of the processes that produce insulin-dependent diabetes mellitus (type I) and non-insulin-dependent diabetes mellitus (type II) are significant. Unlike their younger, juvenile-onset diabetic counterparts, older patients with type II diabetes mellitus usually have sufficient endogenous insulin activity to maintain an anabolic state. They are at lesser risk of ketoacidosis, although relative insulin deficiency in patients with type II diabetes may still produce hyperglycemia sufficiently severe to induce a state of nonketotic hyperosmolar coma. Monitoring of blood sugar may, in fact, be indicated if large amounts of dextrose are infused intravenously as part of perioperative anesthetic and surgical management.[88]

If not associated with abnormalities other than impaired glucose homeostasis, the metabolic consequences of diabetes mellitus itself, regardless of age, do not appear to present a significant surgical risk.[89] In diabetic patients, postoperative morbidity and mortality reflect largely the extent to which various organ functions are impaired,[90] although the disease may be unavoidably associated with poor wound healing.[91] Other than special precautions in the evaluation of the airways of juvenile diabetics of short stature,[92] there is no anesthetic protocol or technique specifically indicated by the underlying metabolic dysfunction characteristic of this disease. The effect of anesthetics on insulin release per se appears to be less important than the overall metabolic state and the degree of neuroendocrine stress. Facilitation of gastric emptying with metoclopramide or other agents may, however, be appropriate as a measure to reduce the possibility of regurgitation and aspiration in patients with diabetes-induced gastric paresis.[93]

Although a primary goal of chronic medical therapy, control of glucose within narrow limits is of uncertain value in the acute management of diabetic patients, except in pregnancy[94] or when the likelihood of perioperative cerebral ischemia is high.[95] The risk of "tight" control reflects the possibility that continued administration of insulin may produce severe hypoglycemia and subsequent nervous system injury. Unlike the situation in other organs, the movement of glucose into brain and spinal cord is accomplished by an insulin-independent mechanism of facilitated molecular transport that requires the presence of a concentration gradient between plasma and tissue glucose. Insulin overdosage creates, in effect, a carbohydrate "steal" syndrome that deprives nervous system tissues of their essential metabolic fuel. Although several conventional regimens for the administration of insulin and glucose are used in contemporary practice,[96] the common principle of management remains the consistent supply of adequate amounts of both insulin and glucose to diabetic patients perioperatively.

Obesity

Factors predisposing to the development of type II diabetes are increased body lipid fraction, a phenomenon associated to some extent with normal physiologic processes of aging, but most notably a function of overt obesity. In its most common form, obesity is a state of primary hyperalimentation. Increased body mass associated with mild or moderate obesity (20% to 40% above ideal body weight) probably does not increase perioperative risk. Morbid obesity, two or more times ideal body weight, produces additional hormonal and metabolically mediated changes in gastrointestinal function that do, however, alter the anesthetic plan significantly.

In obese patients, liver mass and splanchnic blood flow are significantly increased.[97] There is increased plasma cholinesterase[98] and mixed-function microsomal enzyme activity,[31] suggesting a significant degree of direct hepatocellular stimulation; obese patients may therefore be at somewhat higher risk of halothane hepatitis. Obese patients also have increased volume and acidity of gastric secretions.[99] Intragastric pressure and the frequency with which gastroesophageal reflux occurs are also higher than in nonobese patients.

The metabolic requirements imposed by a state of obesity also generate increased demands for cardiac output and for pulmonary gas exchange. These physiologic needs may not be adequately met because of weight-related impairment of cardiovascular homeostasis, deconditioning, loss of lung volume, and increased work of breathing. Perioperative gas exchange may be grossly inadequate without supplementation of inspired oxygen tensions. Chronic hypoxemia due to pickwickian (obesity hypoventilation) syndrome produces pulmonary vasoconstriction, vascular congestion, and pulmonary vascular hypertension. These changes in pulmonary hemodynamics ultimately lead to right ventricular dysfunction and failure, although they may improve markedly in response to weight loss.[100]

In morbidly obese patients with QT abnormalities of electrocardiographic morphology, the incidence of sudden perioperative death from cardiac dysrhythmias is 40 times that occurring in age-matched nonobese subjects.[101] Cardiovascular monitoring during and after surgery, therefore, may require more attention than that indicated solely by the surgical procedure. Pharmacokinetic considerations suggest that both the uptake and excretion of potent inhalational anesthetics should be prolonged in obese patients because of impaired gas exchange and increased cardiac output. However, narcotic-based anesthetics do not appear to have clinically significant advantages in either ease of management or overall safety.[102]

Intestinal Obstruction

A variety of anatomic, mechanical, and neoplastic events can produce intestinal obstruction requiring surgical intervention. Regardless of cause, the acute disruption of intestinal function generally results in intraluminal sequestration of fluid. Nausea, vomiting, and restriction or absence of oral fluid intake under these circumstances lead to generalized dehydration and to a circulating hypovolemia. Clinical signs of arterial hypotension, oliguria, and systemic acidosis suggest inadequate tissue perfusion and a pathophysiologic transition to anaerobic metabolism in some tissues. Hypokalemia and hypochloremia occur in proportion to the extent that loss of electrolytes into intestinal or gastric secretions remains unrecovered.

When intestinal obstruction occurs as part of a subacute syndrome of malignancy, malnutrition, and cachexia, hypoalbuminemia and severe weight loss have grave prognostic implications: perioperative mortality under these circumstances may exceed 40%[103] unless total parenteral nutrition is established preoperatively[104] and during convalescence from surgery.[105] The choice of anesthetic agents does not appear to influence outcome in patients with intestinal obstruction with or without generalized malnutrition, although nitrous oxide is generally avoided because of the possibility of further enteric distention following its diffusion into the volume of intraluminal gas.[106]

Intestinal Tumors

Some gastrointestinal tumors have specific qualities that may complicate anesthetic management intraoperatively. Carcinoid tumors were once thought to be benign, serotonin-secreting lesions[107]; however, they are now known to be metastatic and, like the amine precursor uptake and decarboxylation (APUD) tissues from which they are derived, they also synthesize and release prostaglandins, histamine, calcitonin, and the bradykinins.[108] APUD tissues are widely distributed in the gastrointestinal tract, lungs, thymus, and pancreas. They appear to function physiologically as a newly recognized component subdivision of the autonomic nervous system that produces more sustained, hormonally mediated cardiovascular effects than those of the shorter-acting classic sympathetic and parasympathetic divisions.[109]

Serotonin, responsible for the typical presenting symptom of diarrhea in patients with carcinoid tumors, rarely causes systemic vascular effects intraoperatively because it is cleared efficiently from the portal circulation by the liver.[110] Serotonin-induced arterial hypertension usually indicates, therefore, the presence of posthepatic metastatic lesions.[111] Cardiovascular instability may respond under these circumstances to antiserotonin agents such as cyproheptadine or to somatostatin analogues.[112] In contrast, when abrupt arterial hypotension, cutaneous flush, and tachycardia occur during surgical resection of the gastrointestinal tract, they generally reflect the hemodynamic consequences of the release of bradykinins or of prostacyclin.[113] This phenomenon is commonly seen in response to surgical traction on the mesentery and intestinal viscera, even in patients without known APUD lesions.[114]

Delayed Gastric Emptying

Virtually all patients with debilitating illness, intra-abdominal pathology, obesity, pregnancy, perioperative pain, and even generalized anxiety can be assumed to have both increased volume and acidity of gastric contents. Although a recent meal rich in animal fats or alcohol certainly further depresses gastrointestinal motility and impairs gastric emptying, prohibiting all oral intake for 8 hours before surgery does not appear to be superior to a protocol that permits the ingestion of clear liquids preoperatively.[115] Obesity, pregnancy, and other sources of increased abdominal pressure disrupt the competence of the gastroesophageal sphincter and further increase the risk of regurgitation and pulmonary aspiration of gastric contents (see Chapter 11).

The anesthetic plan for any patient with suspected impairment of gastroesophageal sphincter function or depressed gastrointestinal motility who requires general anesthesia should be designed to minimize the time elapsed between loss of consciousness and tracheal intubation. A rapidly executed or "crash" intravenous induction sequence is required because pharyngeal constrictor reflexes, suppressed by loss of consciousness,[116] may no longer prevent the flow of gastric contents from the esophagus into the pharynx in patients subject to gastric reflux. Consequently, the "full stomach" anesthetic induction includes the Sellick maneuver: the application, by an assistant, of direct compression of the upper end of the esophagus by external digital pressure on the cricoid cartilage of the larynx.[117] This action maintains a physical barrier to further reflux of gastric contents until the trachea has been intubated.

Additional measures to minimize the possibility of pulmonary injury from aspiration of gastric contents in patients with depressed gastrointestinal motility include the use of cimetidine or other antagonists of histamine to reduce gastric acidity,[118] or the pharmacologic acceleration of the process of gastric emptying and elevation of gastroesophageal sphincter pressures with metoclopramide.[58] Oral antacids also elevate pH but increase total gastric volume, and may be sufficiently irritating to cause a pneumonitis if inhaled.[119] Patients with markedly impaired cardiovascular homeostasis who will not tolerate the rapid intravenous injection of induction agents without arterial hypotension, or those who may be difficult to intubate promptly, are candidates for anesthetic approaches that include tracheal intubation prior to loss of consciousness.

SUMMARY

Changes in hepatic, metabolic, and splanchnic function are less discrete and more difficult to measure than perioperative physical and physiologic alterations of cardiovascular and pulmonary function. Perioperative hyperglycemia, intolerance of a carbohydrate load, and reductions of gastrointestinal motility probably reflect stress-related increases in sympathoadrenal state rather than the direct consequences of anesthesia or the agents with which it is produced. Nevertheless, narcotics do potentiate visceral atony, and hepatic blood flow and tissue oxygenation are both significantly reduced during and after anesthesia and surgery. These changes are reversible, occur with both general and regional anesthesia, and do not appear to cause hepatocellular injury unless they are amplified by coincident arterial hypotension or hypoxemia.

None of the anesthetic agents in current use are themselves direct hepatotoxins. However, there is justifiable concern that the metabolic by-products of either reductive or oxidative hepatic pathways may produce hepatocellular injury, especially in patients with enhanced enzymatic activities. Consequently, the synthesis of a chemical structure for inhalational anesthetics that is subject to minimal degrees of hepatic biotransformation has become an important goal of clinical pharmacologists. Inhalational anesthetics may be associated with rare forms of postanesthetic hepatic necrosis that are triggered by an immune mechanism established after prior exposure.

The consequences of liver failure are as extensive as the metabolic and synthetic functions of this organ. Coagulopathy, disorders of electrolyte, renal, and neurologic functions, altered cardiovascular and body water homeostasis, and impaired pulmonary gas exchange are clinically significant. The functional reserve of hepatic tissues is sufficiently great, however, that these changes occur only after there has been massive loss of liver tissue. Enzymatic studies used in the evaluation of liver failure may indicate the nature of the disease process, but rarely provide quantitative information regarding the overall state of hepatic tissue function. The adequacy of albumin and coagulation protein synthesis may prove more useful in the assessment of liver function and functional reserve.

The duration of effect for all anesthetic drugs requiring hepatic clearance is prolonged in patients with liver failure because of the loss of functional hepatocellular mass or reduced liver blood flow. Inhalational anesthetics provide constant pharmacokinetics, but require careful attention to cardiovascular side effects and precise monitoring of fluid balance. The priorities of the anesthetic plan for patients with diabetes mellitus are to avoid neurologic injury from hypoglycemia and to maintain sufficient insulin and glucose that either ketone formation or a state of hyperosmolar dehydration is avoided. In most patients intragastric pressure falls after anesthetic induction. The risk of regurgitation and aspiration of gastric contents during induction of anesthesia is significantly increased, however, in patients with delayed gastric emptying, impaired gastroesophageal sphincter functions, or increased volume or acidity of gastric contents due to obesity, pregnancy, or other factors.

REFERENCES

1. Gelman S, Longnecker DE: Isoflurane and hepatic oxygenation. *Anesthesiology* 1988; 69:639–640.
2. Biebuyck JF: Anesthesia and hepatic metabolism: Current concepts of carbohydrate homeostasis. *Anesthesiology* 1973; 39:188–198.
3. Stoelting RK: Metabolic effects of anesthetics. *Int Anesthesiol Clin* 1980; 18:53–69.
4. Brown BR Jr: Enzymatic activity and biotransformation of anesthetics. *Int Anesthesiol Clin* 1974; 12:25–34.
5. Conney AH, Davison C, Gastel R, et al: Adaptive increases in drug-metabolizing enzymes induced by phenobarbital and other drugs. *J Pharmacol Exp Ther* 1960; 130:1–8.

6. Strunin L: Preoperative assessment of the patient with liver dysfunction. *Br J Anaesth* 1978; 50:25–31.
7. Starker PM, Gump FE, Askanazi J: Serum albumin levels as an index of nutritional support. *Surgery* 1982; 91:194–199.
8. Elwyn DH, Bryan-Brown CW, Shoemaker WC: Nutritional aspects of body water dislocations in postoperative and depleted patients. *Ann Surg* 1975; 182:76–85.
9. Gingerich R, Wright PH, Paradise RR: Inhibition by halothane of glucose-stimulated insulin secretion in isolated pieces of rat pancreas. *Anesthesiology* 1974; 40:449–452.
10. Biebuyck JF: Effects of anesthetic agents on metabolic pathways: Fuel utilization and supply during anesthesia. *Br J Anaesth* 1973; 45:263–268.
11. Houghton A, Hickey JB, Ross SA: Glucose tolerance during anaesthesia and surgery: Comparison of general and extradural anaesthesia. *Br J Anaesth* 1978; 50:495–499.
12. Becker LD, Paulson BA, Miller RD, et al: Biphasic respiratory depression after fentanyl-droperidol or fentanyl alone used to supplement nitrous oxide anesthesia. *Anesthesiology* 1976; 44:291–296.
13. Stoeckel H, Hengstmann JH, Schuttler J: Pharmacokinetics of fentanyl as a possible explanation for recurrence of respiratory depression. *Br J Anaesth* 1979; 51:741–745.
14. Schemel WH: Unsuspected hepatic dysfunction found by multiple laboratory screening. *Anesth Analg* 1976; 55:810–812.
15. Viegas O, Stoelting RK: LDH5 changes after cholecystectomy or hysterectomy in patients receiving halothane, enflurane, or fentanyl. *Anesthesiology* 1979; 51:556–558.
16. Virtue RW, Payne KW: Postoperative death after Fluothane. *Anesthesiology* 1958; 19:562–563.
17. Summary of the National Halothane Study. Possible association between halothane anesthesia and postoperative hepatic necrosis. *JAMA* 1966; 197:775–788.
18. Strunin L, Davies JM: The liver and anaesthesia. *Can Anaesth Soc J* 1983; 30:208–217.
19. Rehder K, Forbes J, Alter H, et al: Halothane biotransformation in man: A quantitative study. *Anesthesiology* 1967; 38:711–715.
20. Plummer JL, Hall PM, Jenner MA, et al: Hepatic effects of repeated halothane anesthetics in the hypoxic rat model. *Anesthesiology* 1987; 67:355–360.
21. Brown BR Jr, Gandolfi AJ: Adverse effects of volatile anesthetics. *Br J Anaesth* 1987; 59:14–23.
22. Klatskin G, Kimberg DV: Recurrent hepatitis attributable to halothane sensitization in an anesthetist. *N Engl J Med* 1967; 280:515–522.
23. Helfrage S, Ahlgren I, Axelson S: Halothane hepatitis in an anesthetist. *Lancet* 1966; 2:1466–1467.
24. Fee JPH, Black GW, Dundee JW, et al: A prospective study of liver en-

zyme and other changes following repeat administration of halothane and enflurane. *Br J Anaesth* 1979; 51:1133–1141.

25. Thomas FB: Chronic aggressive hepatitis induced by halothane. *Ann Intern Med* 1974; 81:487–489.
26. Paronetto F, Popper H: Lymphocyte stimulation induced by halothane in patients with hepatitis following exposure to halothane. *N Engl J Med* 1970; 279:798–801.
27. Kenna JG, Neuberger J, Mieli-Vergani G, et al: Halothane hepatitis in children. *Br Med J* 1987; 294:1209–1211.
28. Ona FV, Patanella H, Ayub A: Hepatitis associated with enflurane anesthesia. *Anesth Analg* 1980; 59:146–149.
29. Hals J, Dodgson MS, Skulberg A, et al: Halothane-associated liver damage and renal failure in a young child. *Acta Anaesthesiol Scand* 1986; 30:651–655.
30. Bentley JB, Vaughan RW, Miller MS: Serum inorganic fluoride levels in obese patients during and after enflurane anesthesia. *Anesth Analg* 1979; 58:409–412.
31. Walton B, Simpson BR, Strunin L, et al: Unexplained hepatitis following halothane. *Br Med J* 1976; 1:1171–1176.
32. Combes B: Halothane-induced liver damage—an entity. *N Engl J Med* 1969; 280:558–559.
33. Larson CP, Mazze RI, Cooperman LH, et al: Effects of anesthetics on cerebral, renal, and splanchnic circulations: Recent developments. *Anesthesiology* 1974; 41:169–181.
34. Gelman SI: Disturbances in hepatic blood flow during anesthesia and surgery. *Arch Surg* 1976; 111:881–883.
35. Epstein RM, Deutsch S, Cooperman LH, et al: Splanchnic circulation during halothane anesthesia and hypercapnia in normal man. *Anesthesiology* 1966; 27:654–661.
36. Leaman DM, Levenson L, Lelis R, et al: Effect of morphine on splanchnic blood flow. *Br Heart J* 1978; 40:569–571.
37. Cooperman LH: Effects of anaesthetics on the splanchnic circulation. *Br J Anaesth* 1968; 44:967–970.
38. Domschke S, Domschke W, Bloom SR, et al: Vasoactive intestinal peptide in man: Pharmacokinetics, metabolic and circulatory effects. *Gut* 1978; 19:1049–1053.
39. Carlei F, Lygidakis NJ, Speranza V, et al: Neuroendocrine innervation of the hepatic vessels in rat and in man. *J Surg Res* 1988; 45:417–426.
40. Price HL, Deutsch S, Davidson IA, et al: Can general anesthetics produce splanchnic visceral hypoxia by reducing regional blood flow? *Anesthesiology* 1966; 27:24–32.
41. Benumof JL, Brookstein JJ, Saidman LJ, et al: Diminished hepatic arterial flow during halothane administration. *Anesthesiology* 1976; 45:545–551.
42. Libonati M, Malsch E, Price HL, et al: Splanchnic circulation in man during methoxyflurane anesthesia. *Anesthesiology* 1973; 38:466–472.

43. Schurizek BA, Kraglund K, Andreasen F, et al: Gastrointestinal motility and gastric pH and emptying following ingestion of diazepam. *Br J Anaesth* 1988; 61:712–719.
44. Ahn H, Bronge A, Johannsson K, Ygge H, et al: Effect of continuous postoperative epidural analgesia on intestinal motility. *Br J Surg* 1988; 75:1176–1178.
45. Nimmo WS, Wilson J, Prescott LF: Narcotic analgesics and delayed gastric emptying during labour. *Lancet* 1975; 1:890–893.
46. Anderson R, Krohg K: Pain as a major cause of postoperative nausea. *Can Anaesth Soc J* 1976; 23:366–369.
47. Muir JJ, Warner MA, Offord KP, et al: Role of nitrous oxide and other factors in postoperative nausea and vomiting: A randomized and blinded prospective study. *Anesthesiology* 1987; 66:513–518.
48. Comroe JH, Dripps RD: Reactions to morphine in ambulatory and bed patients. *Surg Gynecol Obstet* 1948; 87:221–224.
49. Dent S, Ramachandra V, Stephen CR: Postoperative vomiting: Incidence, analysis and therapeutic measures in 3,000 patients. *Anesthesiology* 1955; 16:564–572.
50. Bellville JW, Bross IDJ, Howlands WS: Postoperative nausea and vomiting. IV. Factors related to postoperative nausea and vomiting. *Anesthesiology* 1960; 21:186–193.
51. Alexander GD, Skupski JN, Brown EM: The role of nitrous oxide in postoperative nausea and vomiting. *Anesth Analg* 1984; 63:175.
52. Mendelson CL: The aspiration of stomach contents into the lungs during obstetric anesthesia. *Am J Obstet Gynecol* 1946; 52:191–193.
53. Bannister WK, Sattilaro AJ: Vomiting and aspiration during anesthesia. *Anesthesiology* 1962; 23:251–264.
54. Wynne JW, Modell JH: Respiratory aspiration of stomach contents. *Ann Intern Med* 1977; 87:466–474.
55. Andersen N: Changes in intragastric pressure following the administration of suxamethonium. *Br J Anaesth* 1962; 34:363–365.
56. Muravchick S, Burkett L, Gold MI: Succinylcholine-induced fasciculations and intragastric pressure during the induction of anesthesia. *Anesthesiology* 1981; 55:180–183.
57. Smith G, Dalling R, Williams TIR: Gastro-oesophageal pressure gradient changes produced by induction of anaesthesia and suxamethonium. *Br J Anaesth* 1978; 50:1137–1142.
58. Brock-Utne JG, Rubin J, Downing JW, et al: The administration of metoclopramide with atropine. *Anaesthesia* 1976; 31:1186–1190.
59. Drummond GB, Park GR: Changes in intragastric pressure on induction of anaesthesia. *Br J Anaesth* 1984; 56:873–879.
60. Rubin J, Brock-Utne JG, Greenberg M, et al: Laryngeal incompetence during experimental "relative analgesia" using 50% nitrous oxide in oxygen. *Br J Anaesth* 1977; 49:1005–1008.
61. Turndorf H, Rodis ID, Clark TS: "Silent" regurgitation during general anesthesia. *Anesth Analg* 1974; 53:700–703.

62. Kang YG, Martin DJ, Marquez J, et al: Intraoperative changes in blood coagulation and thromboelastographic monitoring in liver transplantation. *Anesth Analg* 1985; 64:888–896.
63. Papper S: Hepatorenal syndrome. *Contr Nephrol* 1980; 23:55–74.
64. Harville DD, Summerskill WJH: Surgery in acute hepatitis: Cause and effect. *JAMA* 1963; 184:257–261.
65. Kardy KJ, Hughes ESR: Laparotomy in viral hepatitis. *Med J Aust* 1968; 1:710–712.
66. Calacresi P, Belmann WH: Portacaval and protopulmonary anastomoses in Laennec's cirrhosis and in heart failure. *J Clin Invest* 1957; 36:1257–1265.
67. Pugh RNH, Murray-Lyon IM, Dawson JL, et al: Transection of the oesophagus for bleeding oesophageal varices. *Br J Surg* 1973; 60:646–649.
68. Klotz U, Avant GR, Hoyumpa A, et al: The effect of age and liver disease on the disposition and elimination of diazepam in adult man. *J Clin Invest* 1975; 55:347–359.
69. Williams RL: Drug administration in hepatic disease. *N Engl J Med* 1983; 309:161–162.
70. Pandele G, Chaux F, Salvadori C, et al: Thiopental pharmacokinetics in patients with cirrhosis. *Anesthesiology* 1983; 59:123–126.
71. Foldes FF, Swerdlow M, Lipschitz E, et al: Comparison of the effects of suxamethonium and suxethonium in man. *Anesthesiology* 1956; 17:559–568.
72. Ghonheim MM, Pandya H: Plasma protein binding of thiopental in patients with impaired renal or hepatic function. *Anesthesiology* 1975; 42:545–549.
73. Abrams RE, Hornbein TF: Inability to reverse pancuronium blockade in a patient with renal failure and hepatic disease. *Anesthesiology* 1975; 42:362–364.
74. Han YH: Why do chronic alcoholics require more anesthesia? *Anesthesiology* 1969; 30:341–342.
75. Takki S, Tammisto T: The effect of operative stress on plasma catecholamine levels in chronic alcoholics. *Acta Anaesthesiol Scand* 1974; 18:127–132.
76. Wolfson B: Alcohol. *Semin Anesth* 1984; 3:242–250.
77. Welch HF, Welch CS, Carter JH: Prognosis after surgical treatment of ascites. *Surgery* 1964; 56:75–82.
78. Waterman PF: Anaesthesia for liver transplantation—a model for the anaesthetic management of end-stage hepatic failure. *Can Anaesth Soc J* 1983; 30:534–538.
79. Borland LM, Martin DJ: Anesthesia considerations for orthotopic liver transplantation, in Brown BR (ed): *Anesthesia and Transplantation Surgery*. Philadelphia, FA Davis, 1987, pp 157–182.
80. Rosoff L, Zia P, Reynolds TB, et al: Studies of renin and aldosterone in cirrhotic patients with ascites. *Gastroenterology* 1975; 69:698–705.
81. Rosenberg PH, Oikkonen MP, Orko RH, et al: A transplanted liver rap-

idly begins to metabolize enflurane in humans. *Anesth Analg* 1984; 63:1131–1132.

82. Marquez J, Martin D, Virji MA, et al: Cardiovascular depression secondary to ionic hypocalcemia during hepatic transplantation in humans. *Anesthesiology* 1986; 65:457–461.

83. McCammon RL, Stoelting RK, Madura JA: Effects of butorphanol, nalbuphine, and fentanyl on intrabiliary tract dynamics. *Anesth Analg* 1984; 63:139–142.

84. Radnay PA, Duncalf D, Novakovic M, et al: Common bile duct pressure changes after fentanyl, morphine, meperidine, butorphanol, and naloxone. *Anesth Analg* 1984; 63:441–444.

85. Dundee JW, McLeery WC, McLoughlin G: The hazard of thiopental anesthesia in porphyria. *Anesth Analg* 1962; 41:567–574.

86. Parihk RK, Moore MR: Anesthetics in porphyria: Intravenous induction agents. *Br J Anaesth* 1975; 47:907.

87. Watson CF: The problem of porphyria. *N Engl J Med* 1976; 263:1205.

88. Walts LF, Miller J, Davidson MB, et al: Perioperative management of diabetes mellitus. *Anesthesiology* 1981; 55:104–109.

89. Galloway JA, Shuman CR: Diabetes and surgery. A study of six hundred sixty-seven cases. *Am J Med* 1963; 34:177–191.

90. Lawrie GM, Morris GC, Glaeser DH: Influence of diabetes mellitus on the results of coronary bypass surgery. *JAMA* 1986; 256:2967.

91. Goodson WH III, Hunt TK: Wound healing and the diabetic patient. *Surg Gynecol Obstet* 1979; 149:600–608.

92. Salzarulo HH, Taylor LA: Diabetic stiff joint syndrome as a cause of difficult endotracheal intubation. *Anesthesiology* 1986; 64:366–368.

93. Thomas DJ: Diabetic gastroparesis. *Anaesthesia* 1984; 39:1143.

94. Goldman JA, Dicker D, Feldberg D, et al: Pregnancy outcome in patients with insulin-dependent diabetes mellitus with preconceptional control—a comparative study. *Am J Obstet Gynecol* 1986; 155:293–297.

95. Sieber FE, Smith DS, Traystman RJ, et al: Glucose: A re-evaluation of its intraoperative use. *Anesthesiology* 1987; 67:72–81.

96. Petty C, Cunningham NL: Insulin absorption by glass infusion bottles, polyvinylchloride containers and intravenous tubing. *Anesthesiology* 1974; 40:400–404.

97. Fisher A, Waterhouse TD, Adams AP: Obesity: Its relation to anaesthesia. *Anaesthesia* 1974; 30:633–647.

98. Bentley JN, Borel JD, Vaughan RW, et al: Weight, pseudocholinesterase activity, and succinylcholine requirement. *Anesthesiology* 1982; 57:48–49.

99. Vaughan RW, Bauer S, Wise L: Volume and pH of gastric juice in obese patients. *Anesthesiology* 1975; 43:686–689.

100. Sugerman HJ, Baron PL, Fairman RP, et al: Hemodynamic dysfunction in obesity hypoventilation syndrome and the effects of treatment with surgically induced weight loss. *Ann Surg* 1988; 207:604–613.

101. Drenick EJ, Fisler JS: Sudden cardiac arrest in morbidly obese surgical patients unexplained after autopsy. *Am J Surg* 1988; 155:720–726.

102. Cork RC, Vaughan RW, Bentley JB: General anesthesia for morbidly obese patients—an examination of postoperative outcomes. *Anesthesiology* 1981; 54:310–313.

103. Hickman DM, Miller RA, Rombeau JL, et al: Serum albumin and body weight as predictors of postoperative course in colorectal cancer. *J Parent Ent Nutr* 1980; 4:314–316.

104. Myller JM, Dienst C, Brenner U, et al: Preoperative parenteral feeding in patients with gastrointestinal carcinoma. *Lancet* 1982; 1:68–71.

105. Yamada N, Koyama H, Hioki S, et al: Effect of postoperative total parenteral nutrition (TPN) as an adjunct to gastrectomy for advanced gastric cancer. *Br J Surg* 1983; 70:267–274.

106. Eger EI II, Saidman LJ: Hazards of nitrous oxide anesthesia in bowel obstruction and pneumothorax. *Anesthesiology* 1965; 26:61–66.

107. Stone HH, Donnelly CC: The anesthetic significance of serotonin-secreting carcinoid tumors. *Anesthesiology* 1960; 21:203–212.

108. Miller JD: Carcinoid syndrome and the APUD concept. *Semin Anesth* 1984; 3:228–236.

109. Whitman JG: APUD cells and apudomas. *Anaesthesia* 1977; 32:879–888.

110. Jones RM, Knight D: Severe hypertension and flushing in a patient with a non-metastatic carcinoid tumour. *Anaesthesia* 1982; 37:57–59.

111. Mason RA, Steane PA: Carcinoid syndrome: Its relevance to the anaesthetist. *Anaesthesia* 1976; 31:228–242.

112. Marsh HM, Martin JK, Kvols LK, et al: Carcinoid crisis during anesthesia: Successful treatment with a somatostatin analogue. *Anesthesiology* 1987; 66:89–91.

113. Pace-Asciak CR, Carrara KC: Evidence suggesting a systemic antihypertensive role for PGI2. *Prostaglandins* 1978; 15:704.

114. Seltzer JL, Goldberg ME, Larijani GE, et al: Prostacyclin mediation of vasodilation following mesenteric traction. *Anesthesiology* 1988; 68:514–518.

115. Hutchinson A, Maltby JR, Reid CRG: Gastric fluid volume and pH in elective inpatients. Part 1: Coffee or orange juice versus overnight fast. *Can J Anaesth* 1988; 35:12–15.

116. DeWeese EL, Sullivan TY: Effects of upper airway anesthesia on pharyngeal patency during sleep. *J Appl Physiol* 1988; 64:1346–1353.

117. Salem MR, Sellick BA, Elam JO: The historical background of cricoid pressure in anesthesia and resuscitation. *Anesth Analg* 1974; 53:230–232.

118. Weber L, Hirshman CA: Cimetidine for prophylaxis of aspiration pneumonitis: Comparison of intramuscular and oral dosage schedules. *Anesth Analg* 1979; 58:426–427.

119. Bond VK, Stoelting RK, Gupta CD: Pulmonary aspiration syndrome after inhalation of gastric fluid containing antacid. *Anesthesiology* 1979; 51:452–453.

9

Renal Function and Body Fluid Compartments

Like other major organs, the kidneys are the site of many essential processes. Their primary vital function, however, is maintenance of stable body salt and water stores, the osmotically constant physiologic environment that is the "internal sea" essential for optimal cellular and tissue function. Mechanical and hormonal renal mechanisms compensate for variability in dietary salt and water intake and for inevitable fluctuations in the rate at which water is lost from the body. In addition, pressure- and volume-sensing and osmotically stimulated components of the autonomic nervous system adjust peripheral and renal vascular resistance to minimize gross disruption of blood volume homeostasis after physical trauma or surgery.

Renal metabolism and blood flow also largely determine acid-base status, the adequacy of excretion of nitrogenous waste products, the elimination of xenobiotics, and the mineral balance needed for stable skeletal composition. The sections that follow provide an overview of the relationship between the neurohumoral pathways involved in renal control of salt and water balance, tonicity, and effective arterial blood volume. In addition, this chapter reviews the extent to which these mechanisms are altered by anesthesia and anesthetic agents, as well as the anesthetic implications of renal dysfunction and failure.

RENAL FUNCTION

Within the complexity of the microarchitecture of renal tissue is the anatomic basis for efficient filtration of plasma and the active and selective secretion or reabsorption of solute. Both functions are needed for precise regulation of urinary salt and water excretion. The essential repetitive renal subunit is the nephron. This structure is an intimate juxtaposition of specialized vascular elements that are arranged in parallel with tubular epithelial columns to create, conduct, and concentrate glomerular ultrafiltrate, transforming plasma into the tubular fluid that ultimately becomes urine.

The Glomerulus

The glomerular capillaries in which renal plasma flow (RPF) is filtered are located in the renal cortex; associated tubular components of the nephron extend down into the renal medulla. The two million nephrons contained within a pair of normal human kidneys appear, microscopically, to be identical. However, the juxtamedullary nephrons, those with glomeruli near the cortical-medullary border, may play a more important role in salt conservation and determination of maximal urinary concentrating ability than do more superficial nephrons.[1] The deeper medullary zones are particularly salt rich and contain the very long and specialized tubular segments of juxtamedullary nephrons from which large volumes of filtrate are reabsorbed. Sodium and other solutes are also selectively withdrawn or added here to determine the final composition of urine. Richly innervated juxtamedullary nephrons appear to be less responsive to changes in RPF than are their counterparts in the renal cortex,[2] but they are more closely regulated by osmotic factors, especially changes in serum sodium concentration.[3]

A glomerular basement membrane provides the physical barrier needed for hydrostatic filtration of plasma delivered to the nephrons by renal perfusion. The large volumes of urinary tubular fluid formed at net filtration pressures as low as 6 or 8 mm Hg suggest that the basement membrane has extraordinarily great permeability to water.[4] In fact, the hydraulic permeability of this structure appears to be quite variable, under hormonal control by antidiuretic hormone (ADH, or vasopressin) and by parathyroid hormone (PTH). Molecules smaller than 40 Å pass through the basement membrane easily, but filtration of large molecules usually indicates glomerular injury. Gross protein loss into tubular fluid suggests extensive endothelial damage and disruption of the normal electronegativity that prevents extravasation of large, charged molecules.

Renal Blood Flow

Renal blood flow (RBF) traverses both glomerular and nonglomerular vascular channels: there are normally no true intrarenal shunts. RBF provides nutrition and oxygenation for renal tissues and the hydraulic physical basis for the passive process of filtration that largely determines the volume and the initial composition of tubular fluid.[5]

Fluid formation within the glomerulus does not require the local expenditure of metabolic energy, but active transport of sodium and urea from tubular fluid into medullary areas maintains their high local tonicity. Additional energy is consumed by the secretory processes used to eliminate nonvolatile acids and other small molecules. Eighty percent of the oxygen consumed by renal tissues is used for active tubular transport of sodium and other solutes. Although arteriovenous differences in oxygen content are modest in the kidney, the rate at which this organ is perfused is sufficiently high that bilateral renal oxygen consumption, like RBF, is about one fifth of that of the body as a whole.[2]

Glomerular Filtration

The difference between the hydrostatic pressure within the glomerular capillary and the sum of the hydrostatic pressure within Bowman's space and capillary oncotic pressure determines the net pressure available for glomerular ultrafiltration and the generation of tubular fluid. Ultrafiltration pressure declines progressively from the incoming, or afferent, end of the capillary until it is effectively nil at the efferent, or outgoing, terminus. At typical glomerular capillary hydrostatic pressures of 45 mm Hg (Fig 9–1), net ultrafiltration pressure in the middle of the capillary is about 8 mm Hg.[4] The large volume of plasma that is filtered despite this low pressure gradient, about 160 to 180 L per day, reflects both high intrinsic permeability to water and a glomerular capillary surface area that approaches 1.5 m^2 in the average adult.

Control of Renovascular Resistance and Glomerular Filtration Rate

Even more remarkable than the amount of glomerular filtration that occurs is its constancy. Despite unavoidable variations in arterial blood pressure, RBF and RPF remain relatively stable because renal vascular resistance, within the cortical nephrons in particular, is actively and continuously adjusted at the level of the afferent glomerular arteriole. Autoregulation of renal blood flow appears to be an intrinsic myogenic phenomenon similar to, but less rapid and precise than, that which determines cerebral autoregulation.[6] Neurally mediated control of the renal vasculature could, however, be effected by either sympathetic or parasympathetic pathways: both are easily identified anatomically in renal tissues. Nevertheless, under basal conditions, there is lit-

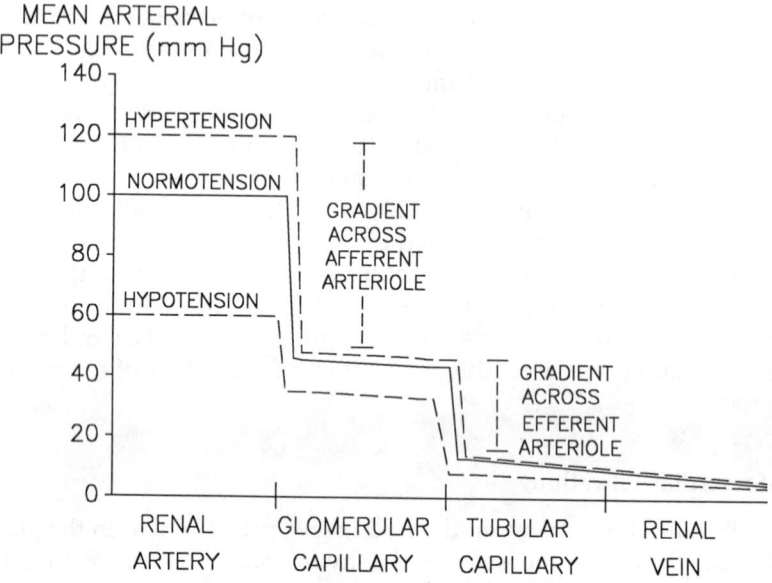

FIG 9–1.
Blood pressure gradients across afferent and efferent renal glomerular arterioles during normotensive, hypertensive, and hypotensive conditions. Marked variations in the caliber of the afferent arteriole generate a variable pressure gradient that compensates for fluctuations in renal artery pressures, maintaining constant the hydraulic pressures available for filtration of plasma and the formation of tubular fluid.

tle evidence that resting vascular tone is neurally or adrenergically maintained.[7]

Increases in renovascular resistance (RVR) occur as part of the pathologic syndromes of chronic arterial hypertension or pre-eclampsia,[8] during short-term generalized increases in sympathoadrenal outflow, or as part of the compensatory hemodynamic response to circulating hypovolemia and arterial hypotension,[9] particularly if associated with reduced left atrial pressure.[10] The renal vasculature is, in fact, predominantly an α-adrenergic vasoconstrictor system, although renovascular smooth muscle has abundant dopaminergic receptor sites and some β-adrenergic responsiveness.

RVR is probably near minimal values at blood pressures just below those of normal arterial pressure, but increases markedly when the kidney participates in generalized catecholamine-mediated sympathoadrenal responses. These properties appear to protect the fragile glomerular capillary filtration apparatus from hydrostatic damage due to arterial hypertension. They also subject the kidney to the risk of ischemic injury during arterial hypotension or prolonged states of stress.

α-Agonist activity in the renal vasculature is normally moderated by the counteracting renal vasodilator effects of localized dopamine and endogenous prostacyclin release.[11]

Renovascular resistance is determined almost entirely by the diameters of the afferent and efferent glomerular capillary arterioles. Within a range of mean arterial blood pressure from 80 to about 180 mm Hg, the absolute and relative diameters of these vascular structures, therefore, determine both glomerular capillary flow and the pressure within the filtration apparatus, respectively. Consequently, both RPF and glomerular filtration rate (GFR) are intrinsically autoregulated and relatively independent of systemic blood pressures.

When systemic arterial pressure approaches the lower limit of effectiveness for renovascular autoregulation, the predominant site of vascular resistance, as judged by the pressure gradient across the glomerular arterioles, shifts from the afferent to the efferent site (see Fig 9–1). Subsequent maintenance of intraluminal capillary pressures at near-normal values despite decreased RPF is accompanied by increases in the fraction of RPF that is filtered. Increased filtration fraction, therefore, augments the effectiveness of renovascular autoregulation and further minimizes fluctuations in the rate of tubular fluid formation even when RBF itself has begun to decline because of arterial hypotension. Changes in glomerular capillary permeability may play a significant role in this compensatory mechanism.[4]

Under most conditions the kidney reabsorbs a constant fraction, at least 99%, of the sodium that is filtered. The mechanism for the "glomerulotubular balance" that maintains sodium reabsorption in proportion to the filtered load remains poorly understood. The daily volume of filtered plasma is four to five times that of total body water, however, so that even with this degree of efficiency an additional mechanism for stabilization of GFR is required to minimize the possibility of net sodium loss. Total sodium reabsorption ultimately reflects additional factors that interact to "fine-tune" total body sodium homeostasis, although virtually all adaptive responses to hyponatremia, contracted plasma volume, or reduced plasma osmolality involve direct or indirect increases in afferent glomerular arteriolar tone. This mechanism reduces GFR and renal medullary blood flow, further minimizing both sodium filtration and its subsequent excretion into urine.[3]

Tubular Reabsorption

Under normal conditions the proximal tubule provides for the isosmolar reabsorption of large volumes of filtered plasma. With some modulation by natriuretic hormone, PTH, and perhaps catecholamines, this segment of the nephron is responsible for reabsorption of 60% to 70% of all filtered sodium, potassium, and water, and as much as 90% of filtered bicarbonate. In addition, the proximal tubule is the site at which glucose, amino acids, and divalent ions reenter the peritubular circulation. The proximal tubule is also responsible for secretion of hydrogen ions and a variety of organic acids and bases.[12]

An additional one fourth to one third of filtered sodium and potassium undergo reabsorption further along the nephron in the thin or ascending limb of Henle's loop, another site at which divalent cations are reabsorbed. From this point onward, the functional characteristics of the tubular components of the nephron change from those of high-volume water and solute transport against low electrochemical gradients, to those providing for both the active and the passive movements of small volumes of water and solute against large osmotic and electrochemical gradients.

Zones of hypertonicity established with sodium and urea in the extremely vascular renal medulla provide a "countercurrent multiplier" effect that permits final passive adjustments of urine osmolality under hormonal control.[13] The distal and collecting tubules and the collecting ducts into which they coalesce are the anatomic sites at which water is passively reabsorbed from tubular fluid under the control of ADH. Most of the small fraction of filtered sodium not already reabsorbed in bulk isosmotic form in the proximal tubules is selectively and actively exchanged for hydrogen ions and potassium under the influence of aldosterone, and calcium and phosphorus are also reabsorbed here.

Tubular Secretion

The kidneys not only regulate the volume and composition of body fluids by maintaining salt and water homeostasis but also fulfill essential excretory functions. Urea synthesized in the liver from ammonia and other nitrogenous by-products of protein and amino acid metabolism is filtered, along with other small molecules, into tubular fluid. One half of the filtered load of urea is excreted; the remainder is reabsorbed and concentrated into renal medullary tissues to facilitate the osmotic dehydration of tubular fluid as it passes through the medullary renal zones.

Consequently, inadequate urea production due to hepatic failure or dietary protein or amino acid deficiency may limit urinary concentrating ability. Ammonia itself is an important buffer, required for efficient excretion of hydrogen ions into tubular fluid. Generated within renal tubular epithelium by the metabolism of glutamine, ammonia facilitates renal excretion of the nonvolatile acids produced by the metabolism of a wide range of organic substances.

Additional "titratable" acid is carried into urine in combination with phosphate. The primary determinant of metabolic acid-base status remains the plasma concentration of bicarbonate, however.[14] Carbonic anhydrase catalyzes the combination of water and carbon dioxide in renal tissues to produce carbonic acid. Subsequent dissociation of this molecule generates bicarbonate, mostly retained in tissues and in plasma, and hydrogen ions, which are then secreted into tubular fluid and buffered there by ammonia. Almost all filtered bicarbonate is reabsorbed from the proximal tubule, although the process appears to vary in effectiveness in direct proportion to arterial carbon dioxide tensions. Acidification of urine is also needed to maintain total body stores of potassium, since there is reciprocal exchange of these two cations in the renal tubules.

Renin and the Juxtaglomerular Apparatus

Other renal functions, although not directly related to salt and water excretion, nevertheless contribute to the homeostasis of oxygen transport to all organ systems by influencing control of circulating blood volume. The erythropoietin required to maintain hemoglobin at normal levels is of renal origin. In addition, the juxtaglomerular apparatus (JGA) of the kidney is the unique source of renin, a powerful intrarenal and systemic vasoconstrictor substance and mediator of body fluid and tissue composition.

The JGA is a cluster of closely associated cells derived from both afferent renal arteriolar endothelium and distal tubular epithelium. It is the anatomic site of synthesis, release, and feedback control for this proteolytic enzyme: renin converts a hepatically synthesized polypeptide into angiotensin I, which is then further catabolized in the lung into angiotensin II. A powerful vasoconstrictor, angiotensin II is also a stimulant for the secretion of aldosterone, which initiates sodium retention in the distal tubule.[15]

The enzyme that converts angiotensin I to angiotensin II is present in renal as well as in pulmonary tissues. It may be a hormonal component of the intrarenal control mechanism that autoregulates RBF by varying RVR in response to changes in renal artery pressure, or to variations in urine flow through the distal tubules. Changes in the geometry of the cells of the JGA produced by distention or collapse of the walls of the afferent glomerular arteriole or the distal tubule link renin secretion mechanically to renal perfusion and GFR. Renin production by the JGA granular cells, in fact, is the rate-limiting step in the renin-angiotensin sequence, since the polypeptides it produces are degraded promptly within the kidney itself.[16]

Consequently, the JGA is in appropriate anatomic, physiologic, and biochemical proximity to the general status of the nephron to provide an effective feedback control mechanism for renin-modulated RVR.[17] Activity of this system appears to be stimulated further by adrenergic mechanisms[17, 18] and interrupted by β-adrenergic blockade,[15] a characteristic useful in the treatment of systemic hypertension caused by derangement of the renin-angiotensin mechanism. Local synthesis and release of prostacyclins may act to limit renin-mediated vasoconstriction and to minimize the risk of ischemia during periods of intense renin-angiotensin activation.[11, 19, 20]

HOMEOSTASIS OF BODY WATER AND OSMOLALITY

The regulation of both extracellular fluid volume and tissue osmolality is accomplished through multiple feedback control systems for sodium and for water balance, respectively. Renal tubular mechanisms for filtration, secretion, and reabsorption are effector components in both systems. However, the complex afferent and integrative pathways of these systems, although interrelated, are physiologically distinct (Fig 9–2).

Assuming modest dietary salt intake, maintaining the volume of the sodium-rich extracellular fluid (ECF) requires stable GFR and reabsorption of almost all filtered sodium, conditions provided by the mechanisms for autoregulation of renal blood flow and persistence of glomerulotubular balance, described earlier in this chapter. Minute changes in the extent to which even a fraction of 1% of filtered sodium is conserved ultimately determine the efficacy of body sodium homeostasis and the ability of the kidney to excrete a sodium load, or to restore a sodium deficit.

Effective Arterial Blood Volume

Because it is the primary solute of plasma and other components of ECF, sodium largely determines ECF volume and effective arterial blood volume (EABV), a conceptual merging of blood volume, interstitial fluid, and other ECF compartments that exist in dynamic equilib-

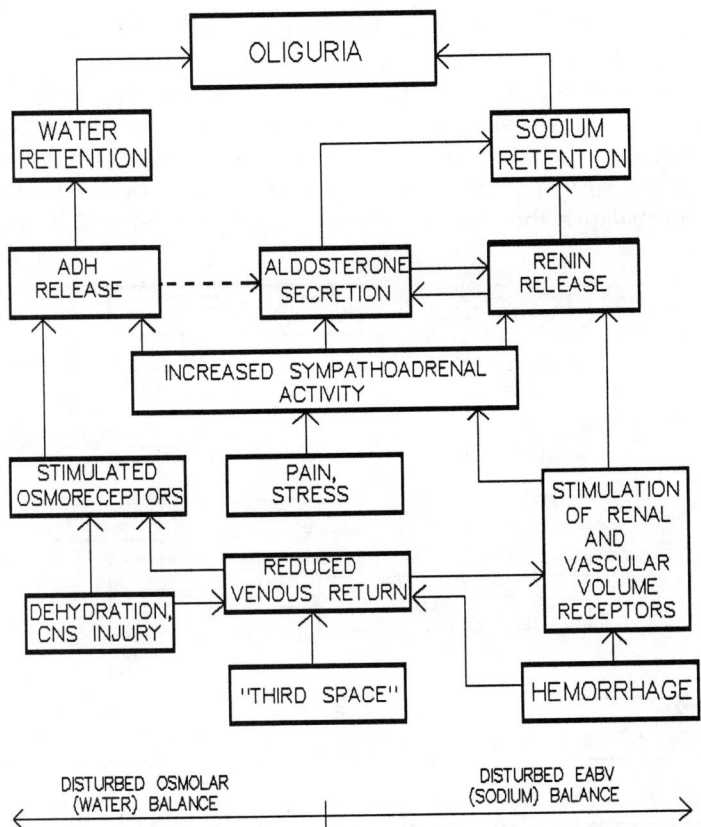

FIG 9–2.
Interaction of mechanisms for homeostasis of effective arterial blood volume *(EABV)* and plasma osmolality. These mechanisms primarily promote retention of salt and of water, respectively. Disturbance of either system initiates a sequence of compensatory mechanisms that ultimately produce oliguria, especially in a setting of enhanced sympathoadrenal tone and tissue injury. *Dashed line* indicates the relative inhibition of aldosterone effect by antidiuretic hormone *(ADH).*

rium. Arterial baroreceptors provide indirect monitoring of body fluid volumes, responding to the dynamic changes in hydrostatic pressure within the cardiovascular system that are ultimately determined by intravascular and cardiac chamber volumes. The precise regulation of sodium concentration, and therefore of EABV, is finally achieved through renal mechanisms, however.

The two essential central determinants of sodium, ECF, and EABV homeostasis are the activity of the JGA-renin system, which is a final common pathway for multiple inputs from both intrarenal and extrinsic sources, and the secretion of aldosterone produced by stimulation of the adrenal cortex by adrenocorticotropic hormone (ACTH) (Fig 9–3). The hierarchy of input to the JGA is not well understood. Renal prostaglandins, prostacyclin in particular, appear to contribute an important antagonist action, offsetting renal vasoconstriction in response to deficits of EABV, but may also have intrinsic natriuretic properties that counterbalance the intense sodium retention produced by aldos-

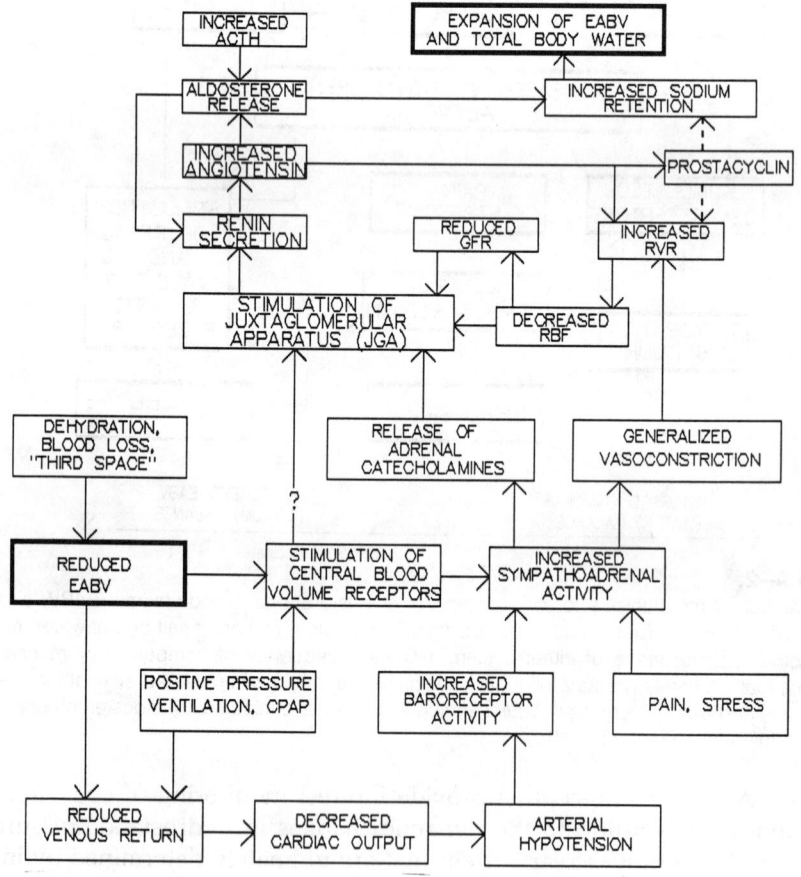

FIG 9–3.

Homeostasis of total body water and effective arterial blood volume *(EABV)*. Increases in renovascular resistance *(RVR)* produce decreased renal blood flow *(RBF)* and reduced glomerular filtration rate *(GFR)*. These changes stimulate the juxtaglomerular apparatus *(JGA)* and activate the renin-angiotensin-aldosterone system. *Dashed lines* indicate competing vasodilator effects of prostacyclin that reduce the likelihood of renin-induced renal ischemia during this sequence of events.

terone.[21] A mineralocorticoid hormone, aldosterone, acts at distal tubular sites and also participates in a positive feedback loop with renin. This enhances the "gain" of this control system: contraction of ECF and EABV accelerates the rate at which sodium is retained and EABV ultimately reexpanded.

The JGA responds to nonrenal as well as to renal output. Generalized sympathoadrenal stimulation triggered by pain or psychologic stress, or the initiation of an autonomic stress response to arterial hypotension, activates the renin-angiotensin system. A more direct link between intracardiac blood volume, mechanoreceptors in the left atrium, and the JGA may provide an additional mechanism by which blood volume homeostasis is maintained. Failure of β-adrenergic blockade to alleviate arterial hypertension in some patients despite reductions in plasma renin secretion suggests a relative deficiency of renal prostacyclin due to intrinsic renal disease or to the renal dysfunction associated with toxemia of pregnancy.[22]

Osmolar Homeostasis

The function of body tissues is exquisitely sensitive to osmolar gradients. Plasma and tissue osmolalities are therefore tightly controlled by a complex system of autonomic and neurohumoral pathways (Fig 9–4). The regulation of body water balance by renal mechanisms is determined largely by the activity of central nervous system osmoreceptors. These specialized hypothalamic sensor cells initiate the release of ADH from neurohypophyseal stores and also generate a sensation of thirst in response to increases in serum osmolality as small as 1%.

The short half-life of ADH ensures rapid responsiveness to changing states of hydration. The expression of the full range of achievable circulating ADH concentrations over a range of plasma osmolality that is less than 20 mOsm also provides a high level of gain, ensuring prompt restoration of normal tonicity.[23] ADH increases the permeability of collecting tubules to water and increases its passive osmotic movement into the hypertonic renal medulla, thus reducing urinary volume and increasing the residual concentration of solute in tubular fluid. The active mechanisms that maintain high renal medullary osmotic concentrations ensure the movement of this additional retained water into peritubular plasma, and subsequently into venous return.

ADH plays a central role in the normal homeostasis of ECF composition, but it may also contribute to a syndrome characterized by severe disruption of body water and solute balance. Syndromes of inappropriate ADH secretion (SIADH) are associated with various forms of cen-

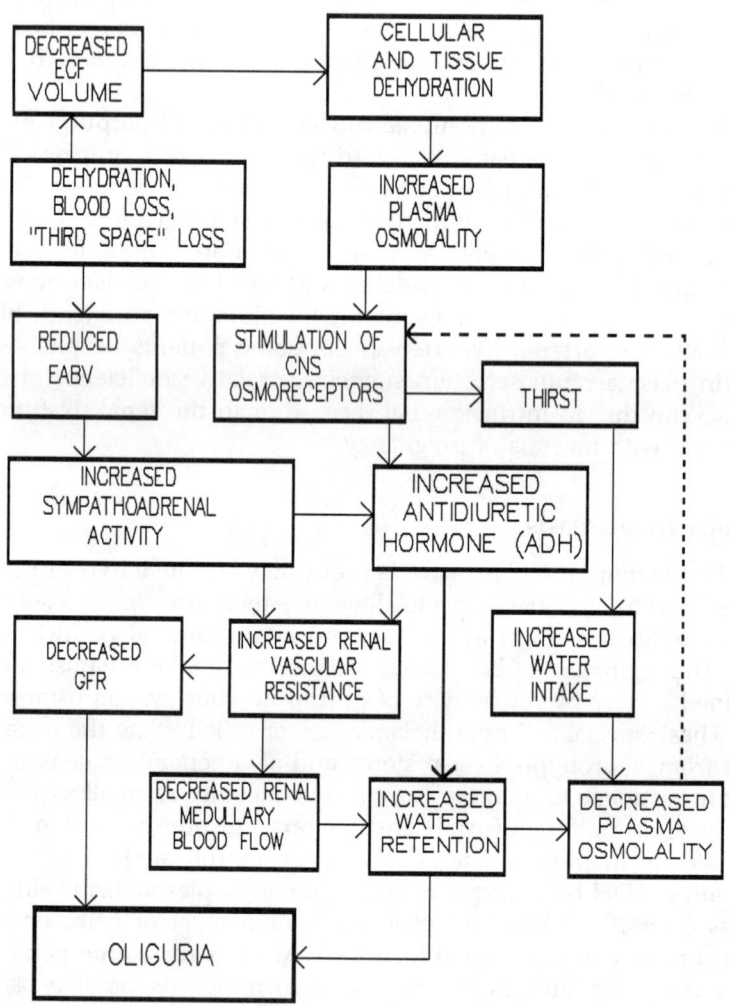

FIG 9–4.
Homeostasis of tissue and plasma osmolality. Hypertonicity and decreased volume of extracellular fluid *(ECF)*, reduced effective arterial blood volume *(EABV)*, or a fall in glomerular filtration rate *(GFR)* can all trigger a sequence of responses leading to increased retention of water and stimulation of intake by enhanced sensation of thirst. Falling plasma osmolality exerts an inhibitory effect *(dashed line)* on central osmoreceptors that suppresses pituitary secretion of antidiuretic hormone *(ADH)* and thereby accelerates loss of free water from the distal tubule.

tral nervous system injury. Exaggerated vascular sensitivity to the vasoconstrictor effects of this hormone may contribute to the severe arterial hypertension that characterizes preeclampsia and eclampsia of pregnancy.[24] Under normal conditions, however, the actions of ADH as a generalized vasoconstrictor appear to be offset by local effects of prostaglandins[25] and produce only minor adjustments of regional renal blood flow. The most important physiologic aspects of this hormone are its ability to alter permeability to water at glomerular and tubular sites and to inhibit the release of renin, limiting the salt retention produced by this hormone.

In general, deficits of ECF or a reduction in EABV initiate aldosterone and renin secretion and a sequence of other sodium-retaining responses. After restoration of ECF or EABV, adjustments of tissue and plasma osmolality are accomplished primarily by variations in circulating concentrations of ADH. In effect, ECF volume is maintained through alterations of sodium balance, and its composition subsequently adjusted by changes in the rate of water intake and excretion. In the hierarchy of autonomic control, volumetric (sodium) homeostasis appears to be accorded the higher priority: acute isosmolar volume deficits produce immediate and marked increases in both the activity of the renin-aldosterone axis and in the rate of secretion of ADH. In fact, both systems are fundamentally interrelated because they share baroreceptor input, responsiveness to the prevailing level of sympathoadrenal activation, the reciprocal interaction between ADH and the renin-angiotensin system, and the frequency with which oliguria is a final common pathway of the compensatory response (Fig 9–2).

TESTS OF RENAL FUNCTION

Glomerular Filtration Rate

The great redundancy of renal tissue provides sufficient functional reserve that less than one half of the normal complement of nephrons is required for clinically normal function. Reductions in GFR, however, occur in direct proportion to the number of functioning nephrons (Fig 9–5). The ability to handle a salt or water challenge may be reduced in patients with renal insufficiency, even though serum creatinine, blood urea nitrogen (BUN), and even baseline urine flow rates are generally maintained within normal limits until two thirds of the renal tissue mass has become dysfunctional. Decreased skeletal muscle mass in el-

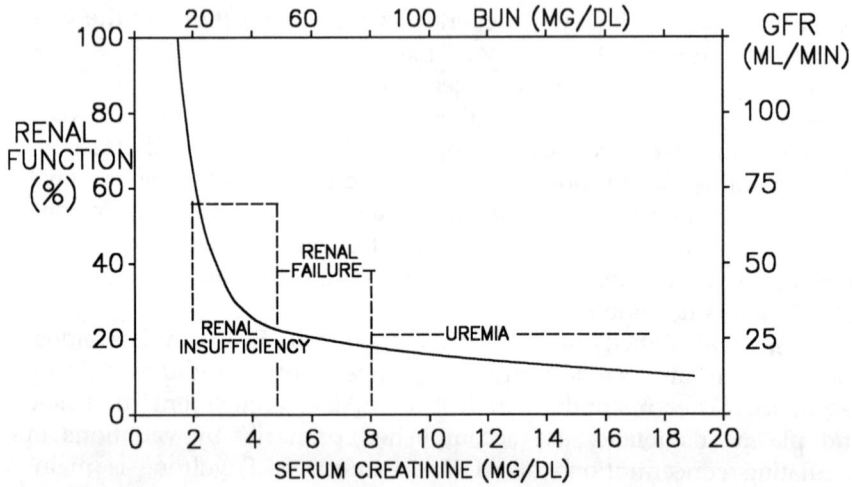

FIG 9–5.
Nonlinear relationship between serum creatinine or blood urea nitrogen *(BUN)* concentrations and renal function as quantified by glomerular filtration rate *(GFR)*. Renal failure implies creatinine values greater than 5 mg/dL; uremia is defined as values greater than 8 mg/dL. Normal creatinine and *BUN* values do not necessarily indicate normal renal function or full renal functional reserve.

derly patients may also reduce creatinine load sufficiently to mask significant renal impairment. Consequently, considerable renal compromise can be overlooked clinically if no measurements of GFR are available. Creatinine clearance, a less accurate reflection of GFR than inulin clearance, is nevertheless a more practical technique in the clinical setting.[26]

GFR may be estimated indirectly through serial measurements of creatinine, but these require correction for age, weight, and state of hydration. Serum creatinine concentrations reflect the balance between creatinine generated by muscle metabolism and its subsequent renal filtration and urinary excretion. Because there is active tubular secretion of creatinine, the relationship between serum creatinine and GFR resembles a hyperbola, with creatinine levels rising minimally until a marked compromise in renal function has occurred. Given the wide range of normal creatinine values encountered clinically, only serial measurements or simultaneous determinations of GFR are likely to detect mild to moderate renal impairment in patients who do not have an obvious history of renal dysfunction at initial presentation.[27]

Blood Urea Nitrogen

BUN reflects dynamic equilibrium between renal function, protein metabolism, and the state of overall hydration. Increased ADH secretion in response to rising plasma osmolality enhances the medullary reabsorption of urea and improves the efficiency with which water is retained and the urine maximally concentrated. This mechanism produces a reduction in the overall amount of nitrogenous waste that is excreted, however, and BUN may rise markedly under these conditions, even in patients with normal renal function. A similar situation may occur with increased dietary protein intake, or after the breakdown of large amounts of blood or other protein-containing tissues in the course of recovery from trauma or sepsis.

These errors can be minimized by evaluating the ratio of BUN to serum creatinine: ratios greater than 10 suggest increased urea formation, or a concentrating effect due to dehydration. A lower ratio implies declining hepatic synthesis of urea from ammonia, increased creatinine after an extensive muscle injury, or a dilutional effect related to overhydration or the inappropriate secretion of ADH.

Tubular Functions and Urine Volume

The assessment of renal tubular function is limited primarily to measurements of the specific gravity or osmolality of urine. Because of the wide variety of inputs that mediate the continuous adjustment of total body water and of plasma osmolality, the response of the renal tubules to a water load or to severe water deprivation provides less ambiguous information regarding renal function than do simple spot checks of urine specific gravity. The only continuous monitor of renal function currently practical for routine intraoperative management, however, is assessment of volumetric urinary output.[26]

The presence of urine flow itself, by definition, confirms the existence of some degree of renal plasma flow, although it is not directly indicative of the extent to which renal perfusion meets the metabolic requirements of these tissues. Oliguria may be an appropriate response of normal kidneys to acute isosmolar depletion of EABV, but must be considered indicative of renal dysfunction until proved otherwise.

The likelihood of renal ischemia can be excluded largely by confirmation of adequate urine flow and cardiac output in conjunction with normal arterial blood pressure. Even when renal blood flow is adequate for metabolic requirements, however, urine flow may cease during controlled hypotensive anesthetic techniques if vasodilator agents produce glomerular pressures too low for net filtration of renal plasma. Failure to resume normal urine flow once arterial blood pressure has returned to normal levels and cardiovascular homeostasis has been re-established, however, suggests renal injury and intrinsic insufficiency. This diagnosis can be confirmed by subsequent comparisons of urinary and plasma solute concentrations that show an inappropriately dilute urine. Although the value of diuretic agents for prophylaxis against re-nal insufficiency remains controversial, lack of diuresis in response to these drugs after a period of oliguria suggests that a state of acute renal failure has, in fact, occurred.

Renal Insufficiency and Failure

The complexity of the vascular and tubular structures within the kidney provides numerous opportunities for damage, dysfunction, and failure of this organ system. Acute renal insufficiency (ARI) and acute renal failure (ARF) differ only in the degree of functional disruption. ARI is applied to states of inadequate urinary concentration and mild elevation of creatinine or BUN; ARF describes a more general deterioration of renal function and a loss of biochemical homeostasis.[28]

ARF usually implies not only an inadequate rate of urine formation but also compromised excretion of metabolic by-products, and electrolyte and acid-base abnormalities. Traditionally, ARF has been subdivided, according to the presumed cause, as renal (intrinsic or parenchymal), prerenal (ischemic), or postrenal (extrinsic, or obstructive). Modifying these categories further are additional descriptors of the abnormal rates of urine flow with which they may be associated: oliguria (50 to 400 mL/day), anuria (less than 50 mL/day), or polyuria (greater than 2,500 mL/day).

Acute Tubular Necrosis

The most common yet complex form of perioperative ARF is acute tubular necrosis (ATN), recently termed *vasomotor nephropathy* to emphasize the role of afferent arteriolar vasoconstriction in this disorder. About one half of all cases of ARF are related to trauma or surgery; fully 80% of these probably reflect ischemic damage to renal tubular cells because of inadequate renal perfusion during hypovolemic or cardiogenic shock states.

The mechanism by which renal dysfunction is perpetuated even after restoration of RBF remains controversial. A unitary theory of ATN suggests that ischemic damage to both tubular and capillary endothelial cells is involved.[29] Injured vascular smooth muscle cells swell, reducing luminal arteriolar diameter, increasing RVR, and limiting RPF (Fig 9–6). Leakage of calcium from adjacent injured cells may produce localized afferent arteriolar vasospasm in the remaining functional nephrons.

Simultaneously, production of metabolic energy under anaerobic or hypoxic conditions may be inadequate to support the essential solute pumping functions of the tubular epithelium, producing cellular swelling and edema that further obstruct the flow of tubular fluid. Finally, the back-leakage of filtered plasma may damage the glomerular capillary itself. ARF or ATN due to nephrotoxins or to intrarenal tubular obstruction by crystals of precipitated drug, or by massive myoglobinemia or hemoglobinemia, could conceivably initiate a similar sequence of events.

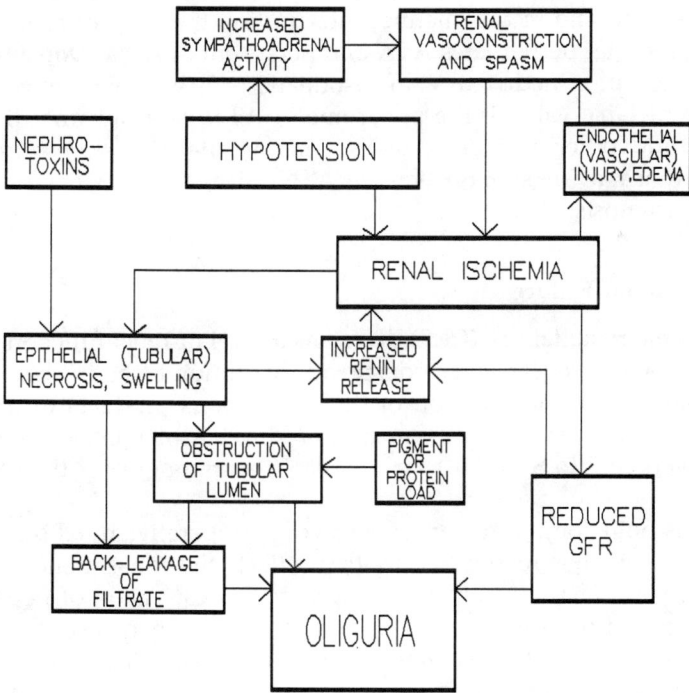

FIG 9–6.
Pathogenesis of oliguria in acute tubular necrosis (ATN) due to ischemic or toxic insult. Vascular and tubular injury are interrelated by mechanical, metabolic, and neurohumoral mechanisms that eventually serve to perpetuate renal dysfunction long after the original insult has been removed.

In its earliest stages, ATN, especially if nonoliguric, may be reversible.[29, 30] Prolonged reduction of urine flow or delay in treatment, however, is associated with high mortality, especially in elderly patients or in those with multiple organ system disorders.[26] Prevention of this syndrome by the continued maintenance of adequate renal perfusion and arterial oxygenation is far more efficacious than attempts to limit or reverse the renal injury with which it is associated. Once an ischemic renal insult has occurred, prompt restoration of adequate renal perfusion and oxygenation remains the cornerstone of current therapy if the ATN is due to prerenal causes.

Furosemide and ethacrynic acid are "loop" diuretics that inhibit reabsorption of chloride and sodium from the ascending limb of Henle's loop; in patients with ATN, they may reestablish urine flow and limit tubular damage due to stasis and subsequent tubular collapse. Mannitol also maintains the flow of tubular fluid, retaining water osmotically within the tubular lumen, suppressing the release of renin from the JGA, and in this manner interrupting the cycle of renal vasoconstriction that perpetuates ATN and persistent oliguria. Dopamine to produce receptor-mediated renal vasodilation[31] is widely employed but of unpredictable value if the syndrome of ATN is far advanced. Gentamicin and other aminoglycosides demonstrate direct renal tubular toxicity that may be synergistic with ATN, increasing injury and influencing prognosis.

Chronic Renal Failure

Chronic renal failure (CRF) describes a level of renal function inadequate to avoid severe and widespread disruption of body solute and water balance or the retention of the nitrogenous products of protein metabolism. Severe renal dysfunction produces azotemia (serum creatinine levels of 2 to 8 mg/dL), or uremia (creatinine greater than 8 mg/dL).[32]

If it is not a long-term consequence of perioperative renal ischemia, CRF is essentially a medical entity that reflects the consequences of infectious, inflammatory, hypertensive, or toxic destruction of nephrons by a variety of nonsurgical disease processes. CRF may also be due to the vascular and metabolic changes associated with diabetes mellitus, polycystic renal disease, autoimmune or collagen disorders, or numerous other, less common sources of renal injury. When present as a pre-existing medical condition, CRF complicates perioperative management and may predispose to additional renal compromise intraoperatively because it increases susceptibility to ischemia and to the direct toxicity of organic or inorganic substances.[33]

Even extensive renal tissue loss does not appear to disrupt glomerulotubular balance. The components of each nephron are part of an interactive and functionally integrated unit that maintains a constant reabsorbed fraction of filtered sodium unless nephron loss is sufficiently severe to reduce GFR to less than 40 mL/min.[34] With continued decline of renal function, however, the total amount of sodium filtered is so small that it produces a generalized state of sodium retention and subsequent expansion of EABV. Hormonal mechanisms for volume homeostasis maximize sodium loss under these circumstances by increasing the rate of natriuresis within those nephrons that remain functional, but the total amount of sodium excreted becomes inadequate to reestablish EABV at normal values. Consequently, a new state of dynamic equilibrium is achieved in patients with CRF that is characterized by expanded ECF and chronic arterial hypertension.

Minimal capacity for sodium conservation is a hallmark of CRF because of the continual suppression of sodium-retaining mechanisms in the small remaining number of intact nephrons. Patients with CRF are, therefore, at high risk of water intoxication: the high rate of sodium loss prohibits selective excretion of free water and makes it nearly impossible to handle a water challenge. Low GFR also limits the total volume of tubular fluid that can be formed and therefore reduces the maximal rate at which water can be excreted, regardless of the dilution of tubular fluid.

Water intoxication in patients with CRF may not respond to simple restriction of water intake because these patients have isosthenuria, inability to generate urine with solute concentrations either greater, or less, than those of filtered plasma. Sodium loads are handled as poorly as states of sodium deprivation because solute excretion is severely compromised by markedly reduced GFR. Filtered volumes may decline even further if JGA stimulation is produced by the collapse of distal tubules after severe oliguria; the response may be sufficient to stimulate angiotensin-mediated renal vasoconstriction. Reasonable osmotic balance and homeostasis of EABV, however, are adequately maintained by most patients with CRF if they are provided appropriate, and consistent, dietary salt and water intake.

Filtered sodium is actively reabsorbed, primarily in exchange for potassium. Consequently, the relative natriuresis associated with CRF also produces hyperkalemia resulting from impaired rates of potassium excretion. Like sodium, potassium loads are therefore handled poorly by patients at almost every stage of CRF. Increased fecal potassium loss and reduced fractional reabsorption of potassium from tubular fluid usually maintain adequate basal potassium homeostasis, however, until there has been an almost total loss of renal function.

Metabolic acidosis due to inadequate excretion of nonvolatile acids is also a preterminal phenomenon. In patients with CRF, increased reabsorption of bicarbonate and reduced arterial carbon dioxide tensions compensate for impaired hydrogen-ion excretion and maintain blood pH near normal levels only if there are no imposed acid loads or accelerated losses of bicarbonate from the kidney or the gastrointestinal tract.

Uremia

Uremia (literally, "urine in the blood") appropriately describes the inadequate excretion of metabolic waste products by patients with end-stage renal dysfunction. Although the predominant toxin has yet to be specifically and unequivocally identified,[35] uremia produces a significant and generalized metabolic disruption of cardiovascular, pulmonary, hepatic, gastrointestinal, endocrine, hematologic, and nervous system functions. It is clear that there is disruption of neurohumoral control of body fluid volume, but many hypertensive patients with CRF do not have excessive plasma levels of renin. Either a more complex hormonal mechanism is involved, or arterial hypertension is due primarily to sodium-induced increases in ECF and EABV directly attributable to severe compromise of GFR.

Uremia can produce a cardiomyopathy. The hyperkalemia common in these patients also increases their risk of cardiac dysrhythmias,[36] although increased serum potassium levels do not themselves further depress cardiac contractility.[37] To the contrary, the anemia associated with CRF increases volumetric perfusion requirements superimposed on a pathologic, renally driven increase in the level of sympathoadrenal activity, which usually produces increased cardiac index despite an elevated systemic vascular resistance.

The mechanism by which CRF, but not ARF, produces anemia is complex but almost certainly involves decreased production of erythropoietin because of destruction or the toxic inhibition of the renal parenchyma.[32] It is perpetuated or aggravated by associated toxic hemolytic processes and by deficiencies of iron and other components needed for normal synthesis of hemoglobin.

Pulmonary vascular changes in uremia may either be primary or due to the pulmonary hypertension and congestive heart failure associated with chronic expansion of EABV. Whatever the cause, these changes further compromise the delivery of oxygen to body tissues by reducing the efficiency of molecular gas exchange within the uremic lung. Central nervous system toxicity is also a common feature of end-stage CRF. In addition to the autonomic disruption just described, uremia may also produce motor dysfunction in the form of weakness, tetanus, and tremor, as well as paresthesias and musculoskeletal irritation, including chronic hiccups. Uremic encephalopathy and seizure disorders usually require drug therapy for adequate control.

The gastrointestinal abnormalities seen with uremia also largely reflect a generalized neuropathy, and include nausea, vomiting, anorexia, and the appearance of chronic gastrointestinal inflammation at multiple sites. There may be an additional role played by unexcreted nitrogenous compounds directly. Skeletal abnormalities produced by CRF and uremia include renal osteodystrophy, with reabsorption of bone due to a deficiency of vitamin D, calcium, and phosphates, and an autonomous elevation of parathyroid hormone levels. Coagulopathy, impaired platelet function, and compromised immune responsiveness may also complicate management of patients with renal failure who have become uremic.

PERIOPERATIVE RENAL FUNCTION

Surprisingly little is known about the mechanisms by which general and regional anesthesia alter urine flow or tubular function. The kidney has been treated largely as a "black box," since input and output are measurable. However, there are few continuous indices of the specific alterations, if any, imposed by this environment on the kidneys' ability to handle water or solute, or on changes in renal tissue metabolism.

Variability in the extent to which the kidneys are subject to intense sympathoadrenal stimulation, circulating vasoactive and mineralocorticoid hormone levels, and abrupt changes in vascular and tubular volumes and pressures further complicates the delineation of primary from coincident changes in perioperative renal function. It is equally difficult to distinguish between initial events and subsequent compensatory renal responses to processes such as anesthetic induction or to distinguish them from agent-specific changes due to the direct effects of the anesthetic drugs themselves. Nevertheless, a state of general anesthesia usually produces relative oliguria.[38]

Renal Blood Flow

Although the extent to which urine flow is reduced is highly variable, it is widely assumed to be a consequence of the reductions in RBF that have been reported consistently in anesthetized subjects.[39] RBF usually falls to a lesser degree than does arterial blood pressure, at least in sedated or lightly anesthetized subjects without surgical stimulation.[40]

The decline in RBF during surgical levels of anesthesia, however, is sufficiently great to suggest that the autoregulation of renal perfusion under those circumstances is either rudimentary or easily abolished by the direct effects of many anesthetics.[41] Under these conditions RBF appears to be largely a passive function of arterial pressure. RBF and urinary output may remain significantly reduced even when blood pressure is returned to normal levels, however, if this hemodynamic adjustment is achieved with use of an anesthetic technique that produces generalized increases in sympathoadrenal stimulation and a subsequent elevation of RVR.[42]

Marked increases in RVR and the subsequent reductions of RBF produced by acute stress responses to pain may be moderated by narcotic analgesia.[43] In fact, the pharmacologic sympathectomy of epidural anesthesia has also been shown to minimize reductions in RBF due to sympathetically mediated renovascular constriction, provided that arterial hypotension is avoided.[44] Assuming a benign cardiovascular environment, general anesthesia can be expected to produce a modest decline in RBF of about 20% to 30%, with a lesser reduction of GFR because of increases in filtration fraction.[39, 45]

Direct renovascular dilation by halothane[46] occurs, but this phenomenon does not maintain or increase RPF beyond control levels because this agent also produces some reduction of systemic arterial perfusion pressures. The use of *p*-aminohippurate to measure RPF in the presence of inhalational anesthesia may underestimate RPF significantly.[47] Reports of profound reductions in RBF during apparently uncomplicated general anesthesia[41] may therefore actually reflect technical difficulties in the accurate measurement of renal function during anesthesia.

Other Factors

In general, changes in RBF and GFR are therefore process-specific and largely independent of the anesthetic agent selected. Changes in urine flow rates and composition reflect both the reduced GFR associated with coincident hemodynamic changes and the altered hormonal environment that accompanies pain and perioperative stress. Stimulation of ADH secretion by contraction of EABV or by the neuroendocrine response to pain augments the consequences of reduced RPF and

GFR, and is at least in part responsible for the oliguria and increased urinary osmolality common in anesthetized subjects.[48] The same mechanism may mediate the oliguria of patients requiring postoperative mechanical ventilation.[49]

Another consistent, predictable, but indirect effect of anesthesia on renal function is increased renin secretion and subsequent activation of angiotensin II and release of aldosterone. The secretion of renin from the JGA is not immediate; a prolonged interval is required for both the release of renin and its subsequent disappearance, suggesting that it is a component of a more fundamental, autonomically integrated response to reduced venous return and disturbed cardiovascular homeostasis than other events. Stress-enhanced secretion of ADH from the central nervous system, in contrast, is rapid enough to augment the acute effects of increased sympathoadrenal activity. Together, these two primary processes appear to explain the generalized phenomenon of oliguria associated with anesthesia and surgery when there is no evidence of arterial hypotension, ischemia, or other mechanisms that can reduce RPF.

Anesthetic Nephrotoxicity

Less commonly, anesthetics have direct effects on renal tissues that are manifestations of toxicity. The addition of halogens to the structure of inhalational anesthetic molecules increases their potency and decreases flammability, making them suitable for use in modern operating rooms. However, biotransformation of fluoride-containing agents by hepatic dehalogenation through inducible pathways generates inorganic fluoride, an ionic species that may damage the proximal convoluted segments of the nephron tubule.

The clinical consequence of fluoride toxicity is acute polyuric renal failure due to impaired reabsorption of glomerular ultrafiltrate.[38] Secondarily, abnormally high rates of urine flow through the more distal tubular segments and overwhelm the mechanisms responsible for selective solute reabsorption and secretion. Inability to concentrate urine even in response to a challenge with exogenous ADH has been demonstrated with plasma fluoride levels as low as 30 μmole/L after enflurane anesthesia.[50] The severity of renal injury produced by inorganic fluoride is a function of the local concentration of this ion within the renal tubules. Consequently the nephrotoxic potential of a general anesthetic agent depends on the extent to which its molecular structure is subject to enzymatic defluorination, the inspired concentration and duration of anesthetic exposure, adequacy of prevailing GFR, and the specific activity and induction state of hepatic microsomal pathways.[51]

More than one quarter of the total administered dose of methoxyflurane undergoes hepatic biotransformation, a fraction sufficiently large that high-output renal failure is a predictable consequence of prolonged exposure to this agent.[52] In contrast, less than 5% of enflurane is usually metabolized; generally low, serum fluoride levels are, however, extremely variable. Consequently, this agent is contraindicated in patients with preexisting renal disease in whom low initial GFR may concentrate the fluoride ions in tubular fluid to toxic levels.[53] The induction of hepatic microsomal enzyme pathways by isoniazid, tetracycline, or the enhanced hepatocellular activity associated with obesity may also predispose to nephrotoxic fluoride levels after exposure to clinically appropriate inspired concentrations of enflurane.[54, 55] Neither halothane nor isoflurane generates significant amounts of inorganic fluoride, and thus they do not appear to have nephrotoxic potential.[50, 56]

Postoperative Salt and Water Balance

The extent to which stress-mediated changes in neuroendocrine state dominate renal function and urine formation is dramatically evident in the patterns of salt and water balance seen postoperatively. RBF usually returns promptly to normal levels in normotensive patients with adequate cardiac output. Nevertheless, transient salt and water retention is almost inevitable perioperatively. Pain and anxiety produce continued stimulation of salt- and water-retaining mechanisms, although surgically traumatized tissues do release prostaglandins that promote natriuresis, antagonize the actions of ADH at the collecting tubules,[25] and accelerate the reestablishment of normal intrarenal distribution of blood flow.[19] Perioperative fluid resuscitation with large volumes of albumin or other colloids or inadequate hydration with balanced salt solutions further aggravates salt and water retention,[57] perpetuating postoperative oliguria without improving overall hemodynamics or pulmonary function.[58, 59]

Postoperative oliguria that does not resolve spontaneously usually reflects continuing hypovolemia. Usually, contracted EABV is due to inadequate intraoperative volume replacement, failure to compensate for ongoing loss from drainage from surgical sites, or the internal sequestration of body fluids into the gastrointestinal tract or other body cavities. Postoperative oliguria may have less obvious causes, such as the formation of a functionally isolated "third space" within injured tissues themselves.[60] Extensive soft tissue trauma, inflammation, or surgical manipulation can impair the integrity of local microcirculations, causing net movement of salt-containing fluid into the injured cells and tissues at the expense of EABV. Consequently total body water may increase by as much as one-third, yet still coexist with an underlying functional deficit in circulating blood volume.

If the mechanoreceptors and other mechanisms described that maintain the homeostasis of EABV continue to send a "low volume" signal postoperatively, retention of salt and water, and thus oliguria, may be persistent. Derangement of the input from intrathoracic cardiovascular stretch receptors by positive pressure mechanical ventilation[49] or the liberal use of salt-free intravenous fluids[61] may further aggravate oliguria. The specific form of intravenous fluid volume therapy appears, however, to be secondary in importance to the general restoration of circulatory stability, the maintenance of adequate tissue oxygenation, and the ample repletion of both the solute and the water needed to reestablish normal body composition.

ANESTHETIC IMPLICATIONS OF RENAL DISEASE

The primary guidelines for the design of an anesthetic plan for patients with renal disease are avoidance of agents capable of producing fluoride nephrotoxicity, maintenance of arterial blood pressure within normal limits, use of diuretics to anticipate or treat intraoperative oliguria, and awareness of inevitable alterations of pharmacokinetics. Halothane, isoflurane, a variety of narcotic-based techniques, and regional anesthesia have all been widely and successfully used for patients with CRF, including those receiving a transplanted renal homograft.[62, 63]

No specific agent appears to be demonstrably superior. The value of stimulating dopaminergic receptors in the renal vasculature to improve RBF in patients with renal dysfunction or failure also remains a matter of debate.[64] Droperidol has dopaminergic-stimulating properties and may, in fact, maintain RBF at levels slightly higher than those usually seen during other forms of intravenous anesthesia.[45] Nevertheless, during neuroleptanesthesia there is still a significant reduction in GFR; in addition, suppression of the increased sympathoadrenal tone that precipitates acute renal vasoconstriction may be less complete with this anesthetic approach than when potent inhalational agents are used to create a "deeper" form of general anesthesia.[38] Generous volume resuscitation to stimulate maximum cardiac output and RBF improves renal homograft survival significantly.[65]

With end-stage renal failure, anesthetic management consists largely of dealing with uremia, electrolyte abnormalities, anemia, disturbed body fluid homeostasis, and other sequelae of the primary disease. Aggressive hemodialysis may acutely contract EABV to a degree sufficient to cause circulating hypovolemia and arterial hypotension. Nephrotoxicity of anesthetics is not a concern once endogenous renal function has been lost completely, but postoperative inorganic fluoride production may compromise the survival of the transplanted renal homograft if the anesthetic agent is subject to defluorination. If there is evidence of uremic platelet dysfunction, regional anesthesia may be contraindicated: epidural[66] or subarachnoid hematomas[67, 68] can produce permanent neurologic injury.[69]

Electrolytes

Hyperkalemia is commonly encountered in end-stage glomerular disease. It predisposes to intraventricular conduction block and ventricular fibrillation, especially if acute; serum potassium concentrations that exceed 8 mEq/L increase the likelihood of these potentially fatal cardiac dysrhythmias.[36] The hyperkalemia associated with renal failure may also produce abnormal QRS and T wave morphology, but it does not compromise cardiac contractility unless there is coincident systemic acidosis to pH values below 7.0,[70] or significant hypocalcemia.[71]

Unfortunately both of these conditions are common in patients with renal failure. Calcium and potassium appear to have similarly antagonistic electrochemical actions in the peripheral vasculature as well: peripheral vasospasm is precipitated by hyperkalemia, but moderated by infusions of ionized calcium.[72] Hypocalcemia may have a more prominent role in the cause of cardiac and vascular abnormalities than has previously been appreciated.

Although hypokalemia has also been traditionally associated with cardiac conduction abnormalities,[73] more recent concepts suggest that serum potassium values as low as 2.6 mEq/L are not a perioperative risk factor unless conduction abnormalities are already present before anesthetic induction,[74] or if they are associated with overt stigmata of arteriosclerotic heart disease[75, 76] or the use of digitalis.[77] The acute changes in serum potassium that routinely follow the use of succinylcholine are no more severe in patients with renal failure than they are in patients with normal renal function.[78]

Pharmacokinetic Theory

Because the uptake and excretion of inhalational agents are independent of renal function, they should provide consistent induction of anesthesia and subsequent emergence in patients with renal failure. In contrast, intravenous anesthetics that require renal excretion of the drug itself, or of its primary metabolites, may require adjustments of dosage or timing if their clinical effects are to be comparable with those seen in patients with normal renal function. The pharmacokinetics or molecular distribution of many intravenous drugs after injection into the circulation is determined primarily by the rate and the extent of their distribution into different body tissues, and by the subsequent rate at which those molecules are eliminated into the urine.

The theoretical volume of body tissue in which a drug would be distributed if it achieved a concentration identical to that measurable in plasma is a "distribution volume." The rate at which renal plasma would have to be completely cleared of drug in order to account for the observed decline in plasma drug concentrations is renal "clearance." Together these two factors determine elimination half-life ($t_{1/2\beta}$), the time interval during which there is a 50% reduction in plasma drug concentrations after the rapid initial phase of redistribution has been largely completed.[79] The steady-state volume of plasma to be cleared of drug (VD_{ss}) and the rate at which the process of clearance (Cl) occurs (Fig 9–7) therefore determine the time required for drug elimination.

Elimination half-life is a pharmacokinetic measurement that may not always correspond to the duration of clinical drug effect. It is derived from measurements of plasma drug concentrations, themselves subject to sampling error,[80] and not from measurements of drug concentrations at their primary site of action. Similarly, the distribution volumes reported as part of the pharmacokinetic profile for intravenous drugs represent mathematic analysis and not anatomic compartments.[81] For most drugs, a "best-fit" conceptual model consistent with the observed time course for the decay of plasma drug concentrations requires two or more hypothetical compartments.[82] Although termed "central" and "peripheral," these volumes have no exact anatomic analogs but may correspond to functional concepts of plasma and other freely exchangeable components of ECF, and to intracellular water, or to tissues with varying degrees of lipid content and rates of perfusion, respectively.[83]

In general, the greater the period of observation and plasma sampling, the larger the number of theoretic compartments that must be constructed in order to explain the observed relationship between plasma drug concentrations and time.[84] The net movement of drug molecules between these various compartments eventually declines to a minimal value of pseudoequilibrium, or steady state. Although true equilibrium is rarely achieved, VD_{ss} nevertheless provides a useful

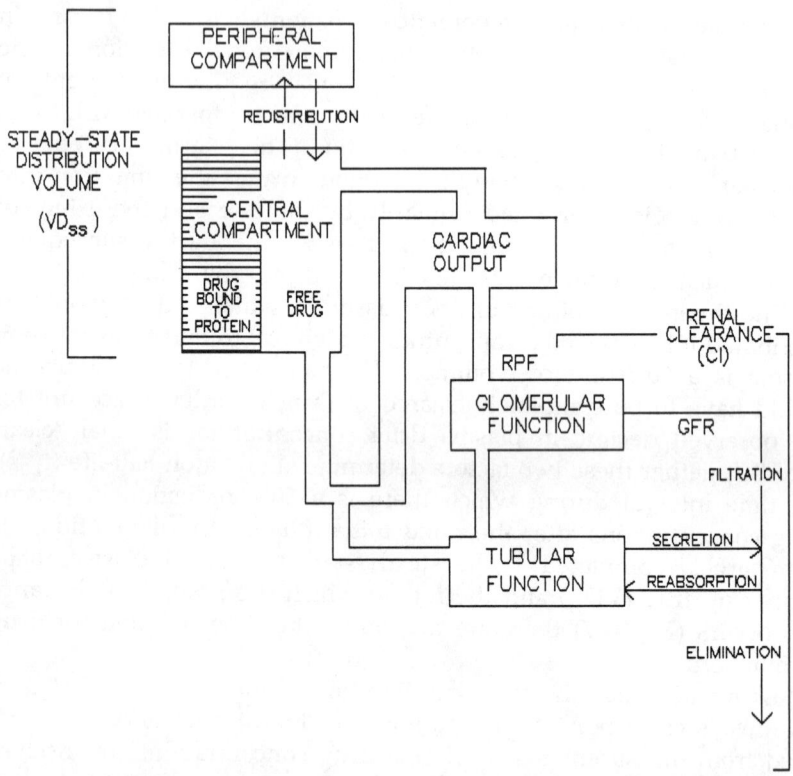

FIG 9–7.
Schematic representation of factors important for drug elimination by renal mechanisms. After intravenous injection, drug concentrations in plasma fall rapidly as "free" (not bound to plasma protein) drug molecules redistribute from the central to the peripheral compartments. This process ultimately establishes the steady-state volume of distribution (VD_{ss}). Simultaneously, cardiac output and vascular determinants of renal plasma flow (RPF) deliver free drug to nephrons where renal elimination occurs by glomerular or tubular processes. Renal clearance (Cl) is therefore determined both by the state of renal tissue function and by the amount of renal plasma flow. The time required for drug elimination is prolonged by either increases in VD_{ss} or by reductions in Cl.

measure of the extent to which drug distribution is altered by renal failure or by other factors that alter body composition.

Clinical Pharmacology in Renal Failure

Narcotics, thiopental, and other potent analgesic and anesthetic agents are predominantly lipid-soluble, distributing themselves preferentially in fatty, rather than in aqueous, tissues. Their actual distribution volumes are therefore changed little by renal failure or other situations that disrupt body water content, although apparent VD_{ss} may be altered if there are marked changes in the extent to which the drug is bound to protein.[85, 86] Drugs that are weak bases appear to be unaffected by reduced protein binding in renal failure, however.[87] Because narcotics and other lipid-soluble drugs require hepatic biotransformation before excretion,[81] their clearance from plasma is also not usually disturbed by renal dysfunction unless cardiac output is severely compromised, or if the water-soluble metabolites of these drugs retain some biologic activity, or the patient has a combined hepatorenal syndrome.[88]

In contrast, the pharmacokinetics of highly charged water-soluble molecules, such as neuromuscular blocking drugs, antibiotics, and other adjuvants, often change significantly and dramatically as a consequence of renal dysfunction (Table 9–1). The primary mechanism is not increased distribution volume, but rather reduced renal clearance and a corresponding prolongation of elimination half-life and clinical drug effect. Renal elimination itself reflects variations in the rates of glomerular filtration, tubular secretion, or reabsorption.[89]

The limiting factor in the clearance of penicillin and hepatically synthesized glucuronide conjugates of lipid-soluble drugs, substances actively excreted by renal tubular mechanisms,[12] is simply renal plasma flow.[90] The rates of renal clearance for most intravenous drugs used for anesthetic management, however, reflect glomerular function and the prevailing rate of GFR. Most nondepolarizing neuromuscular blocking drugs and ganglioplegic agents, neostigmine and other antagonists of neuromuscular blockade, atropine, digoxin, and many antibiotics are cleared largely by a process of filtration.[12]

TABLE 9–1.

Drugs With Prolonged Effect in Patients With Renal Failure Due to Delayed Excretion

Central nervous system depressants
  Haloperidol, methohexital, pentazocine, pentobarbital, phenytoin, various glucuronide
    conjugates
Relaxants/antagonist mixtures
  Atropine, *d*-tubocurarine, edrophonium, gallamine, metocurine, neostigmine,
    pancuronium, pyridostigmine
Antiarrhythmics/antihypertensives
  Diazoxide, digoxin, guanethidine, nitroglycerin, procainamide, quinidine
Diuretics
  Furosemide, hydrochlorothiazide, thiazide
Antibiotics
  Virtually all except isoniazid, rifampin, chloramphenicol

The clearance of *d*-tubocurarine actually parallels changes in GFR precisely.[91] A twofold prolongation of $t_{1/2\beta}$ in patients with CRF has been reported for virtually all nondepolarizing relaxants except atracurium.[92] Gallamine pharmacokinetics are particularly sensitive to renal compromise,[93] and therefore use of gallamine is of major concern in patients with renal failure.[94] Although there is also a fortuitous prolongation of the effects of anticholinesterase drugs used to antagonize nondepolarizing neuromuscular blockade,[95] residual paralysis in patients with renal failure that is resistant to attempted reversal[96] suggests that excretion of the neuromuscular blocking drug remains the predominant factor determining the complete return of neuromuscular function.

Severe renal insufficiency and failure are not in themselves associated with altered pharmacodynamics, or sensitivity to drug effects, unless the patient also has a profound uremic neuropathy or myopathy. Effective plasma concentrations and total loading dosages appear to be the same as in patients with normal renal function, although increases in free fractions of alfentanil, morphine, and thiopental due to reduced protein binding may produce some unexpectedly potent initial drug effects.[86]

Prolonged neuromuscular blockade or other effects associated with the use of water-soluble drugs requiring renal excretion cannot, therefore, be avoided reliably by reduction of initial drug dosage. In general, the most effective clinical strategy for patients with renal failure is to select inhalational anesthetic agents and to use intravenous adjuvants for which the pharmacokinetics are known to be largely independent of renal function.

Transurethral Prostatic Resection

The most common surgical procedures for patients with urinary tract disease are transurethral prostatic resection and treatment of renal or ureteral lithiasis. The anesthetic management of patients undergoing transurethral resection of the prostate (TURP) is uniquely complicated by highly variable, often profound, derangements of water and electrolyte homeostasis. Continuous infusion of glycine irrigant fluid through the prostatic resectoscope may produce net systemic absorption of as much as 2 L of sodium-free water,[97] perhaps one half of this amount within the first 30 minutes,[98] producing hemodynamic signs of volume overload and congestive heart failure.[99]

Water intoxication and dilutional hyponatremia with central nervous system dysfunction under these circumstances are known as the

"TURP syndrome."[100] In addition, glycine itself may be neurotoxic[101] or may produce toxic metabolites[102] that contribute to the clinical symptoms of paresthesia, disorientation, cardiovascular instability, seizures, and coma. Regional anesthesia is most commonly used but does not appear to be demonstrably superior to general anesthesia in terms of outcome.[103] It does, however, facilitate prompt diagnosis and immediate treatment of intoxication due to irrigant absorption or bladder perforation by the resectoscope[104] during TURP.

Therapeutic diuresis induced with furosemide reduces expanded extracellular fluid volumes and facilitates excretion of the excess of water associated with this syndrome. Restoration of plasma sodium concentrations toward normal values with infusions of hypertonic saline is not recommended unless hyponatremia is severe and associated with seizures[105]; overly aggressive manipulation of plasma tonicity may produce a potentially lethal osmotic pontine demyelination syndrome.[106]

Lithotripsy

There is less consensus regarding the most appropriate anesthetic plan for extracorporeal shock wave lithotripsy (ESWL). A relatively new technique that utilizes focused shock waves to fragment renal calculi noninvasively, ESWL can accomplish the spontaneous passage of fragmented renal stones without surgical intervention.[107] The innervation of the renal pelvis, upper ureter, and external upper abdominal wall is easily anesthetized by spinal or epidural techniques.[108] General anesthesia has also been advocated as superior, however, because it provides greater control of patient movement and thereby limits the possibility of injury to adjacent intestinal and pulmonary tissues,[109] especially if used with high-frequency "jet" ventilation patterns.[110]

These theoretical advantages have not been shown to translate directly into improved anesthetic outcome, however.[111] With any anesthetic technique, there remains a significant danger of sequelae from misguided shock waves in patients with paroxysmal atrial tachycardia or other reentry forms of cardiac dysrhythmias,[112] in patients with pacemakers or vascular aneurysms, and in those who are pregnant.

SUMMARY

Normal renal function reflects intricate integration of complex processes of kidney perfusion, glomerular filtration, and active tubular transport. Control of the renal reabsorption of filtered sodium largely determines the homeostasis of extracellular fluid volume. Hormonally mediated variations in tubular permeability to water maintain tissue and plasma osmolality within narrow limits. Urinary excretion is also the major mechanism for the elimination of the nonvolatile acid products of metabolism, of nitrogenous waste products of protein metabolism, and for anesthetic adjuvants, antibiotics, and other water-soluble molecules.

Vascular smooth muscle in the renal circulation has little resting tone but considerable capability for sustained vasoconstriction. This characteristic protects fragile glomerular capillaries from damage during arterial hypertension and maintains filtration pressures in the glomerulus by redistributing vascular resistance from afferent to efferent sites. However, the renal vasculature is therefore largely a participant in, rather than a beneficiary of, the marked increases in systemic vascular resistance produced by generalized sympathoadrenal stimulation. The extent to which renovascular and tubular functions are dominated by the actions of the renin-angiotensin system, aldosterone, prostacyclins, and vasopressin (ADH) reflects the fact that they are components of the hierarchy of stress-related autonomic responses that regulate venous and arterial blood volume, cardiac output, and the metabolic well-being of all tissues.

Anesthetics have diffuse, indirect effects on renal function mediated largely by perioperative activation of sympathoadrenal tone, secretion of ADH, and variations in cardiac output and blood pressure. Renal tubular damage can be produced directly by inorganic fluoride, a consequence of hepatic dehalogenation of methoxyflurane and enflurane. Intraoperative oliguria occurs commonly even with uncomplicated general or regional anesthesia; it appears to be a nonspecific but integrated multiorgan response to perioperative neuroendocrine stress and tissue injury.

Renal failure produces disruption of body salt and water balance and profound biochemical disorders. Inadequate excretion of metabolic waste ultimately poisons every organ system, producing uremia, anemia, neuropathy, encephalopathy, and generalized multiple organ toxicity. Principles of anesthetic management for patients with renal failure are primarily to compensate for widespread organ system dysfunction. In addition, however, the anesthetic plan must avoid superimposing toxic or ischemic conditions that may further compromise residual renal function. Rational use of neuromuscular blocking drugs or other water-soluble agents that undergo excretion by renal mechanisms requires a review of their pharmacokinetic properties and, in most cases, an increase in the interval between repeated dosages to anticipate prolonged clinical effects.

REFERENCES

1. Thurau K: Renal hemodynamics. *Am J Med* 1964; 36:698–719.
2. Bevan DR: *Renal Function in Anaesthesia and Surgery*. London, Academic Press, 1979.
3. Moffat DB: Medullary blood flow during hydropenia. *Nephron* 1968; 5:1–6.
4. Fernandez P, Cox M: Basic concepts of renal physiology. *Int Anesthesiol Clin* 1984; 22:1–34.
5. Elias H, Hossman A, Barth IB, et al: Blood flow in the glomerulus. *J Urol* 1960; 83:790–798.
6. Waugh WH, Shanks RG: Cause of genuine autoregulation of the renal circulation. *Circ Res* 1960; 8:871–888.
7. Kendrick E, Oberg B, Wennergren G: Vasoconstrictor fiber discharge to skeletal muscle, kidney, intestine, and skin at varying levels of arterial baroreceptor activity in the cat. *Acta Physiol Scand* 1972; 85:464–476.
8. Nisell H, Hjemdahl P, Linde B, et al: Sympathoadrenal and cardiovascular reactivity in pregnancy-induced hypertension. *Am J Obstet Gynecol* 1985; 152:554–560.
9. Henrich WL, Pettinger WA, Cronin RE: The influence of circulating catecholamines and prostaglandins on canine renal hemodynamics during hemorrhage. *Circ Res* 1981; 48:424–429.
10. Kahl FR, Flint JF, Szidon JP: Influence of left atrial distension on renal vasomotor tone. *Am J Physiol* 1974; 226:240–246.
11. Margolis BL, Stein JH: The renal circulation. *Int Anesthesiol Clin* 1984; 22:35–63.
12. Prescott LF: Mechanism of renal excretion of drugs (with special reference to drugs used by anaesthetists). *Br J Anaesth* 1972; 44:246–251.
13. Berliner RW, Bennett CM: Concentration of urine in the mammalian kidney. *Am J Med* 1967; 42:777–789.
14. Kliger AS: The role of the kidney in fluid, electrolyte, and acid-base disorders. *Int Anesthesiol Clin* 1984; 22:65–82.
15. Pettinger WA: Anesthetics and the renin-angiotension-aldosterone axis (editorial). *Anesthesiology* 1978; 48:393–396.
16. Blair-West JR, Doghlan JP, Denton DA: Inhibition of renin secretion by systemic and intrarenal angiotensin infusion. *Am J Physiol* 1971; 220:1309–1315.
17. Oparil S, Haber E: The renin-angiotensin system (first of two parts). *N Engl J Med* 1974; 291:389–401.
18. Schrier RW: Effects of the adrenergic nervous system and catecholamines on systemic and renal hemodynamics, sodium and water excretion and renin secretion. *Kidney Int* 1974; 6:291–306.

19. Levenson DJ, Simmons CE Jr, Brenner BM: Arachidonic metabolism, prostaglandins and the kidney. *Am J Med* 1982; 72:354–374.
20. Swain JA, Heyndrickx GR, Boettcher DH, et al: Prostaglandin control of the renal circulation in the unanesthetized dog and baboon. *Am J Physiol* 1975; 229:829–830.
21. Pace-Asciak CR, Carrara MC: Evidence suggesting a systemic antihypertensive role for PGI2. *Prostaglandins* 1978; 15:704–705.
22. Writer WDR: Anaesthetic considerations in high-risk pregnancy. *Can Anaesth Soc J* 1986; 33:S16–S27.
23. Morton JJ, Padfield PL, Forsling ML: A radio-immunoassay for plasma arginine-vasopressin in man and dog: Application to physiological and pathological states. *J Endocrinol* 1975; 65:411–424.
24. Lindheimer MD, Katz AI: Hypertension in pregnancy. *N Engl J Med* 1985; 313:675–680.
25. Anderson RJ, Berl T, McDonald KM: Evidence for an in vivo antagonism between vasopressin and prostaglandin in the mammalian kidney. *J Clin Invest* 1975; 56:420–426.
26. Priebe H-J: Evaluation of renal function. *Int Anesthesiol Clin* 1984; 22:121–135.
27. Charlson ME, MacKenzie R, Gold JP, et al: Postoperative changes in serum creatinine. When do they occur and how much is important? *Ann Surg* 1989; 209:328–333.
28. Mazze RI: Critical care of the patient with acute renal failure. *Anesthesiology* 1977; 47:138–148.
29. Levinsky NG: Pathophysiology of acute renal failure. *N Engl J Med* 1977; 296:1453–1458.
30. Anderson RJ, Linas SL, Berns AS, et al: Non-oliguric acute renal failure. *N Engl J Med* 1977; 296:1134–1138.
31. Frederickson ED, Bradley T, Goldberg LI: Blockade of renal effects of dopamine in the dog by the DA1 antagonist SCH 23390. *Am J Physiol* 1985; 249:F236–F240.
32. Petrie JJB: The clinical features, complications, and treatment of chronic renal failure. *Br J Anaesth* 1972; 44:266–276.
33. Muller MC: Anesthesia for the patient with renal dysfunction. *Int Anesthesiol Clin* 1984; 22:169–187.
34. Weir PHC, Chung FF: Anaesthesia for patients with chronic renal disease. *Can Anaesth Soc J* 1984; 31:468–480.
35. Bergstrom J, Furst P: Uremia toxins. *Kidney Int* 1978; 12:9–12.
36. Ettinger PO, Regan TJ, Oldewurtel HA: Hyperkalemia, cardiac conduction, and the electrocardiogram: A review. *Am Heart J* 1974; 88:360–371.
37. Leight L, Roush G, Rafi E, et al: The effect of intravenous potassium on myocardial contractility and cardiac dynamics. *Am J Cardiol* 1963; 12:686–691.
38. Cousins MJ, Mazze RI: Anaesthesia, surgery, and renal function; immediate and delayed effects. *Anaesth Intensive Care* 1973; 1:355–373.

39. Halperin BD, Feeley TW: The effect of anesthesia and surgery on renal function. *Int Anesthesiol Clin* 1984; 22:157–168.
40. Koeppen BM, Katz AI, Lundheimer MD: Effects of general anesthesia on renal hemodynamics in the rat. *Clin Sci* 1979; 57:469–471.
41. Deutsch S, Goldberg M, Stephen GW, et al: Effects of halothane anesthesia on renal function in normal man. *Anesthesiology* 1966; 27:793–804.
42. Deutsch S, Bastron RD, Pierce EC Jr, et al: The effects of anaesthesia with thiopentone, nitrous oxide, narcotics and neuromuscular blocking drugs on renal function in normal man. *Br J Anaesth* 1969; 41:807–815.
43. Pirano LL, Vatner SF: Morphine effects on cardiac output and regional blood flow distribution in conscious dogs. *Anesthesiology* 1981; 55:236–243.
44. Kennedy WF, Sawyer TK, Gerbershagen HV, et al: Systemic cardiovascular and renal hemodynamic alterations during peridural anesthesia in normal man. *Anesthesiology* 1969; 31:414–421.
45. Jarnberg PO, Santesson J, Eklund J: Renal function during neuroleptanaesthesia. *Acta Anaesthesiol Scand* 1978; 22:167–172.
46. Bastron RD, Pyne JL, Inagaki M: Halothane-induced renal vasodilation. *Anesthesiology* 1979; 50:126–130.
47. Bastron RD, Kaloyanides GJ: Effect of methoxyflurane (MOF) on PAH uptake by rabbit kidney tissue slices. *Am J Physiol* 1974; 227:460–464.
48. Philbin DM, Coggins CH: Plasma antidiuretic hormone levels in cardiac surgical patients during morphine and halothane anesthesia. *Anesthesiology* 1978; 49:95–98.
49. Berry AJ: Respiratory support and renal function. *Anesthesiology* 1981; 55:655–667.
50. Mazze RI, Calverley RK, Smith NT: Inorganic fluoride nephrotoxicity: Prolonged enflurane and halothane anesthesia in volunteers. *Anesthesiology* 1977; 46:265–271.
51. Cousins MJ, Mazze RI: Methoxyflurane nephrotoxicity. A study of dose response in man. *JAMA* 1973; 225:1611–1616.
52. Mazze RI, Shue GL, Jackson SH: Renal dysfunction associated with methoxyflurane anesthesia. *JAMA* 1971; 216:278–288.
53. Eichhorn JH, Hedley-White J, Steinman TI, et al: Renal failure following enflurane anesthesia. *Anesthesiology* 1976; 45:557–560.
54. Mazze RI, Woodruff RE, Heerdt ME: Isoniazid-induced enflurane defluoridation in humans. *Anesthesiology* 1982; 57:5–8.
55. Frascino JA: Tetracycline, methoxyflurane anaesthesia, and renal function. *Lancet* 1972; 1:1127.
56. Mazze RI, Cousins MJ, Barr GA: Renal effects and metabolism of isoflurane in man. *Anesthesiology* 1974; 40:536–542.
57. Lucase CE, Ledgerwood AM, Higgins RF: Impaired salt and water excretion after albumin resuscitation for hypovolemic shock. *Surgery* 1979; 86:544–549.

58. Virgilio RW, Smith DE, Zarins CD: Balanced electrolyte solutions: Experimental and clinical studies. *Crit Care Med* 1979; 7:98–106.
59. Shires GT, Peitzman AB, Albert SA, et al: Response of extravascular lung water to intraoperative fluids. *Ann Surg* 1983; 197:515–519.
60. Shires T, Williams J, Brown F: Acute change in extracellular fluids associated with major surgical procedures. *Ann Surg* 1961; 154:803–810.
61. Hayes MA, Goldenberg IS: Renal effects of anesthesia and operation mediated by endocrines. *Anesthesiology* 1963; 24:487–499.
62. Wyant GM: The anaesthetist looks at tissue transplantation. Three years' experience with kidney transplant. *Can Anaesth Soc J* 1967; 14:255–275.
63. Aldrete JA, Daniel W, O'Higgins JW, et al: Analysis of anesthetic-related morbidity in human recipients of renal homografts. *Anesth Analg* 1971; 50:321–329.
64. Goldberg LI: Cardiovascular and renal actions of dopamine: Potential clinical applications. *Pharmacol Rev* 1972; 24:1–29.
65. Carlier M, Squifflet J-P, Pirson Y, et al: Maximal hydration during anesthesia increases pulmonary artery pressures and improves early function of human renal transplants. *Transplantation* 1982; 34:201–204.
66. Ellison N, Ominsky AJ: Clinical considerations for the anesthesiologist whose patient is on anticoagulant therapy. *Anesthesiology* 1973; 39:328–336.
67. Mayumi T, Dohi S: Spinal subarachnoid hematoma after lumbar puncture in a patient receiving antiplatelet therapy. *Anesth Analg* 1983; 62:777–779.
68. Brem SS, Hafler DA, Van Uitert RL, et al: Spinal subarachnoid hematoma: A hazard of lumbar puncture resulting in reversible paraplegia. *N Engl J Med* 1981; 303:1020–1021.
69. Owens EL, Kasten GW, Hessel EA II: Spinal subarachnoid hematoma after lumbar puncture and heparinization: A case report, review of the literature, and discussion of anesthetic implications. *Anesth Analg* 1986; 65:1202–1207.
70. Goodyear AVN, Goodkind MJ, Stanley EJ: The effects of abnormal concentrations of the serum electrolytes on left ventricular function in the intact animal. *Am Heart J* 1964; 67:779–791.
71. Drop LJ, Laver MB: Low plasma ionized calcium and response to calcium therapy in critically ill man. *Anesthesiology* 1975; 43:300–306.
72. Stanley TH, Isern-Amaral J, Liu W-S, et al: Peripheral vascular versus direct cardiac effects of calcium. *Anesthesiology* 1976; 45:46–58.
73. Holland OB, Nixon JV Kuhnert L: Diuretic-induced ventricular ectopic activity. *Am J Med* 1981; 70:762–768.
74. Vitez TS, Soper LE, Wong KC, et al: Chronic hypokalemia and intraoperative dysrhythmias. *Anesthesiology* 1985; 63:130–133.
75. Stewart DE, Ikram H, Espiner EA, et al: Arrhythmogenic potential of diuretic induced hypokalemia in patients with mild hypertension and ischaemic heart disease. *Br Heart J* 1985; 54:290–297.

76. Masterson BJ: Diuretic-associated hypokalemia. *Arch Intern Med* 1985; 145:1966–1967.
77. Harrington JT, Isner JM, Kassirer JP: Our national obsession with potassium (editorial). *Am J Med* 1982; 73:155–159.
78. Koide M, Waud BE: Serum potassium concentrations after succinylcholine in patients with renal failure. *Anesthesiology* 1972; 36:142–145.
79. Hug CC Jr: Pharmacokinetics of drugs administered intravenously. *Anesth Analg* 1978; 57:704–723.
80. Barrett R, Graham GG, Torda TA: The influence of sampling site upon the distribution phase kinetics of thiopentone. *Anaesth Intensive Care* 1984; 12:5–9.
81. Hug CC Jr, Murphy MR, Rigel EP, et al: Pharmacokinetics of morphine injected intravenously into the anesthetized dog. *Anesthesiology* 1981; 54:38–47.
82. Riegelman S, Loo JCK, Rowland M: Shortcomings in pharmacokinetic analysis by conceiving the body to exhibit properties of a single compartment. *J Pharm Sci* 1968; 57:117–123.
83. Ogilvie RI: An introduction to pharmacokinetics. *J Chron Dis* 1983; 36:121–127.
84. Stanski DR, Ham J, Miller RD, et al: Pharmacokinetics and pharmacodynamics of *d*-tubocurarine during nitrous oxide–narcotic and halothane anesthesia in man. *Anesthesiology* 1979; 51:235–241.
85. Gibaldi M: Drug distribution in renal failure. *Am J Med* 1977; 62:471–474.
86. Chauvin M, Lebrault C, Levron JC, et al: Pharmacokinetics of alfentanil in chronic renal failure. *Anesth Analg* 1987; 66:53–56.
87. Jusko WJ, Gretch M: Plasma and tissue protein binding of drugs in pharmacokinetics. *Drug Metab Rev* 1976; 5:43–140.
88. Duchin KL, Schrier RW: Interrelationship between renal haemodynamics, drug kinetics and drug action. *Clin Pharmacokinet* 1978; 3:58–71.
89. Garrett ER: Pharmacokinetics and clearances related to renal processes. *Int J Clin Pharmacol Biopharm* 1978; 16:155–172.
90. Stanski DR, Watkins WD: Pharmacokinetic principles, in Stanski DR, Watkins WD (eds): *Drug Disposition in Anesthesia*. New York, Grune & Stratton, 1982, pp 1–45.
91. Fisher DM, O'Keeffe C, Stanski DR, et al: Pharmacokinetics and pharmacodynamics of *d*-tubocurarine in infants, children, and adults. *Anesthesiology* 1982; 57:203–208.
92. D'Hollander AA, Luyckx C, Barvais L, et al: Clinical evaluation of atracurium besylate requirement for a stable muscle relaxation during surgery: Lack of age-related effects. *Anesthesiology* 1983; 59:237–240.
93. Feldman SA, Cohen EN, Golling RD: The excretion of gallamine in the dog. *Anesthesiology* 1969; 30:593–598.
94. Feldman SA, Levi JA: Prolonged paresis following gallamine: A case report. *Br J Anaesth* 1963; 35:804.
95. Stanski DR, Miller RD, Sheiner LB: Renal function and the pharmacoki-

netics of neostigmine in anesthetized man. *Anesthesiology* 1979; 51:222–226.

96. Miller RD, Cullen DJ: Renal failure and postoperative respiratory failure: Recurarisation? *Br J Anaesth* 1976; 48:253–256.

97. Taylor RO, Maxson RS, et al: Volumetric gravimetric, and radio-isotopic determination of fluid transfer in transurethral prostatectomy. *J Urol* 1958; 79:490–499.

98. Osester A, Madsen PO: Determination of absorption or irrigating fluid during transurethral resection of the prostate by means of radioisotopes. *J Urol* 1969; 102:714–719.

99. Hahn RG: Blood volume during transurethral prostatic resection. *Acta Anaesthesiol Scand* 1988; 32:629–637.

100. Harrison RH, Boren JS, Robinson JR: Dilutional hyponatremia shock: Another concept of the transurethral prostatic resection reaction. *J Urol* 1956; 75:95–110.

101. Wang JM, Wong KC, Creel DJ, et al: Effects of glycine on hemodynamic responses and visual evoked potentials in the dog. *Anesth Analg* 1985; 64:1071–1077.

102. Hoekstra PT, Kahnoski R, McCamish MA: TBR: Transurethral prostatic resection syndrome—a new perspective: Encephalopathy with associated hyperammonemia. *J Urol* 1983; 130:704–707.

103. McGowan SW, Smith GRN: Anaesthesia for transurethral prostatectomy. *Anaesthesia* 1980; 35:847–853.

104. Kenton HR: Perforation in transurethral operations; techniques for immediate diagnosis and management of extravasations. *JAMA* 1950; 142:798–801.

105. Ayus JC, Krothapalli RK, Arieff AI: Treatment of symptomatic hyponatremia and its relation to brain damage. *N Engl J Med* 1987; 317:1190–1195.

106. Sterns RH, Rigg JE, Schochet SS Jr: Osmotic demyelination syndrome following correction of hyponatremia. *N Engl J Med* 1986; 314:1535–1542.

107. Gissen D: Anesthesia for extracorporeal shock wave lithotripsy. *Semin Anesth* 1987; 6:57–60.

108. Abbott MA, Samuel JR, Webb DR: Anaesthesia for extracorporeal shock wave lithotripsy. *Anaesthesia* 1982; 40:1065–1072.

109. Lingeman JE, Newman D, Mertz J, et al: Extracorporeal shock wave lithotripsy: The Methodist Hospital in Indiana experience. *J Urol* 1986; 135:1134–1137.

110. Perel A, Hoffman B, Podeh D, et al: High frequency positive pressure ventilation during general anesthesia for extracorporeal shock wave lithotripsy. *Anesth Analg* 1986; 65:1231–1234.

111. Zeitlin GI, Roth RA: Effect of three anesthetic techniques on the success of extracorporeal shock wave lithotripsy in nephrolithiasis. *Anesthesiology* 1988; 68:272–276.

112. Walts LF, Atlee JL: Supraventricular tachycardia associated with extracorporeal shock wave lithotripsy. *Anesthesiology* 1986; 65:521–523.

10

Blood and Endocrine Function

Traditionally, anesthesiologists have assessed blood pressure and other physical determinants of organ perfusion to determine the well-being of their anesthetized patients. More recently, with widespread availability of technology permitting analysis of inspired and arterial respiratory gases, the content of blood has become an issue of increasing interest. Blood is not a body fluid passively delivering dissolved substances; it is a complex and highly specialized tissue.

Suspended in plasma, a combination of cellular and noncellular elements confer to blood unique physical properties that facilitate its manifold functions of transport, metabolism, and hemostasis. Blood is fluid but not amorphous; it is capable of coagulating locally into a semisolid mass in a controlled and self-limited manner. Like all tissue specimens, blood removed for in vitro analysis continues to consume metabolic substrate and to generate carbon dioxide, lactate, and other metabolic end products.

The sections of this chapter provide a general overview of the transport of metabolic and hormonal substances by blood, as well as its role in immune defense and the maintenance of cardiovascular homeostasis. These functions complement many of the mechanisms for homeostasis of effective arterial blood volume (EABV) and total body water described in Chapter 9. In addition, the effects of anesthetic agents, the perioperative environment, and congenital and acquired hematologic and endocrine disorders will be summarized, along with a perspective on their impact upon the design of the anesthetic plan.

BLOOD AS A TISSUE

The catastrophic consequences of even short-term deficiencies of tissue oxygenation make oxygen transport of fundamental importance to any consideration of blood and its role in metabolic homeostasis. The physical solubility of oxygen in plasma is limited, not remarkably different from that in other fluids containing protein. It provides for the carriage of less than 2% of arterial oxygen at ambient oxygen partial pressures. The synthetic noncellular perfluorochemical blood substitutes currently available appear to be little better at providing oxygen carriage when used in subtoxic concentrations.[1] An increase in oxygen partial pressure in a hyperbaric oxygen environment, however, does produce a proportional increase in dissolved molecular oxygen that may be sufficient to establish a therapeutic rationale for treatment of gangrene, or in other situations where even small improvements in oxygen tension may be beneficial.

Oxygen-Hemoglobin Dissociation

Under normal atmospheric pressures, the 200 to 250 mL of oxygen consumed at rest each minute by an adult of average body weight is supplied almost entirely as a result of its carriage in blood by hemoglobin. This protein-iron pigment complex is packaged within the erythrocytes which normally comprise about one half of circulating blood volume. There is a nonlinear, freely reversible relationship between oxygen partial pressures and the extent to which erythrocyte hemoglobin exists in combination with this gas. In fact, the complex shape of the oxygen-hemoglobin dissociation curve ensures the efficient application of the unique properties of hemoglobin over the narrow range of oxygen partial pressures that correspond to the gas tensions normally found within the lung and in peripheral body tissues. Unlike other oxygen-carrying pigments such as myoglobin (Fig 10–1), the relationship between oxygen partial pressure and degree to which hemoglobin is saturated with oxygen is optimal not for maximal saturation at low partial pressures, but for unloading of oxygen from capillary blood and into the tissues of the microcirculatory beds, where it is consumed.[2]

The precise sequence of amino acids within the globin protein com-

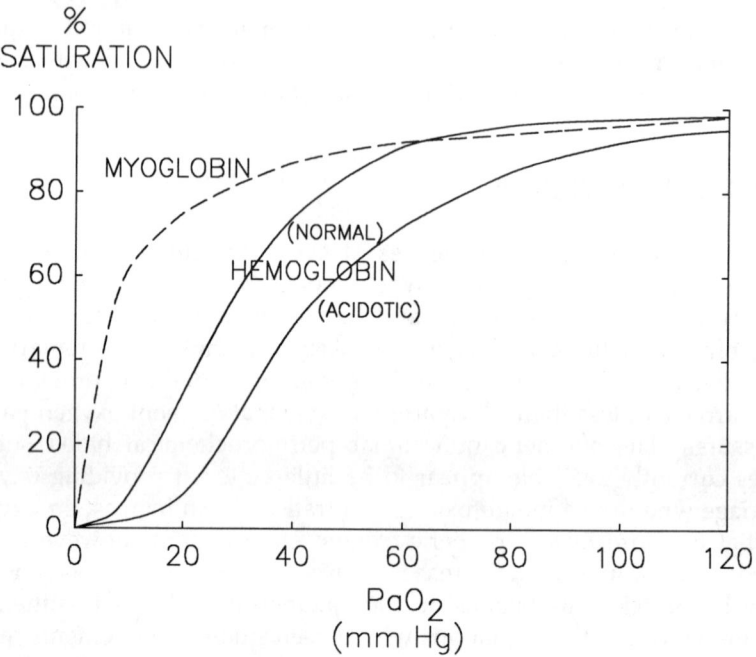

FIG 10–1.

Oxygen dissociation characteristics for myoglobin and for adult hemoglobin in normal and in acidotic blood. The high affinity of myoglobin ensures high saturation at ambient levels of tissue oxygen tension, but allows the release of molecular oxygen during the profound tissue hypoxia common in exercising skeletal muscle. In contrast, hemoglobin provides optimal volumetric oxygen unloading at ambient tissue partial pressures. Acidosis-induced configurational changes in hemoglobin subunits produce a "right shift," increasing the rate of "extraction" of molecular oxygen in poorly perfused tissues without further compromising tissue oxygen tensions.

ponent of normal adult hemoglobin determines the interaction between the subunits of this macromolecule, a phenomenon responsible for the precise characteristics of oxygen affinity. Because the movement of oxygen from blood into tissues is determined directly by oxygen partial pressure gradients, the steep slope of the relationship facilitates the movement of large amounts of molecular oxygen into tissues in response to small decreases in tissue oxygen tensions. The midpoint, or P_{50} value, is the oxygen partial pressure required for 50% saturation of hemoglobin with oxygen; it defines the relative position of this relationship for different types of hemoglobin and therefore determines the metabolic oxygen tension set-points for aerobic equilibrium in tissues.[3]

Variability of oxygen unloading in vivo largely reflects adjustments of the P_{50} characterized as leftward or rightward shifts of this curve. P_{50} is altered by erythrocyte 2,3-diphosphoglyceride (2,3-DPG) concentrations, body and tissue temperatures, and acid-base status. These factors determine the affinity of hemoglobin for oxygen both directly and indirectly: metabolic acidosis within erythrocytes stimulates local production of 2,3-DPG, thereby increasing P_{50}. This reduces the affinity of hemoglobin for oxygen and facilitates its availability to tissues during conditions of hypoxemia or anemia. The resultant phenomenon of "increased oxygen extraction" by peripheral tissues is still a passive process of molecular diffusion along partial pressure gradients, but the net amount of oxygen transferred from blood to tissue is increased because of the lower venous saturation associated with reduced affinity of hemoglobin for oxygen.

Intrinsic genetic or environmentally induced alterations of the structure or the quantity of globin subunits may also alter the normal oxygen-hemoglobin dissociation relationship. Cigarette smoking or other sources of chronic exposure to carbon monoxide not only reduce intracellular 2,3-DPG but also transform significant amounts of hemoglobin to carboxyhemoglobin, a configuration useless for oxygen transport.[4] In addition, the slope of the overall dissociation curve is depressed by carbon monoxide exposure; it becomes more hyperbolic and therefore less efficient in volumetric oxygen transport over the narrow range of oxygen partial pressures prevalent in body tissues.[3]

At ambient pressures equivalent to 1 atm or less, the amount of oxygen contained in arterial blood is, for all practical purposes, limited by hemoglobin concentration and the extent to which this molecule is saturated with oxygen. Oxygen-carrying "capacity" is maximal oxygen content when oxygen partial pressure is sufficiently high (150 mm Hg or more) to ensure complete saturation of hemoglobin.[5] Although measurements of actual arterial oxygen content and cardiac output can be used to estimate systemic oxygen transport (STo_2),[6] the delivery of oxygen to peripheral tissues can be determined only by simultaneous assessment of arterial and venous oxygen content, permitting calculation of the actual quantity of oxygen removed from arterial blood.[7] Systemic oxygen delivery is the most essential, but also the most complex, parameter of oxygen transport by blood: it reflects cardiovascular performance, pulmonary gas exchange, metabolic state, and the qualitative and quantitative characteristics of hemoglobin.

Carbon Dioxide and Other Substances

The transport of carbon dioxide in blood from the microcirculation to the lungs for subsequent excretion is less complex. Although its solubility in plasma is 20 times that of oxygen, carbon dioxide is nevertheless largely carried in blood indirectly, as bicarbonate.[8] Carbon dioxide produced by metabolic processes in tissue diffuses rapidly into the erythrocytes of blood traversing the microcirculation. There it is hydrated to carbonic acid, which subsequently dissociates, forming bicarbonate and hydrogen ions in a process accelerated enzymatically by carbonic anhydrase.

Rapid movement of bicarbonate into plasma in exchange for chloride ions (the "chloride shift") ultimately results, however, in the distribution of more than two thirds of the 200 mL of carbon dioxide produced each minute into the plasma, rather than the cellular fraction, of whole blood. A small but significant amount of carbon dioxide is also carried within erythrocytes as carbamino-hemoglobin, or in plasma as the carbamino form of various proteins. The tendency of desaturated hemoglobin to act as a buffer for osmotically active species within erythrocytes actually produces sufficient swelling of these cells to raise the venous hematocrit a few percent above that measured in arterial blood.

Hormones and Stress

Other essential transport functions provided by the circulation of blood include the distribution of nutrient substances and cofactors required for normal metabolism. Blood also carries the hormonal substances that act as diffuse "slow-response" messengers, augmenting and sustaining the rapid, neurally mediated reflex autonomic responses occurring after disturbances of the internal environment. In addition to producing catecholamine release from the adrenal glands and from postganglionic sympathetic neurons, afferent input from pain and other less-specific somatoreceptors travels through cortical and brain stem pathways to the anterior hypothalamus. There it is processed and integrated (Chapter 2), subsequently generating the complex neurohumoral central nervous system responses to stress.[9]

Although not always defined in a consistent manner, the "neuroendocrine stress response" includes the release of a variety of neurohumoral substances from the pituitary gland. These hormones exert profound effects on the cellular activity of diverse tissues. Adrenocorticotropic hormone (ACTH), a short-lived polypeptide, is released within seconds of a generalized sympathoadrenal response. Subsequently, within minutes, it increases the production of aldosterone and cortisol by the adrenal cortex. Growth or somatotrophic hormone (STH) is also released in response to physical stress and autonomic stimulation.[10] Increases in circulating follicle-stimulating hormone (FSH) and in luteinizing hormone (LH) are also sustained, but less dramatic, under these circumstances.[11] Antidiuretic hormone (ADH) and aldosterone, discussed in the previous chapter, are secreted after tissue injury, or in response to virtually any form of generalized sympathoadrenal stimulation.[12]

Stress does not, however, trigger the release of thyroid-stimulating hormones (TSH) from the anterior pituitary gland. In fact, there may be a hormonally mediated depression of thyronine (T_4) deiodination, the process that normally generates the metabolically active version of this hormone, triiodothyronine (T_3). Stress may also enhance the utilization of alternate synthetic pathways to generate a metabolically inert variant of this hormone, "reversed T_3."[9]

Prostaglandins enhance the neuroendocrine activity associated with sympathoadrenal activation due to tissue injury. Anxiety provides further stimulus for their release. The neuroendocrine response to stress is not limited or suppressed by physiologic processes of aging, at least in the absence of disease. In fact, elderly individuals maintain plasma epinephrine and norepinephrine levels that are consistently higher, both at rest and in response to orthostasis, than those of their younger counterparts.[13] Despite these higher circulating catecholamine levels, however, autonomic equilibrium is rarely restored as rapidly or as completely as in young adults; aging reduces ACTH release,[14] impairs autonomic end-organ responsiveness, and alters adrenergic receptor morphology.[15]

Immune Systems

Some of the cellular elements in blood function not as mediators of transport or neurohumoral communication, but rather as the sensors or the effectors of immune responsiveness. The immune system remains incompletely understood because of its complexity and the extent to which its functions are dispersed among many different tissues.[16] Macrophages, monocytes, and the reticuloendothelial cells of the spleen and liver function as accessory components for this system. They capture antigenic fragments and hold them at the cell surface, facilitating the subsequent lymphocyte contact ultimately needed for activation of an immune response.

Cell-mediated immune responses reflect the activity of elements derived from the thymus, the lymphocyte T cells. Noncellular components in blood are also essential to immune responsiveness: circulating antibody proteins are immune globulins, proteins that are activated and released by preprogrammed cells of bone marrow origin, the B cell lymphocytes. Both cellular and noncellular mechanisms may be activated during anaphylaxis, a general mobilization of immune responsiveness triggered by recognition of a previously established antigen. Anaphylaxis culminates in the release of intracellular stores of histamine from mast cells in the lung and in the liver, and the activation of the complement system, which facilitates immune reactions at cell surfaces.

Preoperative interview for a credible history of drug allergy after prior exposure is essential for design of an anesthetic plan, because true anaphylaxis may occur as often as once in every 3,000 hospitalizations. Typically, this event is "all-or-none," independent of the amount of antigen that has been introduced. It is characterized by the consequences of abrupt and generalized release of histamine and other substances with profound effects on smooth muscle: bronchospasm, vasodilation, tissue edema, and other stigmata of impaired capillary integrity may be sufficiently severe to produce life-threatening respiratory and cardiovascular collapse.[17]

Unlike anaphylaxis, *anaphylactoid* reactions are caused by the release of histamine through nonspecific mechanisms that do not require the participation of immune globulins. Variable amounts of histamine release may occur, usually in proportion to the concentration of the triggering agent.[18] The subsequent clinical consequences often suggest participation of the complement system, however, and they may be so severe that they are virtually indistinguishable from those produced by antigen-mediated anaphylaxis.[19, 20] Anaphylactoid responses to intravenous anesthetic drugs are more common than true anaphylactic events. Despite the apparent absence of immune globulin participation, they occur most often in patients who have a preexisting history of allergic atopy, prior drug exposure, or a history of immune disorders.[21]

Isolated cutaneous urticaria and capillary blush without bronchospasm, hypotension, or other signs of systemic histamine release are seen frequently after injection of intravenous anesthetic agents. They may also occur in many patients during periods of emotional stress. Nonsystemic cutaneous responses are probably due to the release of histamine from intradermal sites, apparently by a neuronal or neurohumoral mechanism that remains poorly understood.[18]

HEMOSTASIS

The most dynamic and complex function of blood is the process of hemostasis. This phenomenon encompasses platelet aggregation, blood coagulation, and clot dissolution. Contrary to the implications of the classical concept of a coagulation "cascade," hemostasis is not an episodic and unidirectional event triggered and carried to completion as needed. Instead, coagulation is one extreme of a dynamic, reversible, and continuous equilibrium between coagulation proteins, cellular and tissue elements, cofactors, and vascular structures. This interaction ultimately determines the relative liquidity of this tissue, and thus the ease with which it can be extravasated. Clot dissolution is as important to normal coagulation as is clot formation.[22] Therefore, an overview of platelet function, fibrinogenesis, and fibrinolysis is required to understand the many varieties of coagulopathy encountered in clinical practice.

Platelets and Vascular Integrity

Total vascular integrity would obviate the need for a hemostatic mechanism. The inevitability of tissue injury makes this condition impossible, however, and after the disruption of an endothelial surface by surgery or trauma, a complex but well-ordered sequence of events rapidly minimizes blood loss and provides temporary occlusion of damaged surfaces.[23] Subsequently, dissolution of the hemostatic complex occurs as endothelial integrity is restored. The vascular endothelium provides not only structural support for these processes but also participates actively in the metabolic events of coagulation itself.

Vascular endothelial cells synthesize and secrete into the subendothelium a protein polymer, von Willebrand's factor (factor VIII:vWF). This protein is in close physical association with the collagen that provides the essential structural integrity of the vascular wall. Exposure of the subendothelium to blood by trauma or injury results in immediate aggregation of platelets (thrombocytes) to the disrupted surface, and thus initiates the formation of a platelet "plug," the first stage of hemostasis (Fig 10–2). Factor VIII:vWF, in effect, is both a marker that indicates a breach of endothelial continuity and an essential component of the sequence that initiates hemostasis.

Platelets themselves provide a physical nidus for hemostasis, blocking the area of disrupted endothelium. Like endothelial cells, they also play an active metabolic role in the coagulation process that follows by releasing membrane-bound stores of adenosine diphosphate (ADP). ADP facilitates a secondary aggregation of more platelets, expanding the size of the plug and making platelets star-shaped. This physical transformation physically accelerates deposition of the fibrinogen required for the next phase of hemostasis, coagulation.

Changes in shape of platelets and the contraction of their metabol-

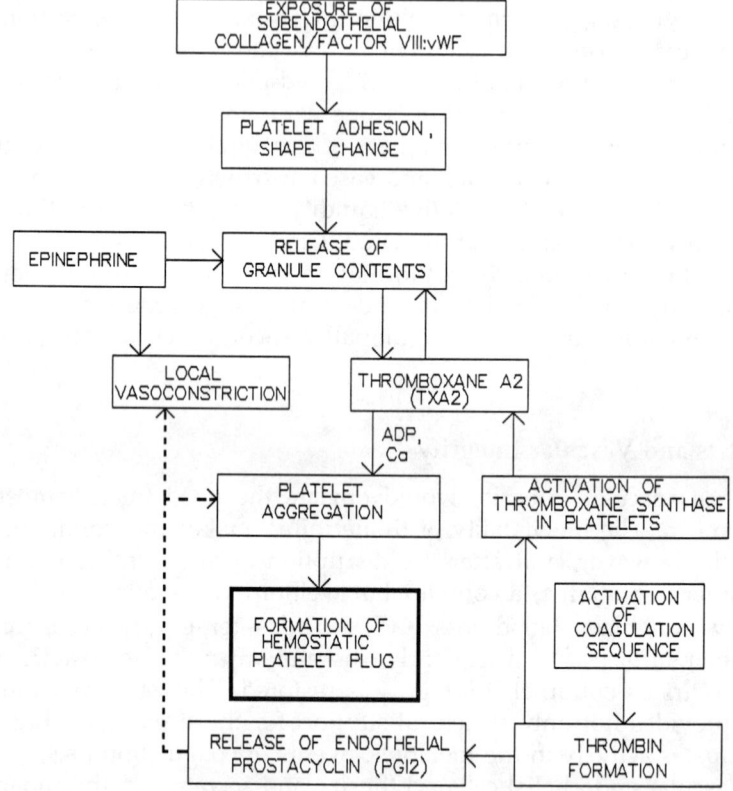

FIG 10–2.
The first phase of hemostasis: formation of the platelet plug. Platelet aggregation and activation occur in response to a breach of endothelial continuity that exposes protein and cellular components of blood to subendothelial tissues. Subsequent aggregation is modulated by the thrombin produced by the process of coagulation and by the systemic release of epinephrine if a generalized sympathoadrenal response to injury is induced. *Dashed lines* indicate inhibitory effects that limit changes to the site of injury.

ically rich granules require calcium and a protein cofactor, calmodulin; platelet aggregation is further enhanced by the local and systemic release of epinephrine. α-Adrenergic activity also produces local vasoconstriction, further packing the hemostatic plug and reducing the arterial pressure that must be contained within the damaged vasculature. Catecholamines may also energize the continuing release of the contents of platelet granules. In addition, activation of enzymes on the platelet membranes generates a prostaglandin, thromboxane A_2 (TXA_2). This substance enhances the release of platelet granules, stimulates platelet aggregation, and may actually enhance local vasoconstriction.[23]

Simultaneous stimulation of the synthesis of prostacyclin (PGI_2) within the vascular endothelium provides a counterbalancing inhibitory effect on platelet aggregation and a local, but powerful, vasodilator influence. Prostacyclin, and perhaps other agents released locally, also confines the extension of the hemostatic platelet plug to the immediate area of endothelial injury. This mechanism appears to be effective in preventing runaway thrombus formation and unnecessary circulatory obstruction once the initial phase of hemostasis has begun.

Coagulation

The initial mechanical occlusion of vascular disruption is provided by the platelet plug, but more sustained hemostasis requires coagulation by polymerization of fibrin at the site of endothelial damage. This process forms clot, the microscopic meshwork needed for secure vascular repair and normal re-endothelialization. The conversion of prothrombin (factor II) to its activated form, thrombin (factor IIa) generates fibrin, the essential step needed for sustained noncellular hemostasis (Fig 10–3). Although many hemostatic disorders reflect platelet dysfunction (thrombocytopathy), virtually all forms of true coagulopathy, whether congenital or acquired, are ultimately characterized by inadequate formation of a fibrin clot.

Prothrombin activation requires one of two interrelated, yet parallel, coagulation sequences involving the "intrinsic" or the "extrinsic" coagulation pathways. Despite the implications of this terminology, all the elements required for fibrin formation by either pathway are included in the composition of normal plasma. Both ultimately involve the activation of factor X (Stuart-Prower factor), essential for the conversion of prothrombin. The pathways differ primarily in the initiation sequence needed for factor activation, however.

Once exposed by vascular disruption, the negatively charged subendothelium "intrinsic" to all vascular tissues rapidly activates factors XI, XII, and kallikrein. In contrast, the "extrinsic" pathway for coagulation is stimulated by the presence of nonspecific phospholipid membrane fragments, elements not normally found in the circulation or on the endothelial surface. These usually appear when shed by damaged cells as a consequence of tissue injury. In the presence of membrane-bound calcium and a large lipoprotein molecule that functions as the ubiquitous "tissue factor" (factor III), these membrane fragments activate factor VII.

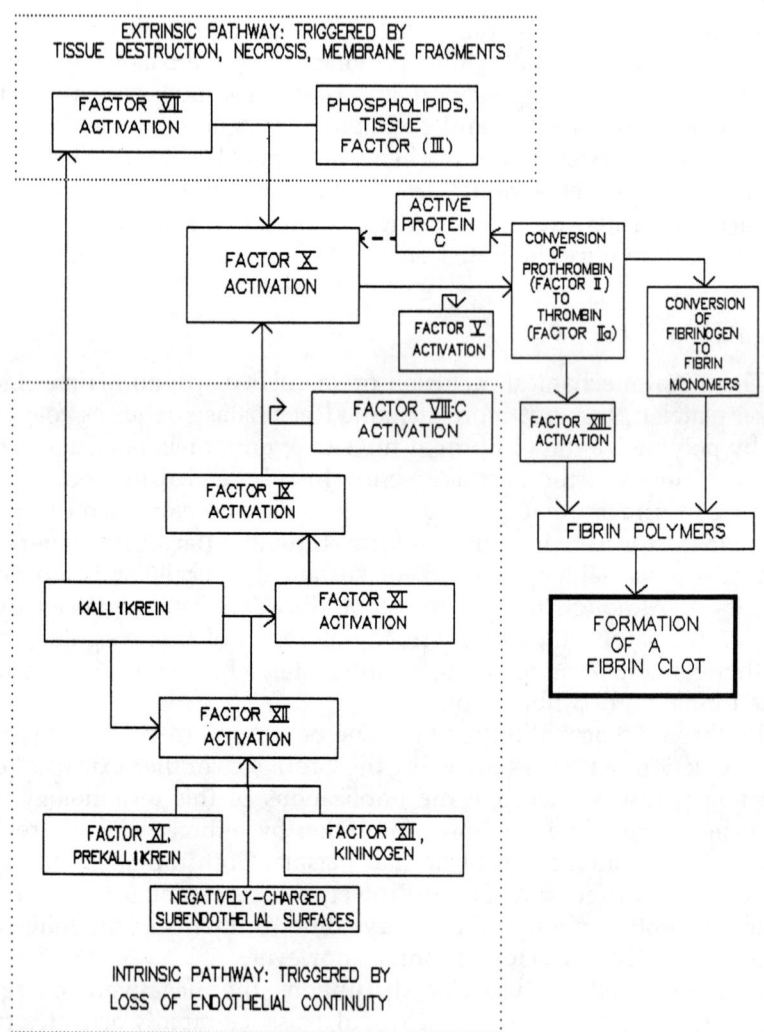

FIG 10-3.
The second stage of hemostasis: coagulation and clot formation. Both the extrinsic and the intrinsic activation sequences share a common pathway of factor activation beginning with factor X and ultimately producing an insoluble cross-linked fibrin meshwork that surrounds the platelet plug. There is some negative feedback *(dashed line)* provided by activation of protein C, which modulates clot formation and usually restricts it to a localized area.

The extrinsic and the intrinsic pathways converge at the point of factor X activation, another membrane-dependent process also requiring calcium. The membrane surfaces required for this common step are provided, in the case of the extrinsic pathway, by the same cell surface fragments produced by cell disruption initiating that pathway. For the intrinsic pathway, the membrane surfaces used are those of the platelets forming the hemostatic plug.

The activation of factor X permits cleavage of physically adjacent prothrombin molecules and subsequent release of thrombin into the immediate vicinity of vascular injury. This, in turn, generates prompt conversion of fibrinogen to fibrin (fibrinogenesis). Elaborate distinctions between the actions of the intrinsic and the extrinsic pathways in vivo are probably not justified: they appear to be activated almost simultaneously after tissue injury, although the extrinsic sequence may produce thrombin and fibrin more rapidly.

There is considerable overlap of these two pathways, and they have a synergistic and complementary relationship. Thrombin appears almost immediately after activation of the extrinsic pathway, and then facilitates the formation of complexes containing activated factor VIII:C on platelet surfaces. This process accelerates the events required for completion of the intrinsic pathway.[22]

Fibrin monomers generated from fibrinogen by the action of thrombin subsequently polymerize in the presence of calcium. When stabilized by activated factor XIII, they form the insoluble cross-linked meshwork described grossly as a "clot." Circulating antithrombin substances inhibit the activation of a coagulation factor in both the intrinsic and the extrinsic pathways, effectively limiting clot formation to the immediate, local area of endothelial injury.

In addition, thrombin itself participates in a negative feedback system for fibrin formation: it activates protein C, an enzyme that scavenges activated coagulation factors distant to the site of tissue injury. Thus during the acute phases of hemostasis, the platelet plug and the encircling fibrin clot continue to provide stable repair of vascular injury, even as the local concentrations of activated coagulation factors are rapidly returned to preinjury levels. This system also avoids generalized changes in the liquidity of blood in noninjured areas.

Clot Dissolution

The third and final major stage in hemostasis is clot dissolution (fibrinolysis). After vascular integrity has been re-established, the restoration of full vascular patency requires fibrinolysis. This process utilizes the action of a proteolytic enzyme, plasmin. In a manner similar to the parallel formation of thrombin via intrinsic and extrinsic pathways, activation of plasminogen to form plasmin can occur through two distinct, but usually simultaneous, processes (Fig 10–4).

The traumatic disruption of injured tissues not only provides phospholipid membrane fragments that trigger the extrinsic coagulation pathway but also releases plasminogen activators from intracellular lysosomes. When tissue disruption is minimal, an alternate mechanism for fibrinolysis is initiated: factor XI is activated by kallikrein generated from prekallikrein at subendothelial surfaces. Plasminogen activator is also produced by intact endothelial cells where, in concert with protein C and antithrombin III, it limits initial clot formation to only those areas in which endothelial integrity has been interrupted. In effect, fibrinogenesis and fibrinolysis are actually initiated simultaneously.

Initial formation of an effective fibrin clot therefore requires local suppression of plasmin formation, a function provided by antithrombin III. Other circulating antiplasmin substances, including α_2-antiplasmin and α_2-macroglobulin, also recombine active plasmin fragments into a single unit identical to the inactive plasminogen molecule. Therefore, fibrin appears to be continually desolubilized and resolubilized without alteration of the consistency of plasma itself until this fragile state of equilibrium is disrupted by exposure to factor VIII:vWF, or to cell membrane fragments. Under these conditions, the zymogens (inactive coagulation factors) are converted to their active configurations and begin to function as enzymes. In the presence of free and membrane-bound calcium and nonendothelial surfaces and platelets, they destabilize this complex system to produce a fibrin clot.

Hypercoagulability

Some hematologic disorders are characterized not by failure of hemostasis, but by inappropriate formation of thrombus. Hypercoagulability is usually a consequence of inadequate fibrinolysis, rather than a state characterized by a surplus of active procoagulant factors.[24] There may be deficiencies of plasminogen activator, or levels of antithrombin III inadequate to inhibit factors X, XI, and XII. Accelerated consumption of antithrombin III during wound healing has been invoked as a possible mechanism to explain impaired fibrinolysis and increased thrombus formation postoperatively.[25]

The physical properties of blood, its viscosity in particular, as well

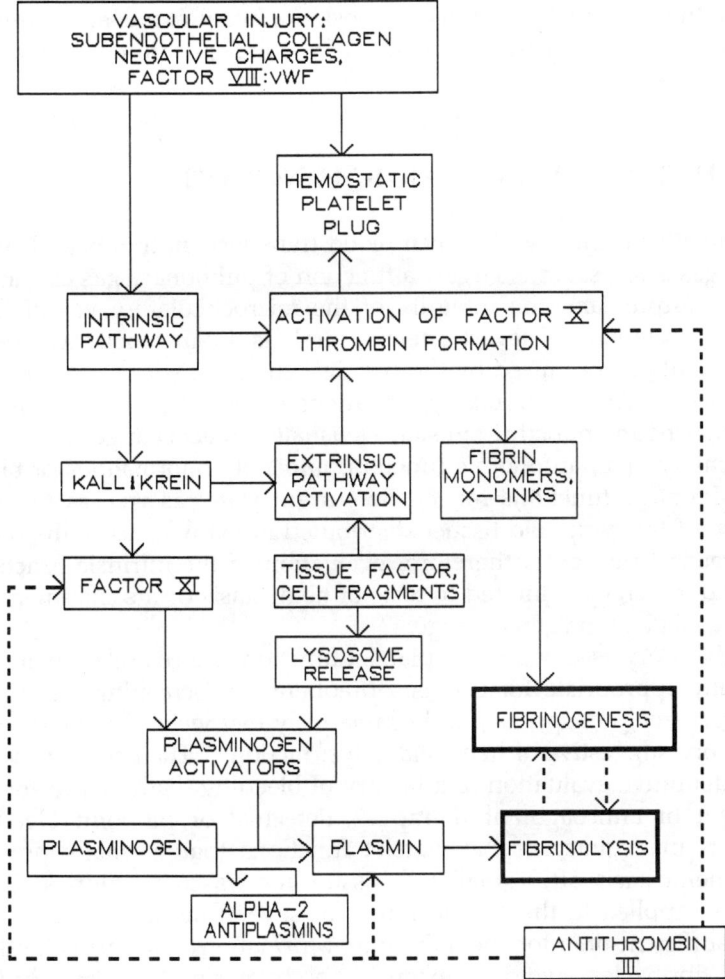

FIG 10–4.
The third phase of hemostasis: equilibrium between fibrinogenesis and fibrinolysis. Extensive interaction between factors that accelerate and inhibit the formation of a fibrin clot restrict its formation to the immediate site of endothelial injury. Dashed lines indicate inhibitory effects that appear to occur sequentially rather than simultaneously (see text).

as disorders of microcirculatory flow patterns also appear to be important in the pathogenesis of thromboembolic disorders after anesthesia and surgery.[26–28] Other factors favoring perioperative thrombosis include chronic endothelial inflammation. Vasculitis may impair local synthesis of plasminogen activator and may disrupt the physical integrity of the endothelial surface, exposing phospholipid structures or causing release of excessive amounts of tissue factor from malignant or necrotic tissues.[25]

EVALUATING HEMATOLOGIC FUNCTION

The effectiveness with which blood transports nutrients and respiratory gases to tissues is largely a function of pulmonary gas exchange, cardiac output, and the integrity of the microcirculatory vasculature. With the exception of severe anemia, rarely is the metabolic well-being of a patient compromised by the physical characteristics of blood or its component elements. Similarly, variations in blood levels of hormones and other neuroendocrine substances usually reflect changes in end-organ activity or in autonomic function, and not abnormalities of blood itself. Immune functions reflect the current state, as well as the past history, of the lymphoid tissues distributed in many areas of the body. For practical purposes, therefore, evaluation of the intrinsic functions of blood generally is limited to tests of hemostasis or measurements of the adequacy of oxygen carriage.

Laboratory assessments of platelet function and coagulation are not generally appropriate for use as a preoperative "screening" test: they are expensive, nonspecific, and of relatively low yield in patients with no history suggestive of hemostatic dysfunction.[29] Their primary value is for definitive evaluation of a history of bleeding diathesis, or for adjustment of anticoagulant therapy.[30] Petechial or pinpoint bleeding suggests inadequacy of the platelet functions that normally provide rapid hemostasis after small soft tissue and vascular injuries. Local pressure applied to the site of injury for several minutes usually provides sufficient time for the subsequent formation of a normal and effective fibrin clot, avoiding extensive ecchymosis. Tests of bleeding time such as the Ivy template provide quantitative, but nonspecific, in vivo assessment of the adequacy of first-stage hemostasis. More specific information regarding the number of platelets (platelet count) or their ability to aggregate and activate (platelet function tests), however, requires in vitro analysis of blood samples.[31]

Acquired Thrombocytopenia and Dysfunction

Acquired disorders of platelet function most commonly reflect the side effects of aspirin, ibuprofen, and perhaps other nonsteroidal anti-inflammatory drugs.[32] These agents disrupt the cyclooxygenase enzyme functions within platelets that are required for synthesis of TXA_2, which mediates localized vasoconstriction, and for the release of platelet granules to facilitate subsequent thrombocytic aggregation. Even normal bleeding time results are greater than the actual time required for hemostasis in vivo because the action of TXA_2 is temperature dependent, and its activity is significantly reduced at ambient skin temperatures. Other less well-understood causes for inadequate platelet function include generalized surgical stress, alcoholism, renal disease, deficiency of vitamin C, malignancy, hypothyroidism, polycythemia vera, hypocalcemia, heparinization, extracorporeal perfusion, and intravenous fluid therapy with solutions containing dextrans or other synthetic colloids.[30, 33–36]

Quantitative, rather than qualitative, platelet deficiencies are common side effects of cytotoxic therapies for malignancy. These drugs depress megakaryocyte precursor cells in bone marrow; malignant cells themselves may also infiltrate the marrow, impairing generation of new platelets. A primary thrombocytopenia may also occur after severe viral illnesses, generalized anemia, or uremia.[34] Excessive filtration of infused blood or generalized hemodilution during massive transfusion of banked blood or other fluids deficient in functioning platelets may lower platelet count,[37] but the ability of the spleen to act as a reservoir for platelets is sufficiently great that dilution itself rarely causes a hemostatic defect.[38]

Thrombocytopenia may also occur as a result of abnormally high rates of platelet destruction in patients with systemic lupus erythematosus, idiopathic thrombocytopenic purpura (ITP), and other autoimmune disorders.[30] Platelets may also be rapidly destroyed by the hemolytic-uremic syndrome, by liver disease with hypersplenism, or by thrombotic thrombocytopenic purpura (TTP).[34] Consumption coagulopathies such as the disseminated intravascular coagulation (DIC) syndrome associated with eclampsia generally include an element of severe thrombocytopenia.[39]

Thrombocytopenia has also been reported after sustained exposure to quinidine, rifampicin, morphine, heroin, and heparin; these drugs can generate an antigenic complex on the platelet surface capable of initiating an immune response that subsequently results in their destruction.[40] Although platelet counts of greater than 100,000/mm^3 are considered to be "normal," hemostasis may not be clinically impaired until levels fall to 50,000/mm^3 or less, provided that platelet function is not impaired (Fig 10–5). Qualitative deficiencies in platelet aggregation may be very subtle, however, and can lead to hemostatic failure even when the platelet count itself is at normal or even higher levels.

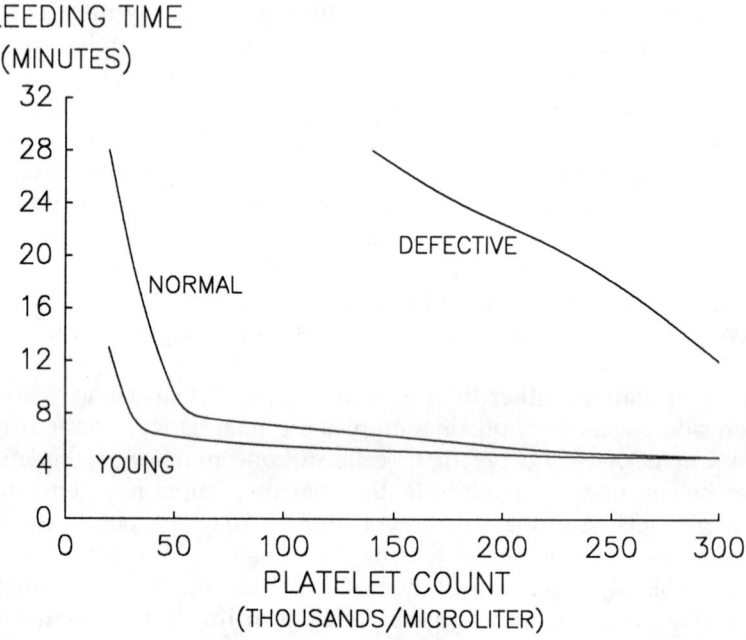

BLEEDING TIME
(MINUTES)

FIG 10–5.
The relationship between the concentration of platelets in peripheral blood and the Lee-White bleeding time is complex. For an abnormally young platelet population, such as would be generated in a patient with ITP, platelet function is somewhat hypereffective, and bleeding time is reduced. When deficiencies of effective platelet function are produced by aspirin, heparin therapy, or uremia, there may be prolonged bleeding times even when platelets are present in normal concentrations.

Congenital Thrombocytopathy

Congenital defects of platelet function are uncommon. Rarest is Bernard-Soulier thrombasthenic syndrome, a defect of platelet aggregation.[41] Most thrombocytopathies encountered are examples of von Willebrand's disease, an entity that includes numerous subtypes; all are characterized by the decreased adherence of platelets to exposed subendothelial surfaces. The mechanisms responsible for these variations include decreased release of factor VIII:vWF from endothelial cells, inadequate polymerization of factor VIII:vWF subunits before their release, or perhaps other abnormalities of this important procoagulant.

In the type IIB variant of this disorder, there may also be a state of relative thrombocytopenia. In other subtypes, there can be a coexisting deficiency of factor VIII:C, especially in patients homozygous for this disorder.[42] Overall, however, this group of autosomal dominant congenital defects of hemostasis can be most accurately characterized as an abnormality of endothelial cell and procoagulant metabolism, rather than a true congenital thrombocytopathy.

Congenital Coagulopathies

An acquired or congenital deficiency of one or more clotting factors produces symptoms of inadequate fibrin formation such as extensive bruising and frequent formation of large hematomas. Although able to form a normal hemostatic platelet plug, patients in whom fibrin formation or clot retraction is inadequate because of congenital or acquired coagulopathy may have persistent bleeding into traumatized joints or soft tissues. They may also suffer potentially life-threatening hemorrhages from large vascular injuries.

Since virtually all clotting factors are normally present in a twofold to threefold excess,[43] a clinically apparent coagulopathy appears only when there has been a severe reduction in one or more of the factors required for clot formation. Hemophilia is now known to describe not one but rather a group of specific, genetically determined deficiencies of procoagulants. Inadequate hepatic synthesis of factor VIII:C appears to play the central causative role in hemophilia A. l-Desamino-8-D-arginine vasopressin (DDAVP; desmopressin) stimulates the synthesis of both factor VIII:C and factor VIII:vWF; it can produce clinical improvements in hemostasis in many hemophiliacs, in some patients with von Willebrand's disease, and even in patients who appear to be hemostatically normal.[44]

Hemophilia B "Christmas disease" is caused by a deficiency of factor IX, a procoagulant required, like factor VIII:C, for completion of the intrinsic coagulation pathway. Other varieties of subtype within the hemophilias may result either from inadequate amounts or from abnormal configurations of one or both of these short-lived coagulation factors.

Acquired Coagulopathies

Acquired coagulopathies, like those that are congenital, reflect inadequate plasma concentrations of procoagulants or cofactors. The mechanism for acquired disorders may be dilution, consumption, or impaired synthesis. Vitamin K plays a central role in the hepatic synthesis of factors II, VII, IX, and X; consequently any form of vitamin K deficiency can limit their production and thereby interrupt the membrane-dependent activation sequence required to form thrombin.

Plasma concentrations of factors II, VII, IX, and X may also be inadequate to support normal coagulation when the enteric absorption of this lipid-soluble vitamin is interrupted by the consequences of biliary tract obstruction.

The anticoagulant effects of coumarin actually reflect its ability to function as a metabolically inactive substitute for vitamin K in the process of hepatic protein synthesis. Similarly, severe hepatocellular disease can be expected to compromise hemostasis by disrupting the coagulation process, since all procoagulants except factor VIII:vWF, derived from endothelial cells, are generated by this tissue.

Tests of Coagulation

Currently available tests of coagulation are not sufficiently specific to define the mechanism of most coagulopathies. Rather, they form the basis for objective confirmation of a diagnosis of coagulopathy, and for the appropriate adjustment of anticoagulant therapy. The prothrombin time (PT) quantitates the time required for generation of a fibrin clot in vitro by means of the extrinsic coagulation pathway when plasma is combined with phospholipid membranes and calcium. Prolongation of the PT occurs with inadequate plasma levels of prothrombin, fibrinogen, or factors V, VII, or X. It is predictably prolonged in patients with hepatocellular disease and in those receiving coumarin-like drugs because of their effects on the synthesis of factors VII and X.

PT may also be abnormal in the presence of large amounts of heparin since this drug interferes with the activation of both prothrombin and factor X.[45] Parenteral vitamin K reverses the effects of coumarin by accelerating hepatic synthesis of vitamin K–dependent coagulation factors at a rate that depends on intrinsic hepatic function. More rapid normalization of PT can be achieved with direct replenishment of deficient procoagulants by transfusion with fresh frozen plasma (FFP) or whole blood.[46]

Partial thromboplastin time (PTT), like PT, measures the time required for fibrin clot formation in vitro. In contrast, however, it is a simulated initiation of factor activation along the intrinsic, rather than the extrinsic, pathway. The membrane fragments with protein components needed to activate factor VII, unique to the extrinsic pathway, are avoided: kaolin provides an artificial, negatively charged surface simulating the subendothelial environment to trigger the intrinsic pathway activation sequence. Consequently, factors V, VIII:C, IX, X, XI, XII, and prekallikrein, as well as prothrombin and fibrinogen, are tested.

Heparin, even in relatively low dosage, inhibits activation of factor IX and thereby prolongs PTT; it may also accelerate the inhibition of thrombin by antithrombin III.[22] The effects of heparin can, like those of coumarin, be reversed with infusion of specific coagulation factors. However, more rapid restoration of clot formation can be achieved with protamine, a naturally occurring, and therefore highly antigenic, antagonist. Used most effectively as part of an activated coagulation time (ACT) or other heparin titration technique,[47, 48] it is frequently employed in patients undergoing major vascular and cardiac surgery, especially those who require full anticoagulation with heparin in order to undergo extracorporeal perfusion.[49]

PT, PTT, and ACT measure only the time required to initiate fibrin formation. The thromboelastogram (TEG) provides direct measurement of the actual mechanical properties of the fibrin clot. The TEG not only quantitates both the dynamics and the structural integrity of the fibrin clot, but also assesses fibrinolysis by monitoring the process of clot dissolution.[50] It thereby facilitates diagnosis of either enhanced, or impaired, fibrinolysis. However, the TEG requires pattern recognition by trained technicians, and the results, unlike those of PT and PTT, cannot be expressed as a single quantitative value. Despite formidable technical details, the TEG has grown in importance because of its value in the management of patients undergoing liver transplantation.[51] Its use has also, however, been described in patients undergoing abdominal surgery[52] or other procedures.[53]

Disseminated Intravascular Coagulation

The most severe form of acute hemostatic abnormality is disseminated intravascular coagulation (DIC). It is a true "consumption coagulopathy," producing thrombocytopenia and disrupting both the first and the second phases of hemostasis (Fig 10–6). A state of hemostatic disequilibrium, DIC is characterized not only by abnormally high local concentrations of coagulation factors, intense thrombus formation, and subsequent fibrinolysis, but also by a diffuse and profound depletion of both the cellular and the protein components required for effective hemostasis.

Vascular endothelial cell damage, extensive nonendothelial injury or necrosis, or the release of procoagulant phospholipid substances may initiate DIC.[54] This disorder can be triggered through either intrinsic or extrinsic coagulation pathways. PT and PTT may be normal, prolonged, or abnormally short, depending on the precise balance between the competing processes of clot formation and dissolution. Spon-

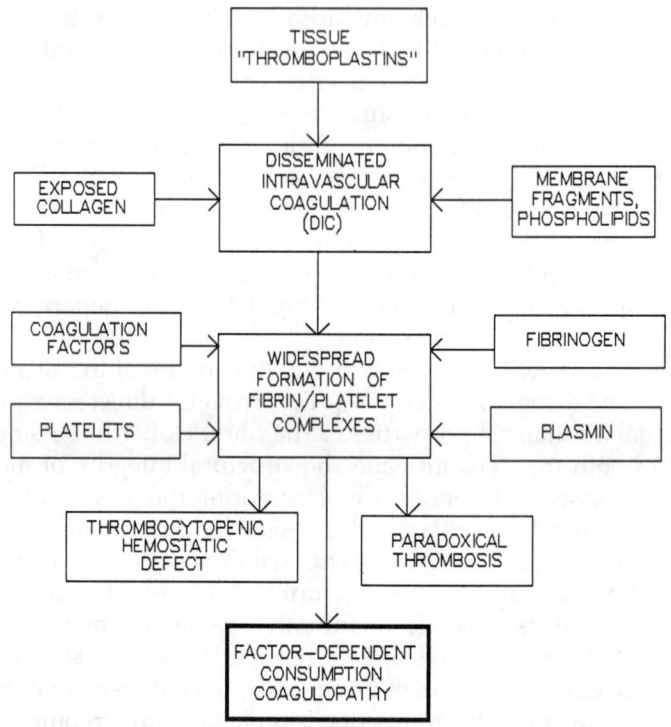

FIG 10–6.

The mechanism of consumption coagulopathy. Release of tissue thromboplastins by a wide variety of foreign materials, physical injuries, and toxins produces disseminated intra-vascular coagulation *(DIC)*. Inadequately modulated systemic formation of fibrin and platelet complexes consumes both the cellular and the plasma protein components needed for normal hemostasis and exhausts the capacity for controlled fibrinolysis.

taneous bleeding from multiple venipuncture and surgical sites is the most common presentation.[55] The clinical diagnosis can be confirmed by laboratory findings of thrombocytopenia, hypofibrinogenemia, or the presence of elevated concentrations of fibrin split products.[39]

Therapy for DIC usually includes replacement of platelets and pro-coagulants simultaneously with intense efforts to eliminate the "trigger" for runaway coagulation, but anticoagulants may be of use if managed by consultants with special expertise. DIC is a major risk factor in obstetric patients with placental abruption, or patients with major trauma, sepsis, and snake bite. It has also been described as a complication of promyelocytic leukemia.[54]

More subtle coagulopathies in which there are laboratory indices consistent with a hemostatic defect but no life-threatening clinical symptoms of hemorrhagic diathesis can occur in pregnant patients with a retained, nonviable fetus, in preeclampsia or eclampsia of pregnancy,[56] after amniotic fluid embolus, or after major blood group incompatibility, head injury, or tissue necrosis due to malignancy. An even milder abnormality occurs commonly after extracorporeal perfusion, heat stroke, thermal burns, or the use of "cell saver" devices to scavenge blood shed during surgery for immediate reinfusion of autologous erythrocytes.

Excessive Fibrinolysis

A coagulopathy due to excessive fibrinolysis may occur without the generalized consumption of components that characterizes DIC. Accelerated fibrin clot dissolution occurs after trauma and extracorporeal transfusion, or after surgery of the urinary tract. Release of plasminogen activators from prostatic tissues or high levels of urokinase derived from lysosomes within renal tubular and endothelial cells normally keep the urinary tract free of fibrin.[57] These substances may also produce sufficient postoperative bleeding after urologic surgery, however, to require the use of an antifibrinolytic agent.[58] ε-Aminocaproic acid (Amicar) may also inhibit excessive fibrinolysis during and after dental procedures in patients with hemophilia.[43] The role of fibrinolysis in non-DIC acquired diffuse coagulopathy, such as may occur immediately after cardiopulmonary bypass, has not yet been clearly established.[59, 60]

Hemoglobinopathies

Unlike the evaluation of plasma proteins, in vitro assessment of hemoglobin is based largely on structure rather than function. Electrophoresis and x-ray diffraction studies have provided extraordinarily detailed analysis of the variations in molecular structure associated with hemoglobinopathies. Under clinical conditions, however, assessment of hemoglobin function is limited primarily to the detection of anemias or to the measurement of oxygen content. The correlation of oxygen partial pressure and hemoglobin saturation across their full range of association and dissociation is obviously not practical in vivo. Rather, the abnormalities of oxygen-hemoglobin affinity characteristic of genetically determined hemoglobinopathies have been studied in laboratory investigations and subsequently extrapolated for clinical application.

If not based on a family history of anemia or hemoglobinopathy, the initial diagnosis of congenitally abnormal hemoglobin structure is usually derived from an extensive evaluation of anemia. Thalassemias are true anemias: they represent a genetic disorder that produces quantitatively inadequate, but qualitatively normal, globin subunits for hemoglobin molecules. In contrast, hemoglobinopathies such as sickle cell disease, or its less severe expression, sickle cell trait, occur because a single amino acid substitution in the polypeptide sequence of the globin subunit chain alters the affinity of this molecule for oxygen. In these disorders, anemia is a secondary phenomenon: the structural damage produced by the characteristic conformational changes that occur in the hemoglobin S of sickle cell disease at low partial pressures of oxygen produces destruction of erythrocytes, significantly compromising oxygen-carrying capacity.[61]

Other hemoglobinopathies involving hemoglobin types C and D may occur in heterozygous combination with the hemoglobin S of sickle cell disease, producing less overt destruction but some degree of decreased erythrocyte flexibility.[62] As a consequence, accelerated erythrocyte surface damage initiates enhanced splenic and reticuloendothelial sequestration and destruction of these cells, producing mild to moderate anemia. When hemoglobin S is heterozygous with normal hemoglobin A, anemia is mild. The consequences of the combination of hemoglobin S with the various thalassemias ("sickle-thal"), however, are usually more severe but variable, and depend on the exact phenotype.

EFFECTS OF ANESTHESIA

Oxygen Transport

Because they exert complex, variable, and frequently profound effects on cardiopulmonary function, the anesthetic state and the drugs with which it is established invariably alter many of the transport functions of blood. Quantitative changes in the total delivery of oxygen and metabolic substrates to tissues, as well as anesthesia-related changes in the carriage and excretion of carbon dioxide and metabolic endproducts, have been described previously. Qualitative changes in the effectiveness of hemoglobin-based oxygen transport and other functions of hemoglobin, however, appear to be far more subtle, and are certainly less well understood.

Anesthesia-induced depression of myocardial and autonomic function may limit the active increases in cardiac output that normally maintain adequate STo_2 with levels of hemoglobin below 9 g/dL.[63] In more mild states of anemia, however, reduced blood viscosity appears to increase cardiac output sufficiently that it effectively compensates for decreased oxygen-carrying capacity on a passive basis alone,[64] maintaining STo_2 at normal levels (Fig 10–7). Anesthesia also reduces total body oxygen consumption significantly, even in anemic subjects.[65] Increased erythrocyte 2,3-DPG production due to enhanced glycolytic metabolism occurs in tissue beds experiencing modest degrees of tissue hypoxia. This facilitates oxygen unloading and probably reestablishes a normal aerobic environment at tissue levels, provided that arterial blood remains fully oxygenated and systemic blood pressure is maintained within reasonable limits.[5] Thus general anesthesia and its effects on hemodynamics should not be associated with tissue

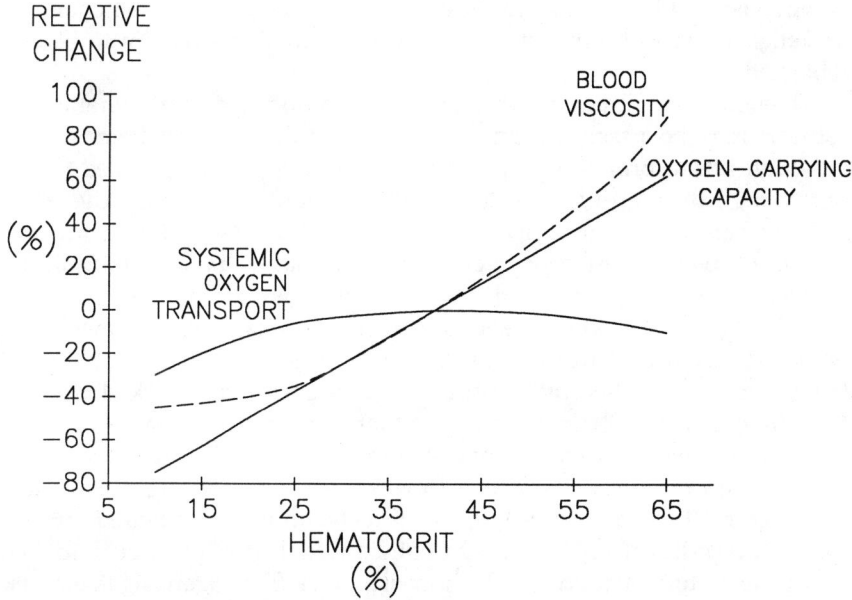

FIG 10–7.
Measured systemic (arterial) oxygen transport (STo_2) in animals is relatively unchanged over a wide range of hematocrit after acute hemodilution or hemoconcentration. In vitro estimates of whole blood viscosity at moderate flow rates and calculations of oxygen-carrying capacity confirm that over this range of hematocrit values these parameters change at rates that offset each other, with a relatively minor net effect on STo_2. All of these estimates assume the maintenance of normothermia, full arterial oxygen saturation, and unhindered spontaneous adjustments of cardiac output by intrinsic mechanisms. STo_2 begins to decrease significantly below hematocrit values of 25% where further reduction of blood viscosity is insignificant relative to the steady decline in oxygen-carrying capacity.

hypoxia or an otherwise abnormal metabolic environment if pulmonary function is adequate and neither cardiovascular depression nor anemia is profound.

Hemostasis

It is not clear to what extent inhalational and intravenous narcotic anesthetics alter platelet function. Enflurane and fentanyl anesthetics appear to produce only insignificant prolongation of bleeding time,[66] although halothane, isoflurane, and nitrous oxide have been shown to interfere with platelet aggregation.[67, 68] Local anesthetic agents can also be shown to inhibit platelet aggregation[69]: regional anesthesia may therefore have value in reducing the incidence of postoperative thromboembolism, although the importance of these relatively small changes and their impact on hemostasis in normal individuals remain to be established.

The incidental hypothermia commonly associated with general anesthesia may be a factor in anesthesia-related disorders of hemostasis, although fibrin formation and polymerization appear to proceed without change during exposure to anesthetic agents. However, the final stage of hemostasis, fibrinolysis, is accelerated during and after inhalational, intravenous, or even regional anesthesia. Enhanced fibrinolysis probably represents a generalized response to perioperative stress, and not a drug-specific phenomenon. In fact, a similar increase in fibrinolytic activity occurs during exercise-induced sympathoadrenal stimulation, and is abolished by epidural anesthesia if neural blockade is sufficiently extensive to eliminate sympathetic outflow.[70]

Altered perioperative fibrinolysis may ultimately lead to other clinically significant problems. Plasma levels of both plasminogen activator and factor VIII:C are increased by catecholamines; sustained or repeated episodes of enhanced sympathoadrenal activity appear to exhaust the factors needed for fibrinolysis before fibrinogenesis itself has been impaired. This may explain why patients are at increased risk of venous thrombosis and thromboembolism after surgery, during hospitalization, or if they are subject to protracted pain or illness.[25] Additional contributions to what may be a multifactorial phenomenon include mechanical or anatomic stasis of blood flow, high hematocrit, and other factors that increase blood viscosity.[26, 27]

In contrast, fibrinolysis is chronically depressed during pregnancy or by the pregnancy-like state associated with oral contraceptive therapy. Predisposition to pathologic venous thrombosis under these circumstances probably reflects relative disequilibrium between clot formation and dissolution. Factors V, VII, VIII, IX, and X are elevated, while plasminogen activators remain depressed.[25] In addition, antithrombin III is low; this substance not only provides negative feedback to limit fibrin formation but also may be required to achieve the full anticoagulant activity of heparin and to ensure its effectiveness in preventing deep-vein thrombosis or in treating DIC.[54] Congenital deficiency of antithrombin III associated with recurrent thromboembolism is, in fact, a rare, but established, disorder.[25]

Immune Competence

The immune responsiveness of lymphocytes grown in culture after harvest from anesthetized patients is normal.[71] Anesthetic agents may therefore have little or no residual effects on this aspect of hematologic function, but anesthesia may increase susceptibility to lethal bacterial infections.[72] It also produces depression of lymphocyte function and immune responsiveness in vivo.[73] Similar predisposition to overwhelming bacterial sepsis and to reduced phagocytic activity occurs after hemorrhagic shock in unanesthetized animals, however.[74, 75]

Stress-related increases in sympathoadrenal tone or other alterations of the neuroendocrine environment are more likely to be directly responsible for depression of immune responsiveness under these circumstances than the direct effects of anesthetics themselves.[76, 77] In fact, the neutrophil-mediated phagocytosis needed for bactericidal immune competence and the activity of lymphocyte "killer cells" are both decreased significantly by elevated plasma glucocorticoids.[78, 79] In addition, human immune competence is impaired routinely after general anesthesia for major surgery, but not when anesthesia is administered solely for short, diagnostic procedures.[80]

Other Functions

Anesthetic toxicity may, however, produce the impairment of other aspects of hematologic function. Clinical concentrations of nitrous oxide oxidize and inhibit vitamin B_{12}, a cofactor needed for the synthesis of thymidine and nucleic acids in bone marrow. The depression of megaloblasts that occurs under these circumstances can be reversed by treatment with folinic acid,[81] although the consequences of this phenomenon are not yet understood. There are even less data available regarding the effect of nitrous oxide on the growth of other bone marrow cells, or on other components of the immune system.

Interference with folate metabolism by nitrous oxide may also have undesirable effects on the activity of other rapidly growing tissues. In laboratory animals nitrous oxide is teratogenic[82] when the fetus is exposed during the first trimester of pregnancy. Retrospective human studies, however, suggest that general anesthesia during early pregnancy does not produce similar effects in humans.[83] Instead, results of large-scale epidemiologic studies show only an increased rate of spontaneous abortion that is statistically, but not clearly causally, related to nitrous oxide exposure.[84] Increased fetal wastage has been observed in animal studies after chronic exposure to nitrous oxide.[85]

Histamine and Endocrines

Transient, dose-related release of cutaneous histamine after intravenous injection of the short-acting induction agents althesin and propranidid, or after alcuronium, a neuromuscular blocking drug, is common, and has in part prevented their introduction into worldwide anesthetic practice.[17] Similar anaphylactoid reactions occur frequently after injection of curare, atracurium, morphine, and thiopental, with variable degrees of subsequent systemic histamine release.[18] These phenomena all represent mast cell destabilization. Because of the variable content of plasma protein fractions, anaphylactoid reactions may complicate homologous blood transfusion.[55]

Secretion of cortisol, catecholamines, aldosterone, growth hormone, and ADH into plasma occurs in direct proportion to the severity and duration of perioperative emotional and physical stress. Perioperative hypercarbia or hypoxia, if sustained, may produce a similar endocrine response.[86, 87] The specific choice of anesthetic agents rarely plays a significant role in this response. Etomidate, however, even after a single dose, can depress cortisol activity and produce acute adrenal insufficiency: it impairs the responsiveness of the adrenal gland to ACTH and depresses the synthesis of cortisol.[88] By interrupting afferent pathways from injured tissues as well as blocking efferent sympathetic outflow, the pharmacologic sympathectomy produced by high epidural or spinal anesthesia functionally isolates the hypothalamus and appears to abolish, at least in part, the neuroendocrine stress response to surgery.[12]

ANESTHETIC CONSIDERATIONS FOR PATIENTS WITH BLOOD AND ENDOCRINE DISORDERS

Thyroid Disease

Major endocrinopathies that require adjustment of the anesthetic plan involve the pituitary, thyroid, or adrenal gland, as well as disorders of pregnancy.[89] Thyroxine (T_4) and, in particular, triiodothyronine (T_3) are potent anabolic hormones essential for normal growth and development. They also play a major role in nervous system function and, in particular, neuroendocrine mechanisms.[90] Primary hyperthyroidism (toxic goiter, or Graves' disease) is intrinsic thyroid hyperplasia, idiopathic or a consequence of pregnancy.[91] Extrinsic, or secondary, increases in thyroid function occur in response to the exaggerated release of TSH in patients with pituitary neoplasm or choriocarcinoma.[92]

Regardless of etiology, hyperactivity of the thyroid gland produces an accelerated metabolic state characterized by increased total body oxygen consumption, increased metabolic rate, and a variety of neurologic and metabolic dysfunctions.[93] The increased demand for cardiac output produces tachycardia and generalized cardiovascular stimulation, and may predispose to dysrhythmias and mitral valve prolapse. Diffuse increases in β-adrenergic receptor activity may play a role in these symptoms, and consequently beta blockade is frequently employed.[92] This therapeutic approach may, however, be contraindicated in the early stages of pregnancy.[94]

Weight loss, diarrhea, heat intolerance, and proximal skeletal muscle weakness are also common, although the mechanism by which they are produced is not well understood. Hyperpyrexia, profound cardiovascular instability, and other life-threatening manifestations of thyroid-induced nervous system toxicity are classically described as "thyroid storm,"[95] a phenomenon that could be triggered by severe illness or the stress of the perioperative environment. Thyroid storm has now been largely eliminated as a clinical problem by effective thyroid suppression using propylthiouracil, iodine, and methimazole.

Hypothyroidism occurs in about 5% of the general population. It is more common than increased thyroid function, but is usually subclinical. When clinically evident, hypothyroidism is associated with depressed metabolic function, bradycardia, cold intolerance, reduced autonomic and ventilatory responsiveness,[96] especially with obesity,[97] and lethargy. Trophic changes in the skin and soft tissues of these patients produce their characteristic "myxedematous" appearance.

Adenomatous goiter is a form of primary hypothyroidism; TSH is elevated, usually by a dietary deficiency of iodine, or by surgical thyroidectomy for hyperthyroidism. Hypothyroidism may also be due to an autoimmune process in which thyroglobulin acts as an antigen; therefore, hypothyroidism may be a symptom of a more extensive autoimmune phenomenon, such as lupus erythematosus or rheumatoid arthritis. In addition, hypothalamic or pituitary dysfunction can impair release of thyrotropic hormones, producing a secondary, or extrinsic, hypothyroidism. Untreated and protracted hypothyroidism may produce increased susceptibility to infection and cardiovascular instability, but thyroid hormone replacement therapy usually reverses hypothyroidism effectively and completely.

In both hyperthyroidism and hypothyroidism, the course of anesthetic management depends largely on the effectiveness of preoperative medical control and the extent to which it has re-established a euthyroid state.[92] β-Adrenergic blockade may suppress evidence of residual cardiovascular and metabolic toxicity in hyperthyroidism, but is not an adequate substitute for preoperative thyroid suppression: in inadequately treated patients, thyroid storm may occur as late as 18 hours after surgery.[93]

Anesthetic requirement is elevated in hyperthyroidism and is reduced by hypothyroidism. In both cases, however, the changes are small enough to fall within the range of variability seen in routine anesthetic practice.[98] Emergence from anesthesia may be somewhat prolonged, and coagulation modestly depressed, in clinically hypothyroid surgical patients.[99] In general, however, the choice of anesthetic agent itself does not appear to exert an important influence on outcome. Because of the site of surgery, mechanical factors play the largest role in perioperative morbidity and mortality: thyroid resection introduces the risk of postoperative airway obstruction by edema of the soft tissues of the neck, hematoma, or as a consequence of laryngeal nerve injury and subsequent vocal cord paralysis.

Parathyroid Disease

Incidental parathyroidectomy during thyroid surgery may produce transient hypocalcemia with sequelae of skeletal muscle tetany, laryngospasm, or seizure activity. Symptoms of hypoparathyroidism usually respond to calcium infusion and to vitamin D, which has effects that are synergistic with even low levels of parathyroid hormone (PTH). Response to PTH infusion itself is delayed, however, and may trigger an immune reaction.[100] In contrast, hyperparathyroidism is characterized by excessive PTH secretion and augmented mobilization of body calcium stores. It may be primary (idiopathic or pregnancy related), secondary (compensatory, associated with increased renal calcium loss), or due to malignancy (pseudohyperparathyroidism).

Classic symptoms of hyperparathyroidism include nausea, weight loss, fatigue, constipation, and painful kidney stones. None of these has a significant impact on the plan for general anesthesia, although both thyroid and parathyroid surgery can be done, if desired, under regional anesthesia with deep sedation.[99] If it produces a significant degree of hypocalcemia, hypoparathyroidism may be associated with profound or prolonged neuromuscular blockade, or inadequate antagonism and return of muscle strength.

Adrenal Disorders

Adrenocortical hyperplasia due to an ACTH-secreting pituitary adenoma (Cushing's disease), or excess glucocorticoid for any other reason, produces significant generalized metabolic and cardiovascular effects. Hypertension, hypokalemia, obesity, muscle weakness, and susceptibility to infection characterize patients with increased cortisol and aldosterone.[89] The adrenal cortex may also be hypertrophied in patients with hyperthyroidism.[93]

Therapeutic or incidental suppression of ACTH or surgical adrenalectomy may produce clinical signs of adrenocortical insufficiency that requires administration of exogenous cortisol. Many patients on chronic steroid therapy, however, maintain good responsiveness to ACTH, and therefore require little additional cortisol.[101] Primary adrenocortical insufficiency (Addison's disease) is less common, and is usually a consequence of the autoimmune or infectious destruction of the adrenal cortex.

Pregnancy

Because pregnancy is characterized by major changes in endocrine balance, it has anesthetic implications that go beyond its occasional association with hyperthyroidism and hyperparathyroidism. Pregnancy alters both the hormonal environment and the responsiveness of many cardiovascular end-organs. During pregnancy, the neurally mediated pathways of the sympathoadrenal axis demonstrate impaired activity,[102] but there is increased vascular responsiveness to ADH.[103] In patients with diabetes mellitus, pregnancy increases the risk of both hypoglycemia and of ketoacidosis because cortisol and prostaglandins have anti-insulin effects.[104]

Preeclampsia and eclampsia appear to have an underlying autoimmune or fetal-immune mechanism: these syndromes are familial, and they are terminated promptly and definitively by the delivery of the fetus and the placenta.[105] During pregnancy, however, there is a generalized and progressive increase in arteriolar smooth muscle tone in eclampsia-susceptible patients that produces profound contraction of blood volume,[106] with a 30% to 40% reduction in plasma volume, low ventricular filling pressures, and abnormally high systemic vascular resistance.[107, 108] Renal blood flow and glomerular filtration are also reduced in preeclampsia and eclampsia. In addition, glomerular capillary damage further aggravates contraction of circulating plasma volume; accelerated protein loss reduces plasma oncotic pressure, thereby further impairing retention of water within the circulation.

The Uteroplacental Barrier

General considerations in the design of the anesthetic plan for pregnant patients, especially those near term, require consideration of the movement of drugs across the uteroplacental barrier (UPB). In early pregnancy the primary concern has been to identify those anesthetic agents, if any, that interfere with normal fetal development, or those that may produce congenital deformities. Once the period of organogenesis within the fetus is completed, however, the risk is not from the toxicity or teratogenicity of anesthetic agents, but rather from the extent to which a newborn infant will share the inevitable depression of respiratory, cardiac, and neurologic functioning produced by anesthetic drugs given to the mother.

Like the blood-brain barrier, the UPB is a functional concept with anatomic analogs. It describes the relative restriction of both active and passive molecular exchange between maternal and fetal blood by the three tissue layers of the placental villi. Small molecules diffuse across the UPB easily, but this lipid barrier hinders the transfer of many anesthetic agents and adjuvants to fetal blood.[109] Because rates of transplacental transport are progressively reduced as molecules increase in size and in their degree of ionization, the passage of neuromuscular blocking drugs is particularly limited.

Although they appear at somewhat lower concentrations in fetal than in maternal blood, all inhalational anesthetics are lipid soluble, and therefore they cross the UPB easily. The delay in equilibrium between maternal blood and fetal nervous system tissues is sufficiently great, however, that anesthetic concentrations are rarely achieved in the newborn during the time elapsed from anesthetic induction to delivery of the infant, provided that relatively low inspired concentrations, about 0.5 minimum alveolar (anesthetic) concentration (MAC), are used for caesarean section. Even nitrous oxide partial pressures in the fetus remain low enough to permit its routine use for general anesthesia under these circumstances, if the baby is delivered within 20 minutes.[110]

Since virtually all intravenous anesthetic agents have central nervous system effects because they possess a significant degree of lipid solubility, some passage from mother to fetus must occur. Equilibrium between maternal and fetal blood concentrations is, in fact, more rapid for intravenous agents than for inhalational anesthetics. High concentrations of these drugs in maternal blood after bolus intravenous administration further accelerate transfer across the UPB. Atropine, scopolamine, barbiturates, phenothiazines, ethanol, paraldehyde, narcotics, and local anesthetics have all been found in fetal blood in clinically significant concentrations.[111] Meperidine is of special concern because it has an unusually long elimination half-life in the newborn.[112] The fraction of drug dosage that is bound to protein in maternal blood may also influence the ease with which these molecules pass across the UPB; a higher degree of binding to maternal protein retards subsequent transfer to the fetal circulation.

Assuming placental perfusion is abundant and intact, fetal oxygenation and carbon dioxide excretion change in proportion to variations in maternal respiratory status. Respiratory gas exchange may be compromised, however, by premature placental separation, maternal hypotension, uterine hypertonicity, vasoconstriction, or mechanical compression or kinking of the umbilical cord. Some limitations on the adequate exchange of respiratory gases between mother and baby may also be imposed in older parturients, especially those with the prolonged gestation of a postmaturity fetus.

In general, however, the primary mechanism by which the anesthetic plan provides for fetal metabolic well-being is the maintenance of normal maternal cardiac output and ventilation. Therefore, the cardiovascular side effects of potent inhalational anesthetics may depress placental blood flow if they produce significant or sustained arterial hypotension in the mother. Except for nitrous oxide, these agents also inhibit uterine motility. They depress the effectiveness of uterine contractions, and may compromise uterine hemostasis after placental separation if inspired concentrations exceed 1.5 MAC.[113]

Rheology of Blood

The complex structure of blood confers characteristic flow properties, or "rheology," which influence the anesthetic management of patients with abnormal types of hemoglobin, or those at the extremes of the normal range for hemoglobin or hematocrit. Unlike a pure fluid, blood has non-newtonian flow properties: its viscosity, or consistency, changes as a function of both the concentration of its cellular elements and the velocity at which it traverses the circulation.

Interactions between erythrocytes to form aggregates (rouleaux) and the electrostatic association of cellular elements, mediated by fibrin, are largely responsible for determining "yield stress," the pressure required to resume blood movement after stasis.[114] Blood viscosity also increases with decreasing temperature, rising significantly even during the relatively mild hypothermia of cardiopulmonary bypass.[27] These mechanical properties of blood are particularly important at the low velocities of flow that exist within the microcirculation. In the microcirculation, a laminar flow pattern "skims" cellular from plasma elements, reducing effective hematocrit in the smallest branches of the tissue exchange beds.

Anemia as a Risk Factor

Blood viscosity affects the hydraulics of the general arterial circulation in two ways. It interacts with systemic vascular resistance to determine total peripheral resistance and, thus, indirectly, arterial blood pressure; it also influences the stroke volume associated with a given level of end-diastolic volume by changing the characteristics of ventricular ejection (Chapter 6). Systemic oxygen transport (STo_2) varies little over the range of hematocrit values from 25% to 45% (Fig 10–7), since decreases in oxygen-carrying capacity are largely offset by the improved hydraulics associated with reduced blood viscosity.[63] Consequently, the classical requirement for a minimum preoperative hemoglobin concentration of 10 g/dL has given way to adoption of a "soft" standard with a more appropriate lower value of 7 to 8 g/dL.[3, 5, 115]

With chronic anemia, development of compensatory microcirculation collaterals may provide an additional element of safety.[116] Hemoglobin values reduced acutely below this level may, however, be associated with significant reductions of STo_2 during anesthesia. They have, in fact, been shown to predict a significant increase in perioperative surgical mortality.[117] Anemia is not the only factor that can compromise systemic oxygen transport severely, however, even in well-oxygenated patients. Both polycythemia and the low flow velocities associated with cardiogenic shock can increase blood viscosity and yield stress, impairing molecular exchange at the capillary level and predisposing to thrombosis in the microcirculation.

Sickle Cell Disease

Similarly, distortion of erythrocyte morphology by variant hemoglobin phenotypes such as the hemoglobin S of sickle cell disease prevents free movement of these cells through capillaries. Obstructed flow may produce the infarcts of spleen, bone, and lung, which characterize the "sickle crisis." The fundamental approach to the design of the anesthetic plan for these patients reflects basic rheologic considerations: ample hydration, oxygenation to minimize erythrocyte sickling because of desaturation, and avoidance of hypothermia or other initiators of vasoconstriction that can reduce velocity of tissue blood flow.[62]

Consequently, the time these patients are at highest risk is not during, but rather after, surgery. Postoperatively, ventilation and oxygenation may be impaired, and hypothermia, shivering, and the full sympathoadrenal response to pain and stress almost always increase systemic vascular resistance.[118] Patients heterozygous for hemoglobin S, however, do not appear to be at similar levels of increased perioperative risk.[119]

Erythrocyte sickling is minimal when less than 30% of the patient's hemoglobin consists of hemoglobin S,[61] but preoperative replacement of abnormal hemoglobin by transfusion with blood of normal hemoglobin A can, if final hematocrit is elevated, actually impair microcirculatory flow and compromise tissue metabolism. Hemoconcentration due to dehydration or endogenous polycythemia can also reduce cardiac index, since autonomic cardiovascular homeostasis utilizes afferent input from a variety of pressure and volume receptors, but is insensitive to flow at the level of the tissue exchange beds themselves.[120] Arterial and cardiac filling pressures that would normally be adequate may not generate sufficient velocity of erythrocyte movement through peripheral tissues under these circumstances. In addition, the increased yield stress produced by elevated blood viscosity may produce a "no-reflow" phenomenon, creating or extending tissue infarction after acute arterial occlusion.[121]

Hemodilution

Intentional hemodilution can be used as an adjunct to extracorporeal perfusion or deliberate (controlled) hypotension, maintaining adequate peripheral oxygen delivery at arterial blood pressure values normally associated with inadequate microcirculatory flow.[7] The reduction in blood viscosity produced by acute hemodilution lowers total peripheral resistance even when systemic vascular resistance remains unchanged. For any given level of arterial pressure, therefore, cardiac output will be higher than that occurring at a normal hematocrit or hemoglobin value. The increase in volumetric blood flow does not completely offset simultaneous loss of oxygen-carrying capacity, but STo_2 remains within 10% of normal values until hematocrit falls below 30%.[122]

Lack of a "compensatory" increase in cardiac output in response to decreased oxygen transport under experimental conditions of methemoglobinemia[123] supports the concept that the increased cardiac output associated with moderate anemia is a mechanical consequence of reduced blood viscosity, and not necessarily an active, autonomic response to metabolic derangement and tissue hypoxia.

Hemodilution may prevent the "no reflow" phenomenon in reperfused tissues that have undergone a prior episode of ischemia.[124] Unlike chronic anemia or acute hypovolemic hemorrhage, there appear to be no changes in the oxygen-hemoglobin dissociation relationship during acute hemodilution with intravenous crystalloid infusion. Since intentional intraoperative hemodilution does not increase STo_2 above normal levels, however, arteriovenous oxygen differences may still be increased postoperatively when tissue demands for oxygen are significantly elevated by shivering or generalized autonomic stimulation.[7]

Transfusion

In those surgical procedures where major bleeding can be anticipated, intraoperative hemodilution is accomplished by elective phlebotomy, either preoperatively or intraoperatively, before the onset of surgical hemorrhage. Three or more units of blood can be obtained from patients scheduled for elective surgery within the month before operation, especially if used in conjunction with iron supplementation. Reinfusion of this autologous blood avoids the risk of infection acquired from the transfusion of homologous blood, limitations imposed by inadequate supplies of rare blood types, or the risk of inadvertent major blood group incompatibility. However, the patient remains equally susceptible to transfusion reactions that are due to clerical error or the mishandling of blood products, and autologous techniques may actually encourage unnecessary blood transfusion.[125]

Considerations of cardiovascular stability usually limit acute intraoperative phlebotomy to two units. In contrast, intraoperative salvage of shed blood with use of an autotransfusion system for continuous collection, washing, and reinfusion of erythrocytes has, in theory, no such obvious limitations. However, unavoidable manipulation and mechanical damage to cellular and protein blood components creates the possibility of air and tissue microemboli and may induce a consumption coagulopathy.[126] Additional concerns regarding intravascular dissemination of tumor and spread of infected material also limit the practical application of this approach to major vascular surgery or to other procedures with well-defined and "clean" sources of surgical blood loss.

When blood from nonautologous donors is used, potential complications of blood transfusion include a wide variety of antigen-mediated and nonspecific immune reactions.[55] In many ways transfusion more closely resembles a tissue graft than a simple volume infusion. Generalized suppression of immune responsiveness by transfusion was, in fact, once utilized to enhance renal homograft survival,[127] but may actually increase mortality in patients with metastatic disease.[128]

Catastrophic, immediate reactions to transfused blood usually represent hemolysis from major blood group incompatibility mediated by the formation of antigen-antibody complexes on erythrocyte surfaces. The rapid lysis of donor cells is further accelerated by the presence of complement in the immune complex. Fatal outcome may occur once in 100,000 transfusions.[115] Free hemoglobin is released into plasma from damaged cells, then into renal tubular fluid, and subsequently produces hemoglobinuria. After hemolytic transfusion reactions, thromboplastin released from damaged erythrocytes may precipitate DIC by providing the phospholipid membrane fragments needed to trigger the extrinsic coagulation pathway. Vasoactive polypeptides can also produce cardiovascular collapse. When transfusion recipients have low levels of antibody, there may be a delayed, postoperative transfusion reaction to intraoperative major group incompatibility. Antibody within donor plasma can also attack recipient erythrocytes, with similar results.

Other forms of host reactions to transfused blood do not involve blood group incompatibilities. Donor white cells in transfused plasma can release pyrogens, precipitating a febrile transfusion reaction. Host antibodies may attack donor platelets. Antigenic moieties in transfused plasma or in the residual plasma of packed erythrocytes may induce an anaphylactoid response, with nonspecific histamine release. None of these complications of blood transfusion have been eliminated by the widespread adoption of component therapy. This approach maximizes the availability of specific blood components, but does not minimize the risk associated with blood transfusion.[46]

With adequate safeguards to ensure blood group compatibility and screening to exclude infected blood, transfusion of blood and its components in response to appropriate indications (Table 10–1) remains effective and relatively safe; fewer than 1 in 600 patients have clinically

TABLE 10-1.

Perioperative Indications for the Use of Blood Products*

Deficiencies of Oxygen Transport	Etiology	Component Preferred
Symptomatic chronic anemia	Hemolysis; renal failure; chronic bleeding; bone marrow depression; hemoglobinopathy; inadequate transfusion; phlebotomy	Packed RBC
Hypovolemia	Hemorrhage; dehydration	Plasma expander/ crystalloid
Acute anemia and hypovolemia	Sustained hemorrhage; surgical bleeding	Whole blood or RBC with plasma expanders
Hemostatic defects		
Severe thrombocytopenia	Radiation or chemotherapy; leukemia; massive transfusion; DIC	Platelet concentrate
Symptomatic thrombocytopathy	Aspirin or heparin therapy; renal failure; congenital disorders	Platelet concentrate; desmopressin (DDAVP)
Coagulopathies		
Factor VIII deficiency	Hemophilia A; von Willebrand's disease	Factor VIII concentrate (AHF); cryoprecipitate, DDAVP
Factor V deficiency	Congenital	FFP
Deficiency of factors II, VII, IX, or X	Hepatic failure; hemophilia B	Factor IX complex; FFP; plasma; vitamin K
Hypofibrinogenemia	Congenital; DIC	Cryoprecipitate; plasma
Consumption coagulopathy	Disseminated intravascular coagulation (DIC)	Platelet concentrate; FFP; plasma; heparin

*DIC = disseminated intravascular coagulation; FFP = fresh frozen plasma; RBC = red blood cells.

significant transfusion reactions.[55] Massive transfusions of blood in amounts 1½ times or greater than the circulating blood volume of the patient[129] may, however, produce a dilutional coagulopathy or transient hypocalcemia because of the large amount of citrate contained in blood preservatives.

Infusion of hematologic debris, including microaggregates and fibrin, is also of concern because of the consequences of their deposition in the pulmonary circulation.[130] They can be removed from infused blood with fine mesh blood filters designed for this purpose,[131] but these devices also reduce platelet concentrations significantly when used with blood that is fresh or only a few days old.[37] These microfilters are also expensive and limit maximum infusion rate; thus, they have been recommended only for the transfusion of multiple units of blood, or if the blood components are at the limits of their viability and may contain large amounts of debris.[132]

SUMMARY

Blood is not a body fluid, but a complex tissue that provides both passive transport and many active intrinsic functions essential to body metabolism. The normal characteristics of the oxygen-hemoglobin dissociation relationship maximize delivery of oxygen to peripheral tissues despite the relatively small partial pressure gradient that exists between them and arterial blood. In the small vessels of the microcirculation, volumetric blood flow and flow velocity are influenced greatly by the rheology of blood, which largely depends upon hematocrit and temperature.

Hemodilution, whether intentional or inadvertent, reduces blood viscosity and, to a large extent, offsets reduced oxygen-carrying capacity sufficiently to maintain systemic oxygen transport at near-normal levels over a wide range of values for hematocrit. Consequently, minimum acceptable preoperative values for hemoglobin may be considerably lower than has been traditionally maintained, especially if anemia is chronic.

When the integrity of the vasculature is compromised by trauma or surgery, hemostasis is accomplished initially by the formation of a platelet plug. Subsequently, a fibrin meshwork stabilizes the defect. This "clot" is resolubilized in a controlled manner by circulating fibrinolytic agents as vascular healing proceeds. Despite the terminology of coagulation "cascade," the cellular and noncellular components of hemostasis are now thought to participate in a dynamic equilibrium of continuous fibrinogenesis and fibrinolysis that maintains a near-constant liquidity of blood, except in areas in which the endothelial layer has been breached.

Quantitative or qualitative abnormalities of platelets, coagulation factors, or fibrinolytic agents produce a wide variety of congenital or acquired hemostatic disorders. Virtually all are usually treated by the replacement of the deficient procoagulant or anticoagulant factors. Inadequate fibrinolysis can produce pathologic thrombosis, especially in low-flow cardiovascular states; enhanced fibrinolytic activity causes accelerated clot dissolution and may explain some types of persistent postoperative bleeding. Disseminated intravascular coagulation occurs when there has been massive consumption of platelets, fibrinogen, and other coagulation factors. Diffuse fibrinogenesis can be triggered by foreign materials or by extensive tissue injury through either the intrinsic or the extrinsic coagulation pathways.

Design of a successful anesthetic plan for patients with coagulopathies, hemoglobinopathies, endocrinopathies, or pregnancy depends more on the adequate therapy of the underlying disorder than on the specific anesthetic agents selected. Generalized depression of immune responsiveness during and after general anesthesia and surgery appears to reflect the change in neuroendocrine environment associated with perioperative stress. A variety of anesthetic drugs may produce mild, probably transient, depression of bone marrow and platelet function, however. Virtually all anesthetic agents and adjuvants are transferred to some degree from maternal to fetal blood across the uteroplacental barrier, but inhalational anesthetics and neuromuscular blocking drugs can be used safely for obstetric anesthesia provided that the timing and dosage of drug administration are considered appropriately.

REFERENCES

1. Gould SA, Rosen AL, Sehgal LR, et al: Fluosol-DA as a red cell substitute in acute anemia. *N Engl J Med* 1986; 314:1653–1656.
2. Perutz MF: Stereochemistry of cooperative effects in haemoglobin. *Nature* 1970; 228:726.
3. Gillies IDS: Anaemia and anaesthesia. *Br J Anaesth* 1974; 46:589–602.
4. Lawther PJ, Commins BT: Cigarette smoking and exposure to carbon monoxide. *Ann NY Acad Sci* 1970; 174:135–147.
5. Allen JB, Allen FB: The minimum acceptable level of hemoglobin. *Int Anesthesiol Clin* 1982; 20:1–22.
6. Finch CA, Lenfant C: Oxygen transport in man. *N Engl J Med* 1972; 286:407–415.
7. Laks H, Pilon RN, Kovekorn WP, et al: Acute hemodilution: Its effect on hemodynamics and oxygen transport in anaesthetized man. *Ann Surg* 1974; 180:103–109.
8. Kinney JM: Transport of carbon dioxide in blood. *Anesthesiology* 1960; 21:615–633.
9. Salo M: Endocrine response to anaesthesia and surgery, in Watkins J, Salo M (eds): *Trauma, Stress and Immunity in Anaesthesia and Surgery*. London, Butterworth, 1982, pp 141–173.
10. Wright PD, Johnston IDA: The effect of surgical operation on growth hormone levels in plasma. *Surgery* 1975; 77:479–486.
11. Oyama T, Toyota M, Shinozaki Y, et al: Effects of morphine and ketamine anaesthesia and surgery on plasma concentrations of luteinizing

hormone, testosterone and cortisol in man. *Br J Anaesth* 1977; 49:983–990.

12. Kehlet H: Influence of epidural analgesia on the endocrine-metabolic response to surgery. *Acta Anaesthesiol Scand* 1978; 70(suppl):39–42.
13. Young JB, Rowe JW, Pallotta JA, et al: Enhanced plasma norepinephrine response to upright posture and oral glucose administration in elderly human subjects. *Metabolism* 1980; 29:532–539.
14. Strong R: Neurochemistry of aging: 1982–1984. *Rev Biol Res Aging* 1985; 2:181–196.
15. Heinsimer JA, Lefkowitz RJ: The impact of aging on adrenergic receptor function. *J Am Geriatr Soc* 1985; 33:184–188.
16. Nossal GJV: The basic components of the immune system. *N Engl J Med* 1987; 316:1320–1325.
17. Levy JH: Allergic reactions during anesthesia. *J Clin Anesth* 1988; 1:39–46.
18. Moss J, Rosow CE: Histamine release by narcotics and muscle relaxants in humans. *Anesthesiology* 1983; 59:330–339.
19. Nordstrom L, Fletcher R, Pavek K: Shock of anaphylactoid type induced by protamine: A continuous cardiorespiratory record. *Acta Anaesthesiol Scand* 1978; 22:195–201.
20. Madowitz JS, Schweiger MJ: Severe anaphylactoid reaction to radiographic contrast media. *JAMA* 1979; 241:2813–2815.
21. Watkins J: Anaphylactoid reactions to I.V. substances. *Br J Anaesth* 1979; 51:51–60.
22. Roath S, Francis JL: Normal blood coagulation, fibrinolysis, and natural inhibitors of coagulation. *Int Anesthesiol Clin* 1985; 23:23–35.
23. Mackie IJ, Pittilo RM: Vascular integrity and platelet function. *Int Anesthesiol Clin* 1985; 23:3–21.
24. Wessler S: The role of hypercoagulability in venous and arterial thrombosis. *Cardiovasc Clin* 1971; 3:2–13.
25. Yardumian A, Machin SJ: Hypercoagulable states. *Int Anesthesiol Clin* 1985; 23:141–155.
26. Dormandy JA, Edelman JB: High blood viscosity: An aetiological factor in venous thrombosis. *Br J Surg* 1973; 60:187–190.
27. Gordon RJ, Ravin MB: Rheology and anesthesiology. *Anesth Analg* 1978; 57:252–261.
28. Kakkar VV: Diagnosis, prevention, and treatment of venous thromboembolism. *Int Anesthesiol Clin* 1985; 23:157–172.
29. Rorher MJ, Michelotti MC, Nahrwold DL: A prospective evaluation of the efficacy of preoperative coagulation testing. *Ann Surg* 1988; 208:554–557.
30. Moir DJ: Investigation of bleeding disorders. *Int Anesthesiol Clin* 1985; 23:37–47.
31. Levine PH: Platelet-function tests: Predictive value. *N Engl J Med* 1975; 292:1346–1347.
32. Giddings JC, Evans BK: Drugs affecting blood coagulation and hemostasis. *Int Anesthesiol Clin* 1985; 23:103–123.

33. O'Brien JR, Etherington M, Jamieson S: Refractory state of platelet aggregation with major operations. *Lancet* 1971; 2:741–743.
34. Slater NGP: Acquired bleeding disorders. *Int Anesthesiol Clin* 1985; 23:73–87.
35. Weinberg AD, Brennan MD, Gorman CA, et al: Outcome of anesthesia and surgery in hypothyroid patients. *Arch Intern Med* 1983; 143:893–897.
36. Harker LA: Bleeding after cardiopulmonary bypass (editorial). *N Engl J Med* 1986; 314:1446–1448.
37. Dunbar RW, Price KA, Cannarella CF: Microaggregate blood filters. *Anesth Analg* 1974; 53:577–583.
38. Reed RL II, Heimbach DM, Counts RB, et al: Prophylactic platelet administration during massive transfusion. *Ann Surg* 1986; 203:40–48.
39. Colman RW, Robboy SJ, Minna JD: Disseminated intravascular coagulation (DIC): An approach. *Am J Med* 1972; 52:679–689.
40. Moss RA: Drug-induced immune thrombocytopenia. *Am J Hematol* 1980; 9:439–446.
41. Tuddenham EGD: Inherited bleeding disorders. *Int Anesthesiol Clin* 1985; 23:61–72.
42. Ruggeri ZM, Mannucci PM, Lombardi R: Multimeric composition of factor VIII:vWF following administration of DDVAP: Implications for pathophysiology and therapy of von Willebrand's disease. *Blood* 1982; 59:1272–1278.
43. Entwistle CC: Clotting factor concentrates. *Int Anesthesiol Clin* 1985; 23:49–59.
44. Mannucci PM: Desmopressin: A nontransfusional form of treatment for congenital and acquired bleeding disorders. *Blood* 1988; 72:1449–1455.
45. Ellison N: Diagnosis and management of bleeding disorders. *Anesthesiology* 1977; 47:171–180.
46. Blumberg N, Laczin J, McMican A, et al: A critical survey of fresh-frozen plasma use. *Transfusion* 1986; 26:511–513.
47. Hattersley PG: Progress report: The activated coagulation time of whole blood (ACT). *Am J Clin Pathol* 1976; 66:899–904.
48. Jobes DR, Schwartz AJ, Ellison N, et al: Monitoring heparin anticoagulation and its neutralization. *Ann Thorac Surg* 1981; 31:161–166.
49. Umlas J, Taff RH, Gauvin G, et al: Anticoagulant monitoring and neutralization during open heart surgery: A rapid method for measuring heparin and calculating safe reduced protamine doses. *Anesth Analg* 1983; 62:1095–1098.
50. Franz RC, Coetzee WJ: The thromboelastographic diagnosis of hemostatic defects. *Surg Annu* 1981; 13:75–107.
51. Kang YG, Martin DJ, Marquez J, et al: Intraoperative changes in blood coagulation and thromboelastographic monitoring in liver transplantation. *Anesth Analg* 1985; 64:888–896.
52. Butler MJ: Thromboelastography during and after elective abdominal surgery. *Thromb Haemost* 1978; 39:488–495.

53. Tuman KJ, Spiess BD, McCarthy RJ, et al: Effects of progressive blood loss on coagulation as measured by thromboelastography. *Anesth Analg* 1987; 66:856–863.
54. Bolton FG: Disseminated intravascular coagulation. *Int Anesthesiol Clin* 1985; 23:89–101.
55. Brzica SM: Complications of transfusion. *Int Anesthesiol Clin* 1981; 19:171–193.
56. Wright JP: Anesthetic considerations in pre-eclampsia and eclampsia. *Anesth Analg* 1983; 63:590–601.
57. Bell WR, Meek AG: Guidelines for the use of thrombolytic agents. *N Engl J Med* 1979; 301:1266–1270.
58. Anderson L: Antifibrinolytic treatment with epsilon-aminocaproic acid in connection with prostatectomy. *Acta Chir Scand* 1964; 127:552–564.
59. Lambert CJ, Marengo-Rowe AJ, Leveson JE, et al: The treatment of post-perfusion bleeding using ε-aminocaproic acid, cryoprecipitate, fresh-frozen plasma, and protamine sulfate. *Ann Thorac Surg* 1978; 28:440–444.
60. Davis RF: The experts opine. *Surv Anesthesiol* 1986; 30:375–382.
61. Bunch C: Abnormal hemoglobins. *Int Anesthesiol Clin* 1985; 23:175–195.
62. Dobson MG: Anesthesia for patients with hemoglobinopathies. *Int Anesthesiol Clin* 1985; 23:197–211.
63. Cromwell JW, Ford RG, Lewis VM: Oxygen transport in hemorrhagic shock as a function of the hematocrit ratio. *Am J Physiol* 1959; 196:1033–1038.
64. Murray JF, Gold P, Johnson BL: The circulatory effects of hematocrit variations in normovolemic and hypervolemic dogs. *J Clin Invest* 1963; 42:1150–1159.
65. Loarie DJ, Wilkinson P, Tyberg J, et al: The hemodynamic effects of halothane in anemic dogs. *Anesth Analg* 1979; 58:195–200.
66. Gotta AW, Gould P, Sullivan C, et al: The effect of enflurane and fentanyl anesthesia on human platelet aggregation in vivo. *Can Anaesth Soc J* 1980; 27:319–322.
67. Ueda I: The effects of volatile general anesthetics on adenosine diphosphate–induced platelet aggregation. *Anesthesiology* 1971; 34:405–408.
68. Fauss BG, Meadows JC, Bruni CY, et al: The in vitro and in vivo effects of isoflurane and nitrous oxide on platelet aggregation. *Anesth Analg* 1986; 65:1170–1174.
69. Borg T, Modig J: Potential anti-thrombotic effects of local anaesthetics due to their inhibition of platelet aggregation. *Acta Anaesthesiol Scand* 1985; 29:739–742.
70. Uppington J: Anesthetic management of patients with coagulation disorders. *Int Anesthesiol Clin* 1985; 23:125–140.
71. Robertson AJ, Gibbs JH, Potts RC, et al: Effect of anesthesia and surgery on the pre-s-phase cell cycle kinetics of mitogen-stimulated lymphocytes of previously healthy people. *Br J Anaesth* 1983; 55:339–347.

72. Hansbrough JF, Zapata-Sirvent RL, Barlte EJ, et al: Alterations in splenic lymphocyte subpopulations and increased mortality from sepsis following anesthesia in mice. *Anesthesiology* 1985; 63:267–273.

73. Slade MS, Simmons RL, Yunis E, et al: Immunodepression after major surgery in normal patients. *Surgery* 1975; 78:363–372.

74. Esrig BC, Frazee L, Stephenson SF, et al: The predisposition to infection following hemorrhagic shock. *Surg Gynecol Obstet* 1977; 144:915–917.

75. Zweibach BW, Benacerraf B: Effect of hemorrhagic shock on the phagocytic action of Kupffer cells. *Circ Res* 1958; 6:83–87.

76. Berenbaum MC, Fluck PA, Hurst NP: Depression of lymphocyte responses after surgical trauma. *Br J Exp Pathol* 1973; 54:597–607.

77. Cullen BF, van Belle G: Lymphocyte transformation and changes in leukocyte count: Effect of anesthesia and operation. *Anesthesiology* 1975; 43:563–569.

78. Fuenfer MM, Olson GE, Polk HC Jr: Effect of various corticosteroids upon the phagocytic bactericidal activity of neutrophils. *Surgery* 1975; 78:27–33.

79. Tonnesen E, Brinklov MM, Christensen NJ, et al: Natural killer cell activity and lymphocyte function during and after coronary artery bypass grafting in relation to the endocrine stress response. *Anesthesiology* 1987; 67:526–533.

80. Vose BM, Moudgil GC: Post-operative depression of antibody-dependent lymphocyte cytotoxicity following minor surgery and anaesthesia. *Clin Exp Immunol* 1976; 30;123–128.

81. Nunn JF, Chanarin I, Tanner AG, et al: Megaloblastic bone marrow changes after repeated nitrous oxide anaesthesia; reversal with folinic acid. *Br J Anaesth* 1986; 58:1469–1470.

82. Lane GA, Nahrwold ML, Tait AR, et al: Anesthetics as teratogens: Nitrous oxide is fetotoxic, xenon is not. *Science* 1980; 210:899–901.

83. Aldridge LM, Tunstall ME: Nitrous oxide and the fetus. *Br J Anaesth* 1986; 58:1348–1356.

84. Baden JM: Mutagenicity, carcinogenicity, and teratogenicity of nitrous oxide, in Eger EI II (ed): *Nitrous Oxide.* New York, Elsevier, 1985, pp 235–247.

85. Mazze RI, Fujinaga M, Rice SA, et al: Reproductive and teratogenic effects of nitrous oxide, halothane, isoflurane, and enflurane in Sprague-Dawley rats. *Anesthesiology* 1986; 64:339–344.

86. Sechzer PH, Egbert LD, Linde HE, et al: Effect of CO_2 inhalation on arterial pressure, ECG and plasma catecholamines and 17-OH corticosteroids in normal man. *J Appl Physiol* 1960; 15:454–458.

87. Dobkin AB, Byles PH, Neville JF Jr: Neuroendocrine and metabolic effects of anaesthesia during spontaneous breathing, controlled breathing, mild hypoxia, and mild hypercarbia. *Can Anaesth Soc J* 1966; 13:130–171.

88. Wagner RL, White PF, Kan PB, et al: Inhibition of adrenal steroidogenesis by the anesthetic etomidate. *N Engl J Med* 1984; 310:1415–1421.

89. James ML: Endocrine disease and anaesthesia: A review of anaesthetic

management in pituitary, adrenal, and thyroid disease. *Anaesthesia* 1970; 25:232–252.

90. Sterling K: Thyroid hormone action at the cell level (2 parts). *N Engl J Med* 1979; 300:117–123; 173–177.

91. Burrow GY: Maternal-fetal considerations in hyperthyroidism. *Clin Endocrinol Metab* 1978; 7:115–125.

92. Roizen MF, Hensel P, Lichtor JL, et al: Patients with disorders of thyroid function. *Anesthesiol Clin North Am* 1987; 5:277–286.

93. Stehling LC: Anesthetic management of the patient with hyperthyroidism. *Anesthesiology* 1974; 41:585–595.

94. Levy CA, Waite JH, Dickey R: Thyrotoxicosis and pregnancy: Use of preoperative propranolol for thyroidectomy. *Am J Surg* 1977; 133:319–321.

95. Mackin JF, Canary JJ, Pittman CS: Thyroid storm and its management. *N Engl J Med* 1974; 291:1396–1398.

96. Zwillich CW, Pierson DJ, Hofeldt FD, et al: Ventilatory control in myxedema and hypothyroidism. *N Engl J Med* 1975; 292:662–665.

97. Levelle JP, Jopling MW, Sklar GS: Perioperative hypothyroidism: An unusual postanesthetic diagnosis. *Anesthesiology* 1985; 63:195–197.

98. Babad AA, Eger EI II: The effects of hyperthyroidism and hypothyroidism on halothane and oxygen requirements in dogs. *Anesthesiology* 1968; 20:1087–1093.

99. Saxe AW, Brown E, Hamburger SW: Thyroid and parathyroid surgery performed under regional anesthesia. *Surgery* 1988; 103:415–420.

100. Nimmadada U, Salem MR, Ivankovich AD: Anesthesia and parathyroid disease. *Semin Anesth* 1984; 3:175–185.

101. Symreng T, Karlberg BE, Kagedal B: TBR: Physiological cortisol substitution of long-term steroid-treated patients undergoing major surgery. *Br J Anaesth* 1981; 53:949–973.

102. Nisell H, Jhemdahl P, Linde B, et al: Sympathoadrenal and cardiovascular reactivity in pregnancy-induced hypertension. *Am J Obstet Gynecol* 1985; 152:554–560.

103. Lindheimer MD, Katz AI: Hypertension in pregnancy. *N Engl J Med* 1985; 313:675–680.

104. Freinkel N, Dooley SL, Metzger BE: Care of the pregnant woman with insulin-dependent diabetes mellitus. *N Engl J Med* 1985; 313:96–101.

105. Massobrio M, Benedetto C, Bertini E, et al: Immune complexes in preeclampsia and normal pregnancy. *Am J Obstet Gynecol* 1985; 152:578–583.

106. Hays PM, Cruikshank DP, Dunn LI: Plasma volume determination in normal and pre-eclampsic pregnancies. *Am J Obstet Gynecol* 1985; 151:958–966.

107. Writer WDR: Anaesthetic considerations in high-risk pregnancy. *Can Anaesth Soc J* 1986; 33:S16–S27.

108. Clark SL, Horentein JM, Phelan JP, et al: Experience with the pulmonary artery catheter in obstetrics and gynecology. *Am J Obstet Gynecol* 1985; 152:374–378.

109. Moya F, Smith BE: Uptake, distribution, and placental transport of drugs and anesthetics. *Anesthesiology* 1965; 26:465–476.

110. Dawes GS: The distribution and action of drugs on the fetus in utero. *Br J Anaesth* 1973; 45(suppl):766–769.

111. Marx GF: Placental transfer and drugs used in anesthesia. *Anesthesiology* 1961; 22:294–313.

112. Caldwell J, Natrianni LJ, Smith RL: Impaired metabolism of pethidine in human neonates. *Br J Clin Pharmacol* 1978; 5:362–363.

113. Munson ES, Embro WJ: Enflurane, isoflurane, and halothane in isolated human uterine muscle. *Anesthesiology* 1967; 46:11–14.

114. Merrill EW: Rheology of blood. *Physiol Rev* 1969; 49:863–888.

115. Consensus conference: Perioperative red blood cell transfusion. *JAMA* 1988; 260:2700–2703.

116. Eckstein RW: Development of intra-arterial coronary anastomoses by chronic anemia. *Circ Res* 1955; 3:306–310.

117. Carson JL, Poses RM, Spence RK, et al: Severity of anemia and operative mortality and morbidity. *Lancet* 1988; 1:727–729.

118. Homi J, Reynolds J, Skinner A, et al: General anaesthesia in sickle cell disease. *Br Med J* 1979; 1:1599–1601.

119. Sears DA: The morbidity of sickle cell trait: Review of the literature. *Am J Med* 1978; 64:1021–1036.

120. Rosenthal A, Nathan DG, Marty A: Acute hemodynamic effects of red cell volume reduction in polycythemia of cyanotic congenital heart disease. *Circulation* 1970; 42:297–301.

121. Kloner RA, Ganote CE, Jennings RB: The "no-reflow" phenomenon after temporary coronary occlusion of methemoglobinemia and anemia. *J Appl Physiol* 1968; 25:594–599.

122. Lundsgaard-Hansen P: Hemodilution—new clothes for anemic emperor. *Vox Sang* 1979; 36:321–336.

123. Murray JF, Escobar E: Circulatory effects of blood viscosity: Comparison of methemoglobinemia and anemia. *J Appl Physiol* 1968; 25:594–599.

124. Fischer EG, Ames A: Studies on mechanisms of impairment of cerebral circulation following ischemia: Effect of hemodilution and perfusion pressure. *Stroke* 1972; 3:538–542.

125. Wasman J, Goodnugh LT: Autologous blood donation for elective surgery; effect on physician transfusion behavior. *JAMA* 1987; 258:3135–3137.

126. Brzica SM, Pineda AA, Taswell HF: Autologous blood transfusion. *Mayo Clin Proc* 1976; 51:723–737.

127. Perloff LJ: The role of blood transfusion in the age of cyclosporine. *Transplant Proc* 1986; 18(suppl 1):29–33.

128. Stephenson KR, Steinberg SM, Hughes KS, et al: Perioperative blood transfusions are associated with decreased time to recurrence and decreased survival after resection of colorectal liver metastases. *Ann Surg* 1988; 208:679–687.

129. Zauder HL: Massive transfusion. *Int Anesthesiol Clin* 1982; 20:157–170.

130. Jenevein EP, Weiss DL: Platelet microemboli associated with massive blood transfusions. *Am J Pathol* 1964; 45:313–321.
131. Reul GJ, Greenberg SD, Lefrak EA, et al: Prevention of post-traumatic pulmonary insufficiency: Fine screen filtration of blood. *Arch Surg* 1973; 106:386–393.
132. Cullen DJ, Ferrara L: Comparative evaluation of blood filters. A study in vitro. *Anesthesiology* 1974; 41:568–583.

11

Anesthesiologist as Consultant: Establishing Priorities to Minimize Risk

The most insidious and dangerous aspect of modern anesthesia is, paradoxically, its apparent safety. The physiologic and pharmacologic principles and details described in the preceding chapters form a basis for decision making that appears to be objective, comprehensive, and complete. The expectation, then, is that a "properly" planned and administered anesthetic should have no unexpected or adverse effects. In fact, there are numerous technical and judgmental processes that must also be skillfully executed if all patients encountered in clinical practice are to be safely anesthetized. Anesthesiology is not a purely scientific discipline; the complexity of disease processes and the virtually infinite variety of physiologic states simply make some things unknowable at the time the anesthetic plan is designed.

Inevitably, as Osler noted, "Errors in judgment must occur in the practice of an art which consists largely in balancing probabilities."[1] The extent to which adverse outcome reflects these "errors in judgment" rather than intrinsic and unavoidable anesthetic toxicity remains, however, a controversial issue.[2] Nevertheless, risk-free anesthesia is the common expectation for healthy patients scheduled for elective surgery.[3] The sections that follow summarize the concept of the anesthesiologist as both practitioner and as consultant, attempting to identify patients at increased risk of adverse outcome, and then modifying the anesthetic plan to minimize perioperative complications.

ACCIDENTS AND THE INTRINSIC RISK OF ANESTHESIA

Perioperative Morbidity and Mortality

Anesthesia-related morbidity and mortality encompass both predictable and unexpected adverse outcome during or after anesthetic administration. Because anesthetic exposure is almost always associated with a surgical procedure, it necessarily occurs in many patients with complex disease processes and intensive coincident drug therapy. It is not always possible, therefore, to distinguish the cause of perioperative problems. In fact, even the term *perioperative* has no uniform definition. At one extreme, the concept of intraoperative "anesthetic death" unrelated to surgery has virtually disappeared: contemporary mechanical and pharmacologic techniques of cardiopulmonary resuscitation (CPR) are sufficiently effective that patients almost always survive long enough to allow transport to postoperative intensive care environments.

In contrast, even subtle forms of behavioral dysfunction or complications that appear days or weeks after anesthetic exposure will be revealed when perioperative assessment of outcome is extended for 3 months or more. An interval of this length also permits complete evaluation of the extent to which a patient returns to the usual level of daily activity, ideally in the patient's normal living environment. In addition, those patients who have suffered inevitably lethal injuries during anesthetic administration yet are the recipients of prolonged life support measures will also be included in the final statistical assessment of perioperative outcome. Although it affords a more accurate determination of the consequences of anesthesia, therefore, the difficult logistics of locating, interviewing and examining patients months after their discharge effectively limits studies of this type.

Most recent analyses of anesthetic outcome review events within 30 days of surgery. This compromise between the practical realities of patient flow and data collection and long-term assessment of patient status is reasonably comprehensive, and should be consistent with the clinical experience of most practitioners. Distinguishing between the anesthetic and surgical components of perioperative morbidity and mortality, however, remains a more difficult, perhaps insoluble, problem.[4] Both classic retrospective and more recent prospective studies suggest that perhaps 20% of all perioperative deaths are "anesthesia related," although there is frequently a further distinction between anesthesia as a primary and as a contributory factor. Even this may be an overestimate of the role of anesthesia in adverse outcomes, since deaths not clearly attributable to other causes usually are assumed to be related to anesthesia until proved otherwise.[5]

Variability in surgical population and in patient physical status, the exact nature and urgency of the operative procedure, hospital facilities, and the era of anesthetic practice that is being surveyed are factors that have produced a tenfold variability in estimates of gross perioperative mortality.[6-8] Consequently, anesthetic management has been estimated as contributing to perioperative death in from 1 in 2,000 to 1 in 85,000 anesthetic administrations.[9] When elective surgical procedures are considered for patients who are not critically ill, however, even the recent estimate of one anesthesia-related fatality for every 75,000 anesthetics may not fully reflect dramatic improvements in outcome because of the implementation of the newest standards for minimum intraoperative monitoring.[10] For complex situations, however, death related to anesthesia appears to occur at least once in every 10,000 anesthetics.[11] The true frequency with which nonlethal complications occur as a consequence of anesthetic management remains unknown because of lack of a mechanism for mandatory reporting of such events.

Unexpected sudden death due to intrinsic cardiac, respiratory, or nervous system dysfunction probably occurs in hospitalized patients at a rate equal to or greater than that experienced by the general population at large. In effect, there must be a minimal or "obligatory" rate of perioperative mortality that is independent of surgical, anesthetic, or other circumstantial factors.[1] Of the 2,000 or more anesthesia-related deaths that occur yearly in the United States, perhaps 100 are, in fact, obligatory and therefore unavoidable under any circumstances.[3] The balance of perioperative anesthetic mortality appears to be due, in about equal parts, to potentially preventable "mishaps" (simple random errors) and to judgmental errors or other patient-specific perioperative mismanagement, the "systematic" errors that result in adverse outcome.[2]

Mishaps

Anesthetic mishaps are true accidents. They are the consequence of human error or mechanical malfunction.[12] They occur largely as the result of a lack of discovery ("surveillance failure"), or because of inadequate response to the discovery of a "simple" incident such as a disconnected hose or a ventilator failure. A simple incident that remains undiscovered may progress to become a "critical" incident that threatens vital functions if it fails to generate an appropriate reaction on the part of the anesthesiologist (Fig 11–1). Mishaps themselves are essentially unpredictable; they rarely occur as a direct consequence of the patient, the surgical procedure, or the anesthetic plan.

Early recognition of simple incidents prevents their evolution into critical incidents and, ultimately, the generation of an anesthetic-related injury. The process linking a simple mishap to adverse patient outcome is accelerated by the pharmacologic and physiologic complexity inherent in an anesthetized patient.[13] The patient, the anesthetic routine, and the operative environment become components in a tightly coupled system in which a single initial failure rapidly disrupts the function of other components. The complexity of the system may obscure the initiating event or make it difficult to interpret promptly. The ease with which the system is disrupted (the "tightness" of the coupling between its components) is further enhanced by the generalized disintegration of autonomic homeostasis produced by anesthesia (see Chapter 4). As the ability of physiologic functions to self-regulate is lost, the survival of the patient becomes increasingly dependent on external control of vital functions and progressively more susceptible to anesthetic mishaps.

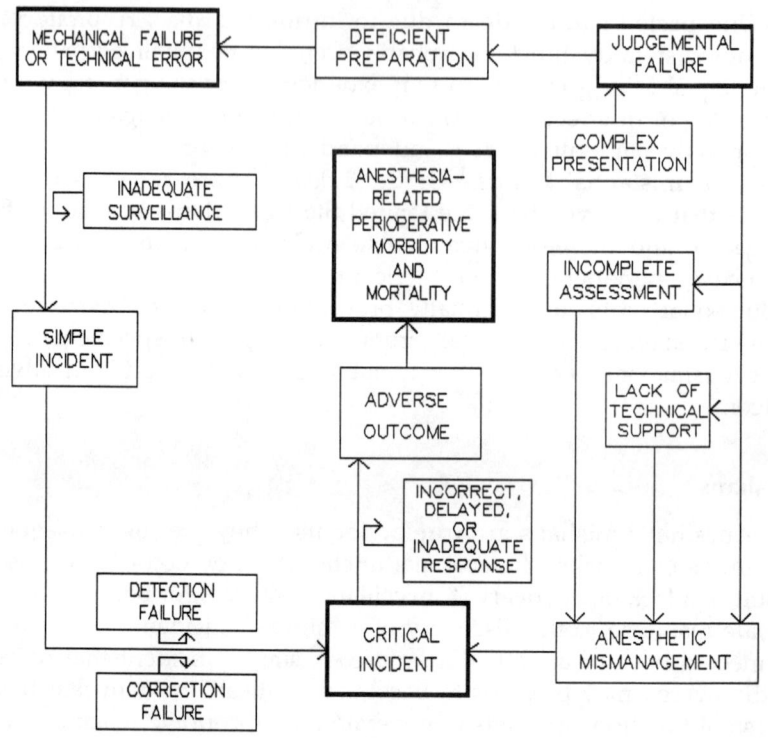

"ACCIDENT OR MISHAP"   "SYSTEMATIC ERROR"

FIG 11–1.
Genesis of adverse anesthetic outcome due to mishaps or systematic errors. Critical incidents are those that potentially compromise vital functions; adverse outcomes occur when critical incidents are not treated in an appropriate or timely manner. Mishaps are largely the consequence of technical complexity; systematic errors occur, in part, because of conceptual complexity in the patient's presentation or because of the demands of the operating room environment itself.

Most simple incidents related to anesthetic administration are corrected promptly and properly. At times of reduced alertness by the anesthesiologist, such as may occur in mid-procedure, however, a response failure is more likely.[14] Speed and effectiveness of an appropriate response may be compromised if the mishap occurs after a prior history of repeated false alarms,[15] or during a rapid sequence of unexpected events. The use of multiple, overlapping monitoring modalities to provide "fail-safe" monitoring for critical ventilation-related parameters may be necessary to supplement simple human vigilance,[3] since this remains the primary source of anesthesia-related morbidity and mortality.[14] However, the growing abundance of variables to be monitored, each with separate alarm mechanisms, may detract from efforts to sustain effective vigilance.[16] Some progress has been made in refining and integrating monitoring and alarm functions into priority-based "smart" warning systems.[17]

Systematic Error

Unlike mishaps, systematic errors are not random events; therefore, their occurrence may not necessarily decline in response to improved monitoring or increased vigilance. Systematic errors occur predictably as a consequence of judgmental decisions regarding choice of anesthetic agents or techniques, or of the execution of various options for monitoring, positioning, or patient disposition. Unlike mishaps, systematic errors are likely to recur when similar decisions are repeated under similar circumstances. There is little evidence that any of the anesthetic agents in current use have sufficient intrinsic cellular or tissue toxicity that their routine contributes to adverse anesthetic outcome, although ester-type local anesthetics may possess an unavoidable element of direct neurotoxicity.[18]

The widespread adoption of pulse oximetry and end-tidal capnography has increased the speed and precision with which simple incidents are discovered, correctly interpreted, and subsequently corrected. Therefore, anesthetic mishaps appear to be occurring with progressively less frequency.[10, 19] Improved monitoring may also reduce the frequency with which critical incidents produce adverse outcome.[20] Systematic errors in the design or the execution of the anesthetic plan remain a persistent element of anesthesia-related morbidity and mortality, however. They arise from ignorance of, or disregard for, established physiologic or pharmacologic relationships. They therefore reflect intrinsic limitations of education, medical knowledge, and human personality, and it is unlikely that they will ever be overcome completely in anesthetic practice.

PATIENTS AT INCREASED RISK

Epidemiologic, retrospective reviews of anesthesia-related morbidity and mortality provide information essential for understanding the factors that contribute to perioperative events. They may also be helpful in refining and improving the design of the anesthetic plan. Of even more value to the patient, and to the physicians responsible for his care, however, is the predictive value of this information for estimating perioperative risk and permitting assessment of the need for increased monitoring or special precautions.

Unfortunately, perioperative and anesthetic risk can currently be defined only in terms of the probability of untoward or adverse outcome. These diffuse numerical estimates of "risk" may actually be uninterpretable by the patient unless they are either prohibitive or virtually nonexistent. However it is asked, the question posed by the patient is not really, "How often, in every 1,000 anesthetics, will cerebrovascular accidents occur?" but rather, "Will I have a stroke during my anesthetic tomorrow?"

Given the current state of our understanding, preoperative assessment of perioperative morbidity and mortality remains largely a matter of identifying patients more likely to suffer specific types of postoperative organ system dysfunction than other patients. Characteristics statistically associated with a high probability of major complications or death are frequently described as "risk factors," but this information does not identify the specific individuals within the "high-risk" group who will, in fact, suffer adverse outcome. Thus the information of most value to the patient in providing an accurate picture of the risks and benefits of surgery for him is, in fact, also the most elusive. Continuing prospective study of factors associated with a high probability of adverse outcome may, however, identify those patients in whom judgmental error is most likely to produce iatrogenic injury. These sources of morbidity and mortality may be eliminated once the major relationships are clearly established and widely appreciated.

The Elderly Patient

In general, overall physical status and activity level, operative site, and preexisting cardiopulmonary disease appear to be the only preoperative factors that currently have consistent predictive value in identifying the high-risk surgical patient. Age itself, long considered to be sufficiently important that some patients were thought to be simply "too old" for elective surgery, is no longer a contraindication to surgical intervention. In fact, age-related disease, rather than age per se, largely determines the increased frequency of complications and mortality apparent in an elderly surgical population.[21] When morbidity and mortality figures for young and elderly adults are reviewed with regard to their relationship to physical status (Fig 11–2), there is little difference, except at the extremes of pathophysiologic complexity produced by multiple organ system failure.[22]

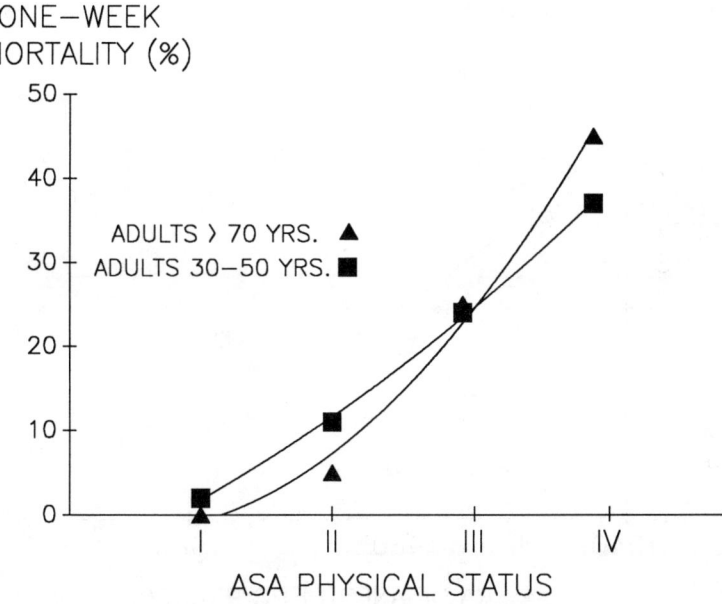

FIG 11–2.
Gross perioperative mortality as a function of American Society of Anesthesiologists (ASA) physical status (PS). Outcome is largely independent of age: patients more than 70 years of age appear to have higher mortality than do young adults only when there is profound or complex organ system dysfunction, as for PS IV. Very high mortality rates shown here reflect a large proportion of emergency surgery and traumatic injury in data obtained by Marx et al[22] from experience in a large municipal hospital.

Fortunately, continuing improvements in diagnosis, management, and treatment of virtually every disease have been self-evident over the past half century. The data for anesthesia-related morbidity and mortality also demonstrate a parallel and substantial improvement in outcome (Fig 11–3); improvements in anesthetic management and perioperative care undoubtedly have contributed to this phenomenon.

The Problem Airway

Preoperative assessment of physical status, even when "vertically" oriented by organ system rather than by chief complaint (see Chapter 1), invariably focuses on disease. Often overlooked are variations in airways anatomy that impose technical difficulties for ventilation or intubation and therefore increase the risk of hypoxemia during anesthetic induction. For example, healthy women undergoing very limited surgical procedures such as early termination of pregnancy have

ANESTHETIC–RELATED
MORTALITY

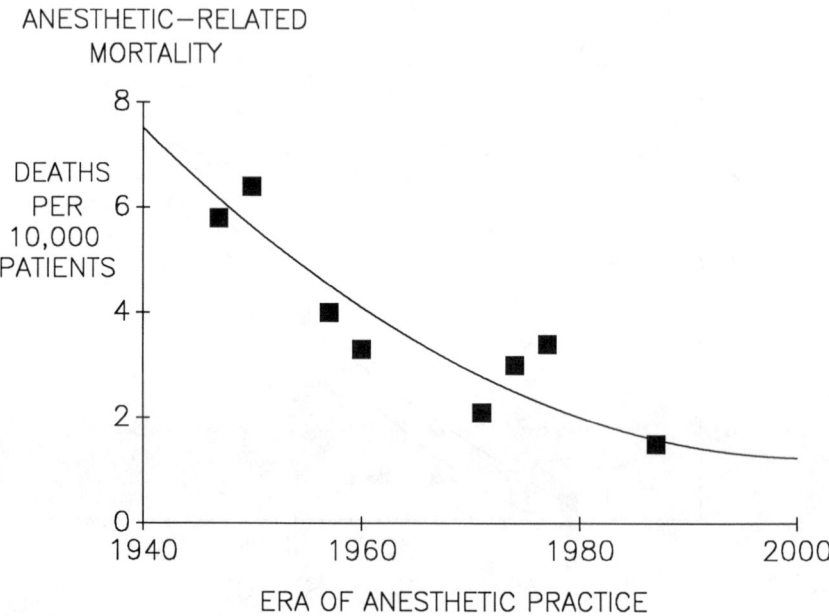

FIG 11–3.
Estimated overall rates of adult perioperative mortality (within 1 week of surgery) directly or primarily attributable to the anesthetic management of combined elective and emergency procedures. Data derived from multiple sources and published reviews.[9, 22, 25, 27]

relatively limited pathophysiology. They are usually fit and active, patients in whom the analysis of cause and effect for adverse outcome is more straightforward than for most surgical patients. Of the rare anesthesia-related mortality that does occur in this patient group, almost 90% of perioperative deaths are directly attributable to respiratory obstruction, failure to ventilate, or other aspects of airway mismanagement.[23] Other studies conducted on a larger scale include a greater number and variety of "risk" factors; similarly, they confirm that failed tracheal intubation, unrecognized esophageal intubation, or inability to ventilate represent the major cause of death and catastrophic injury in contemporary anesthetic practice, both for adults[24–27] and children.[28]

Some errors in "airway management" may be true accidents, random breathing circuit or oxygen supply incidents that have become critical incidents because of inattention or inadequate monitoring.[14, 24] However, the majority of these occurrences appear to be preventable systematic errors that reflect inadequate airway evaluation and surveillance, or other forms of judgmental error.[29] Adverse outcome related to airway mismanagement occurs primarily because of the devastating consequences of nervous system hypoxia. Specific errors include failure to recognize those factors that predispose to difficult ventilation, laryngoscopy, or intubation, or inadequate technical skill in accomplishing tracheal intubation in a timely manner in patients at high risk of aspiration of gastric contents.

Review of the anatomic factors that produce a problem airway suggests that preexisting stridor is an obvious, and onerous, indicator of reduced airway diameter at or near the level of the larynx.[30] Stridor is usually acute, due to laryngeal edema, vocal cord dysfunction, or external compression of the tracheobronchial tree by mediastinal lesions or obstruction by a foreign body. In these patients, tracheal intubation is usually accomplished before anesthetic induction, under well-controlled conditions in the operating room, or during cautious induction of inhalational anesthesia with additional technical assistance available to perform prompt tracheobronchoscopy or tracheostomy, if necessary.

Obesity

Less obvious, and therefore more dangerous, are the nonpathologic variations in upper airway morphology that predispose to difficult ventilation because of soft tissue obstruction (Table 11–1). The extent to which a large, thick tongue or a short cervical spine will compromise

TABLE 11–1.

Preoperative Physical Findings Suggesting Potential for Difficult Intraoperative Airway Management

	Difficult Ventilation by Mask	Difficult Glottic Visualization
Edentulous maxilla and mandible	X	
Obesity	X	X
Large tongue	X	X
Short, thick, or muscular neck	X	X
Limited mouth opening		X
Prominent "buck" teeth		X
Inability to visualize both soft palate and uvula during voluntary mouth opening		X
Short or thick mandible		X
Chin to laryngeal (thyroid cartilage) distance of less than 6 cm		X
Limited cervical spine mobility	X	X
Previous laryngeal or pharyngeal surgery or radiation therapy	X	X

ventilation by face mask in the patient with redundant, fatty facial and neck tissues is frequently underestimated, especially in obese patients.[31] Generalized depression of consciousness during anesthetic induction interrupts the normal reflex pathways that modulate active maintenance of airway patency in many patients, and may produce a marked increase in resistance to airflow in the airway above the level of the larynx.[32]

Soft tissue obstruction after loss of consciousness appears to be further accelerated by the application of topical anesthesia to the pharyngeal musculature. Drug-induced neuromuscular blockade may produce a similarly dramatic and abrupt loss of upper airway muscle tone, precluding effective ventilation by mask unless oropharyngeal and nasal airways or manual elevation of the mandible is used to maintain upper airway continuity.

There may also be a telltale history of extremely stertorous breathing during sleep in patients prone to upper airway obstruction. The "sleep apnea" syndrome described in many obese patients is not, in fact, a condition of apnea: there is no absence of respiratory effort, but rather a condition of recurrent upper airway obstruction during depressed consciousness.[33] Decreased muscle tone in the tongue and pharynx of obese patients produces obstruction to airflow and a rapid fall in arterial oxygenation; hypoxemia, although transient, is sufficiently severe to stimulate both hypoxia-enhanced respiratory drive and a simultaneous sympathoadrenal release of epinephrine during acute obstruction.

The sequelae that follow hypoxia induce a maximum respiratory effort; increased pharyngeal muscle tone returns with partial reawakening, providing temporary resolution of ventilatory obstruction.[34] Characteristically, the patient jerks awake from sleep, begins to ventilate adequately, and then becomes progressively more obstructed as consciousness is once again depressed and upper airway muscle tone begins to diminish, repeating this sequence of events.

Difficult Laryngoscopy

Skeletal and soft-tissue facial anomalies may also complicate airway management. Unlike the soft tissue factors associated with obesity, bony abnormalities of the maxilla, mandible, and cervical vertebrae only rarely limit the ability to ventilate. More frequently, they compromise the direct visualization of the glottis that is needed for safe and expeditious laryngoscopy.[35] Some patients may be simply impossible to intubate by conventional methods; visualization of the larynx and trachea may require use of illuminated fiberoptic devices.[36] Congenital facial anomalies such as micrognathia and Pierre-Robin syndrome[29] or degenerative changes in temporomandibular joint morphology, such as those produced by rheumatoid arthritis,[37] commonly present considerable difficulty when tracheal intubation is attempted.

Visualization of the laryngeal structures by direct laryngoscopy requires approximate alignment of the oropharyngeal and laryngotracheal axes (Fig 11–4). Extension of the neck with slight forward elevation ("sniffing position") and a rearward rotation of the occiput permit easy exposure of glottic structures if mouth opening is adequate, if the tongue can be displaced easily by the laryngoscope, and if the larynx itself is relatively mobile and free to drop "downward," in a dorsal direction. During normal laryngoscopy, elevation of the mandible and the soft tissues of the floor of the mouth by the laryngoscope blade

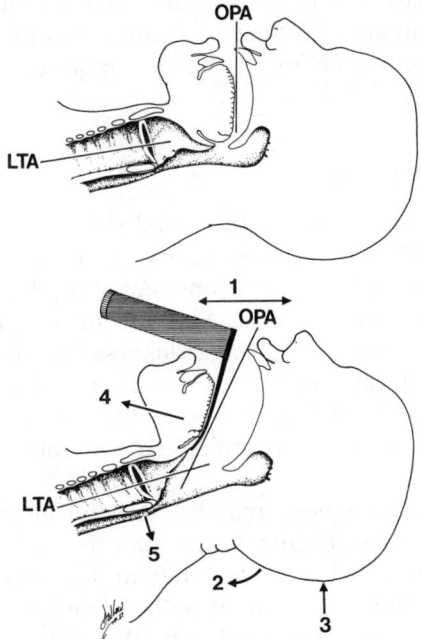

FIG 11–4.
Major factors permitting the alignment of the oropharyngeal axis *(OPA)* and the laryngotracheal axis *(LTA)* for laryngoscopic visualization. Major factors include the following: *1,* adequate mouth opening; *2* and *3,* the anterior and rotational movements of the cervical spine that occur with adequate vertebral motility; *4,* displacement of the tongue and floor of the mouth structures by the laryngoscope blade; and, *5,* downward or dorsal descent of the larynx itself. (Modified from the diagram originally presented by Otto CW: Tracheal intubation, in Nunn JF, Utting JE, Brown BR Jr (eds): *General Anaesthesia,* ed 5. London, Butterworth, 1989.)

permits visualization of the larynx as soon as its longitudinal axis coincides with the line of vision established into the oropharynx.[38]

Any factors that limit the range of available motion normally used to establish either of these visual axes reduce the probability of direct visualization of the larynx. Without exposure of some laryngeal anatomy, at least a glimpse of the arytenoid cartilages, the trachea cannot be intubated under direct vision with certainty. Limited mouth opening, large tongue, short muscular neck, a short or receding mandible, especially if associated with enhanced posterior thickness of the ramus, prominent upper teeth, or the loss of laryngeal mobility after surgery or radiation may compromise direct laryngoscopy.

The extent to which exposure of the uvula can be voluntarily accomplished appears to provide a useful predictor of difficult laryngeal visualization.[39] Inadequate mobility of the cervical spine due to short intervertebral distances or arthritis can also make intubation difficult, however. Increased anterior laryngeal attachment is the most common factor limiting the approximation of the axes required for easy visualization of the glottis.

Airway Management Strategies

Identification of the patient at increased risk of anesthesia-related complications because of a problem airway or challenging laryngoscopy leads directly to important decisions regarding the options for airway management. A patient who is likely to have upper airway obstruction immediately after loss of consciousness requires an anesthetic plan in which tracheal intubation is accomplished before anesthetic induction, or one in which intubation is accomplished immediately after an expeditious induction, without prolonged attempts at ventilation by face mask.

Local and regional anesthesia may be attractive alternatives to general anesthesia under these circumstances, but they add an element of safety only if they are consistent with the surgical procedure and are successfully accomplished. If a patient with a problem airway or difficult intubation experiences acute respiratory depression because of systemic toxicity from the rapid absorption or intravascular injection of the local anesthetics used for regional anesthesia, or if motor blockade produced by regional anesthesia is extensive enough to compromise spontaneous ventilation, the same risk factors that made a plan for general anesthesia complex would again be in effect. Consequently, every plan for anesthesia in a patient in whom ventilation or intubation may be difficult must include full consideration of airway control, even when regional anesthesia is selected.

Awake Intubation

Awake tracheal intubation before anesthetic induction in the patient with a difficult airway can be accomplished atraumatically. Adequate topical anesthesia of the oropharynx and an appropriate degree of general sedation minimize patient discomfort. Passage of a tracheal tube by either nasal or oral routes can be utilized. Because the patient continues to breathe spontaneously, using whatever compensatory mechanisms normally provide him with adequate airway patency, "awake intubations" have a high degree of inherent safety. There is minimal risk of hypoxemia during anesthetic induction, especially if supplemental oxygen is provided to accompany the use of sedative or narcotic drugs.[40] Excessive sedation or topical anesthesia may, however, produce a noticeable loss of upper airway patency in patients who are dependent on reflex pharyngeal mechanisms.

With supplemental oxygen provided, an endotracheal tube can be introduced into the trachea over a directed fiberoptic instrument,[41, 42] with other types of illuminated insertion devices,[43] or guided along a translaryngeal wire that has been inserted retrograde through the cricothyroid membrane.[44] More common is the classic "blind" approach utilizing auscultation of exhaled air flow through the nasally inserted tracheal tube as a guide to proper insertion.[45]

The technical details of an awake intubation depend largely on the experience, training, and equipment available to the anesthesiologist. The essential element in the anesthetic plan is the recognition of factors that portend difficult ventilation or inadequate laryngoscopy and the suitable adjustment of the anesthetic induction sequence. The primary priority is to avoid situations in which the patient is apneic but can be neither intubated nor effectively ventilated by face mask.

Denitrogenation

Some patients have redundant soft tissues of the neck and pharynx that predispose to upper airway obstruction with loss of consciousness, yet they may have adequate fundamental laryngeal and pharyngeal anatomy that poses no problem for effective and rapid laryngoscopy and prompt tracheal intubation. For these patients, an alternative approach to regional anesthesia or to awake intubation is to proceed promptly from spontaneous, awake ventilation with an oxygen-rich mixture directly to full anesthetic induction with neuromuscular blockade to facilitate prompt tracheal intubation.

A rapid intravenous anesthetic induction sequence in patients who have this intrapulmonary oxygen reserve to maintain continuous arterial oxygenation during subsequent apnea eliminates the need for mask ventilation before laryngoscopy.[46, 47] Oxygenation may be adequate for 30 minutes or longer if the patient remains continuously connected to a source of oxygen, but will fall rapidly, in minutes, after removal of the face mask,[48] especially if the patient is obese.[49] Consequently, denitrogenation or "preoxygenation" followed by anesthetic induction is appropriate only when intubation itself is quickly and expertly accomplished. This rapid, or "crash," intravenous anesthetic induction sequence should not be attempted if the fundamental factors determining the ease of intubation are not clearly favorable, if the presence of assistants familiar with the mechanics of laryngoscopy and intubation cannot be assured, or if the predictable cardiovascular consequences of the large doses of intravenous drugs needed for rapid induction will not be tolerated.

A failed intubation in a patient who then cannot be ventilated effectively represents a persistent source of anesthesia-related hypoxic injury that has both technical and judgmental components. Inevitably, however, this event must be seen as a form of anesthetic mismanagement. In many obese patients, the same anatomic factors that make ventilation of the unconscious patient difficult also compromise the ease with which intubation is accomplished.

Especially in combination with pregnancy, obesity poses a particularly difficult combination of factors: the increase in abdominal pressure produced by these conditions reduces the functional residual capacity of the lung, yet increases cardiac output.[50] Therefore, the quantity of oxygen available in the intrapulmonary oxygen reservoirs established before induction by the process of oxygen breathing is reduced, yet the rate at which oxygen is consumed is elevated. Thus, safe apnea time during laryngoscopy is reduced to as little as 90 seconds before conditions of generalized hypoxemia occur. In fact, even a reasonably well-executed and efficient rapid induction sequence often produces transient arterial oxygen desaturation in the pregnant or morbidly obese patient.[48, 49]

INDUCTION FOR "FULL STOMACH" PATIENTS

The high mortality associated with intraoperative pulmonary aspiration of gastric contents during obstetric anesthesia identified the "full stomach" as a major risk factor for anesthesia-related complications. Subsequently, the rapid-sequence induction became a standard of care not only for the parturient, but also for a wide variety of other patients at increased risk for aspiration of gastric contents. In conventional terminology, "full stomach" patients also include those who have ingested food or drink (other than clear liquids) within 8 hours of surgery; patients with nausea, vomiting, or any form of intra-abdominal disease; patients in severe pain, especially if they have already received narcotics[50]; those who are extremely anxious; patients who are obese[51]; patients who are intoxicated; and those patients with hiatal hernia and symptoms of gastric reflux.

Reflux of Gastric Contents

Induction of general anesthesia predisposes to aspiration pneumonitis because three physiologic and anatomic factors that normally preclude this phenomenon are profoundly altered when consciousness is lost. The initial barrier to reflux of gastric contents is the cardia of the stomach.[52] Anatomically, no discrete sphincter is apparent, but the angulation of the cardioesophageal junction and the redundancy of gastric mucosal folds in this area are augmented by the intrinsic tone of gastric smooth muscle to form a zone of high local pressure.

This mechanism normally provides the functional equivalent of a one-way valve, and prevents the movement of gastric contents up into the esophagus under normal circumstances. However, acute gastric distention from illness or injury, or any alteration of the original anatomic relationship between stomach and esophagus, such as may be produced by intestinal obstruction, hiatal hernia, or pregnancy, may result in gastroesophageal reflux. The symptoms of reflux esophagitis that occur under these circumstances are commonly described as "heartburn."

Gastric acid can produce irritation and injury to the esophagus. Gross and continued displacement of gastric contents from the esophagus into the pharynx is usually prevented by the active contraction of the cricopharyngeal muscle at the upper end of the esophagus. If this muscle fails in its function as an upper esophageal sphincter, however, reflex glottic closure, accomplished by the intrinsic muscles of the larynx itself,[53] provides the third, and final, barrier to the aspiration of gastric contents.

Vomiting is a coordinated gastrointestinal reflex phenomenon. Glottic closure by laryngeal mechanisms effectively prevents the aspiration of gastric contents into the tracheobronchial tree during vomiting, even while gastric contents are actively expelled up into the oropharynx. Although normally effective in preventing aspiration, glottic reflexes may be impaired significantly by aging, nervous system dysfunction, intrinsic laryngeal pathology or drug effects.[54]

Because a surgical level of general anesthesia predictably and effectively depresses most reflex activity, actual intraoperative vomiting occurs only during the transitional, hyperreflexive stage of excitement or "disinhibition" associated with anesthetic induction or emergence. The fundamental rationale for a rapid intravenous induction sequence, therefore, is to minimize the risk of vomiting and aspiration by proceeding immediately from the awake state, when glottic reflexes are intact, to a deep level of general anesthesia, in which the complex neural mechanism needed for vomiting has been disabled by generalized nervous system depression.[55]

A rapid anesthetic induction does not, however, eliminate the possibility that gastric contents can be aspirated into the tracheobronchial tree by passive regurgitation of gastric contents. Cephalad reflux of gastric contents will, in fact, occur whenever intragastric pressure (IGP) exceeds the "barrier" pressure that gives the cardioesophageal junction its sphincter-like characteristics. Although succinylcholine-induced fasciculations cause sporadic increases in IGP, but they also produce a parallel and simultaneous rise in lower esophageal muscle tone that maintains an adequate barrier to reflux if the normal anatomic relationship of the cardioesphageal junction remains intact (Chapter 8).

Unfortunately, there is no evidence that the normal relationship between stomach and esophagus is maintained effectively or consistently in patients with acute intra-abdominal pathology. In fact, the frequency with which these patients, as well as obese or pregnant patients, experience symptoms of gastric reflux suggests that it is a mechanism easily and frequently disturbed. Protection against reflux of gastric contents into the hypopharynx is afforded largely by an unconscious, reflexive increase in cricopharyngeal muscle tone and by a preference for a semisitting position. In this posture, a typical vertical gradient between stomach and pharynx exceeds 15 to 20 cm, pressures equivalent to those typical for IGP. Although barrier pressure appears to be reduced significantly by systemic narcotics,[56] they are effectively enhanced by the administration of atropine.[52]

The supine position and induction of general anesthesia therefore eliminate both the gravitational and the cricopharyngeal defense mechanisms, respectively, which normally compensate for inadequate cardioesophageal sphincter function. Anesthetic induction with patients in a technically inconvenient, extreme foot-down tilt was once advocated under these circumstances.[55] The essential component of a contemporary rapid induction sequence, however, is the maintenance of active compression of the upper esophagus by downward digital displacement of the cricoid cartilage of the larynx. Initiated immediately upon loss of consciousness, the "Sellick maneuver" replaces the function of the cricopharyngeal sphincter and may be the only barrier between gastric contents and the tracheobronchial tree in patients in whom the cardioesophageal junction has become incompetent. Pressure on the cricoid cartilage is maintained until a cuffed endotracheal tube has been successfully placed within the trachea, affording sustained protection against the tracheobronchial aspiration of gastric contents during anesthetic induction.

CARDIAC DISEASE AND PHYSICAL STATUS AS RISK FACTORS

The epidemiologic relationship between physical status and anesthetic outcome is both intuitive and statistically well established (Chapter 1). Every anesthetic agent and anesthetic technique depresses or disrupts the function of vital organ systems. Therefore, preexisting disease and impaired organ system functional reserve, even when apparently well compensated, must be considered risk factors predisposing to perioperative organ system failure.[1, 57]

Precise identification of those disease processes associated consistently with adverse outcome could make this form of analysis useful in establishing predictors of patients at high risk of anesthetic complications. Unexpected cardiac arrest during anesthesia and surgery is a relatively rare event that usually occurs in the context of airway mismanagement and subsequent arterial hypoxia.[24] Far more often, perioperative decompensation of myocardial disease is associated with less acute, and more subtle, forms of cardiac morbidity, such as ischemia, infarction, dysrhythmias, or low cardiac output syndromes occurring in the first 48 to 72 hours after surgery.

Preoperative Evaluation

The essential element predictive of perioperative cardiac dysfunction appears to be inadequate ventricular or "pump" function. Preoperative signs and symptoms of grossly impaired myocardial contractility include pulmonary edema, neck vein distention, or an S-3 gallop; there is frequently a history of inability to tolerate even moderate levels of physical exertion. Correlation of these findings with increased risk of postoperative cardiac complications has been established retrospectively with use of multivariate analysis.[58] These aspects of the physical examination and medical history may actually be equivalent in predictive value to the more rigorous estimates of exercise tolerance obtained by stress testing in the cardiology laboratory.[59, 60] In a prospective investigation, however, only a finding that the patient was actually unable to exercise at all predicted cardiac complications consistently in elderly patients who subsequently had noncardiac surgery.[61]

Although traditionally assessed preoperatively by invasive cardiac catheterization techniques, left ventricular ejection fraction (EF) remains the most reliable and objective index of pump function and cardiac functional reserve. EF values of less than 50% usually suggest a need for direct assessment of left ventricular filling pressures by measurement of pulmonary artery wedge pressures obtained with a pulmonary artery (Swan-Ganz) catheter.[60] Estimating the adequacy of venous return and cardiac filling with measurements of right atrial or central venous pressure is unreliable in the presence of this degree of left ventricular dysfunction.[62] EF and left ventricular functional reserve can also be assessed radiographically with multiple uptake gated acquisition (MUGA) scanning. This technique has been used to demonstrate a highly significant correlation between impaired EF, elevated pulmonary artery wedge pressures, and postoperative cardiac mortality.[63]

Routine preoperative screening of cardiac disease with use of electrocardiography (ECG) is safe and generally cost-effective.[64] This information provides little indication of ventricular function, however. Its primary value is for identification of patients with significant coronary insufficiency and for surveillance of perioperative ischemia and myocardial infarction. In combination with a history of ischemic disease, serial ECG assessment is a more specific, but somewhat less sensitive, monitoring modality than repeated measurements of the blood levels of cardiac enzymes such as creatine kinase.[65] Although ECG abnormalities may be nonspecific, the likelihood of recent myocardial infarction in patients with a new ECG configuration apparent from comparison with previous tracings should encourage more detailed and objective assessment of ventricular function before surgery,[58] especially if discovered in patients who have additional risk factors such as extremes of age[66] or diabetes mellitus.[67, 68]

Recent improvements in perioperative management of ischemic heart disease and myocardial infarction appear to have improved outcome significantly. Reinfarction within 3 months of surgery has fallen from almost 30%[69] to less than 10%.[70] A major ischemic event remains associated with an elevated risk of cardiac morbidity and mortality, however, probably because of the frequency with which it is associated with some degree of impaired ventricular function.

Invasive Monitoring

Increasing familiarity and expertise in the insertion of pulmonary artery catheters have made the use of invasive cardiac monitoring routine for patients with established myocardial dysfunction who are undergoing surgery.[71, 72] The pulmonary artery catheter has also become commonplace in preparation for cardiac and major vascular surgery, thoracic procedures, and many forms of upper abdominal surgery in patients who have lesser degrees of cardiovascular disease. Placement of catheters within the pulmonary artery may also be an important part of the anesthetic plan for patients having surgery in the sitting position, or for other patients at high risk of air embolization, since it can be used both to diagnose and to extract bubbles of air or other gases from the pulmonary artery.[73]

In the geriatric surgical population, in particular, preoperative insertion of invasive hemodynamic monitoring has been shown to facilitate the restoration of depleted circulating blood volume and other abnormalities that would otherwise go undiscovered and untreated preoperatively.[66] The measurement of cardiac output by thermodilution techniques and the assessment of the adequacy of tissue perfusion using oximeter-tipped catheters are now also widely practiced.[74] In contemporary practice, there is general familiarity with pulmonary artery catheterization and the clinical application of the information that it can provide regarding left ventricular filling pressures, vascular resistance, and cardiac output.[75] The placement of this catheter within the pulmonary circulation, however, can be associated with potentially lethal perforation and hemorrhage[76-78]; the catheter also represents a foreign body in the cardiac chambers, and may precipitate cardiac dysrhythmias.[79]

Continuous systemic arterial monitoring has also become a minimum standard of care in patients with well-established cardiopulmonary disease. Cannulas of small diameter, especially if left in place for less than 72 hours, rarely produce significant injury. Nevertheless, pain at the site of cannulation, hematomas, and infection still complicate this procedure.[80] Improved techniques, equipment, and maintenance protocols have reduced markedly the frequency of thrombosis and occlusion after cannulation of the radial artery to 1%, or perhaps even less.[81]

Nevertheless, there are specific indications for cannulation of peripheral arteries. Currently they include the expectation of fluctuations in hemodynamics sufficiently dramatic or rapid to require "beat-to-beat" monitoring of arterial blood pressure, the need for repeated analysis of arterial blood specimens for the assessment of pulmonary and metabolic status, the use of techniques of controlled arterial hypotension at levels of blood pressure too low for noninvasive, cuff-based techniques of measurement, and in rare cases, situations in which the physical characteristic of the patient or the site of surgery precludes accurate determination of blood pressure by other techniques.

PULMONARY DISEASE AS A RISK FACTOR

Preexisting pulmonary disease, especially chronic obstructive lung disease (COLD), is the most important factor predisposing to perioperative pulmonary morbidity and mortality.[82, 83] Twenty percent of patients with well-established COLD subsequently experience some form of major postoperative pulmonary complication,[82] and almost 10% may suffer fatal complications if COLD is severe.[84, 85] Restrictive lung disease appears to have less significance as a pulmonary risk factor but is associated with cardiac complications, especially right ventricular failure.[86]

Preoperative Evaluation

Traditional pulmonary function tests (PFTs) quantify the severity of COLD[87, 88] but have little predictive value in identifying those patients who will subsequently experience postoperative ventilatory failure.[89, 90] Prospective studies also suggest that PFTs rarely provide information that alters patient management, nor do they predict the duration of postoperative intubation.[91] Other than provide the anesthesiologist with evidence of a reversible, usually bronchospastic, component of COLD, preoperative PFTs appear to contribute little more to the design of the anesthetic plan than could be contributed by a history of smoking or the obvious clinical signs or symptoms of chronic pulmonary disease.

When preoperative treatment of patients with COLD with bronchodilators, chest physiotherapy, or other forms of treatment fails to produce either objective or subjective improvement in pulmonary function, there may be a threefold increase in the incidence of postoperative pulmonary morbidity of some type.[88] In contrast, a response to these therapeutic maneuvers reduces the incidence of postoperative pulmonary complications, although it does not appear to have any significant influence on the overall rate of postoperative pulmonary mortality.[85]

Surgery and Outcome

The type of surgery performed also is an important co-determinant of the incidence of postoperative pulmonary complications.[82, 85] Proximity of the site of surgery to the respiratory diaphragm and to the lower intercostal muscles disrupts the coordination of complex respiratory muscle patterns. Simple relief of perceived surgical pain with use of regional nerve blocks or infiltration of local anesthetics at the site of surgery reduces the need for parenteral narcotics and minimizes the risk of central respiratory depression, but does not restore normal ventilatory mechanics.[92, 93]

The dramatic fall in vital capacity to a value as little as one third of that measured preoperatively within 24 hours of upper abdominal surgery, therefore, appears to reflect more than "splinting," which is the cessation of voluntary deep breathing because of incisional pain. Upper abdominal or lower thoracic surgery produces a diffuse interruption of the reflex pathways that normally provide coordinated activation and reciprocal inhibition of the musculature of the diaphragm, chest wall, and abdominal wall (see Chapter 7). Even in the absence of pain, fluid overload, central respiratory depression, or other contributory factors, discoordinate breathing patterns appear to play an important, but poorly understood, role in the gross restriction of normal ventilation after surgery in this area.

Intraoperative pulmonary complications, like postoperative complications, largely reflect the consequences of preexisting lung disease. When airway management is technically uncomplicated, there is nevertheless a twofold to fourfold increase in the frequency of hypoxemia or other intraoperative pulmonary complications.[83] Asthmatics and other patients with COLD that is characterized by hyperreactive airways are at increased risk of bronchospasm, especially in response to the airway stimulation produced by tracheal intubation or suctioning. Consequently, bronchodilator therapy, using aerosolized or nebulized β-agonist drugs or, more recently, atropine, is frequently employed before and during anesthetic induction and intubation, and often before extubation.

Inhalational anesthetics may be preferred for general anesthesia of patients who have preexisting COLD because, at least at higher inspired concentrations, these agents blunt the reactivity of bronchial smooth muscle to direct stimulation. They may also reduce resting bronchomotor tone if it is elevated above normal levels.[94] In addition, inhalational anesthetics offer greater flexibility in providing elevated inspired oxygen fractions for patients with COLD: they do not require the simultaneous administration of nitrous oxide, usually included as part of a narcotic-based anesthetic.

Postobstruction Pulmonary Edema

Acute, reflex laryngospasm produced by irritation of the vocal cords may cause obstruction to air movement sufficiently severe to prevent spontaneous or controlled ventilation. In patients who develop laryngospasm immediately after tracheal extubation following surgery, vigorous respiratory efforts generate sustained negative intrathoracic pressures. Very high pulmonary artery pressures may be produced simultaneously because the arterial oxygen desaturation that occurs during this period of obstructed ventilation also stimulates hypoxic pulmonary vasoconstriction.

This sequence of events can produce a postobstructive, noncardiogenic pulmonary edema syndrome in children,[95] and in young adults.[96] Although characterized by copious production of pink, frothy sputum and severe arterial oxygen desaturation, it occurs most commonly in young, healthy patients who do not have preexisting myocardial dysfunction. Therefore, this entity is distinguishable from cardiogenic pulmonary edema due to fluid overload or myocardial failure by its time course and by the clinical setting in which it occurs.[97] Appearing within minutes of an acute upper airway obstruction, the edema then resolves rapidly and spontaneously over a period of a few hours once adequate oxygenation is re-established and, in fact, may be radiologically undetectable within 24 hours.

THE CONSULTANT'S ROLE

Frequently asked to provide expert assessment of "fitness for anesthesia" or the likelihood of complications, the anesthesiologist must review, condense, and crystallize the data available to him. His perspective on the effect of anesthetic agents, surgical injury, and postoperative stress on organ systems and autonomic function is unique. If he were merely a skilled technician, using modern drugs and equipment, an anesthesiologist could usually provide a level of perioperative care that is "state of the art." However, optimal management of a complex or difficult patient, or identification of patients at exceptional risk, requires more than consistent professionalism. These circumstances call upon all the skills of a consultant in anesthesiology: depth and breadth of knowledge, awareness of priorities, ability to assess the relative risk and benefit associated with various anesthetic approaches, and the judgment and skill necessary to design and execute an anesthetic plan uniquely suited to the best interests of every patient.

The anesthesiologist has responsibilities that overlap those of both a primary physician and a consultant; he functions in a manner somewhat different from the other medical specialists contributing to the body of expert opinion available to the surgeon (Fig 11–5). He is also quite different in his responsibilities to the patient than is the surgeon, since he rarely is the primary physician who admits the patient to the hospital, coordinates the patient's day-to-day management, and discharges the patient after recovery from the surgical procedure. Unlike other consultants, the anesthesiologist does not limit himself to formulating assessments of specific medical issues at the surgeon's request.

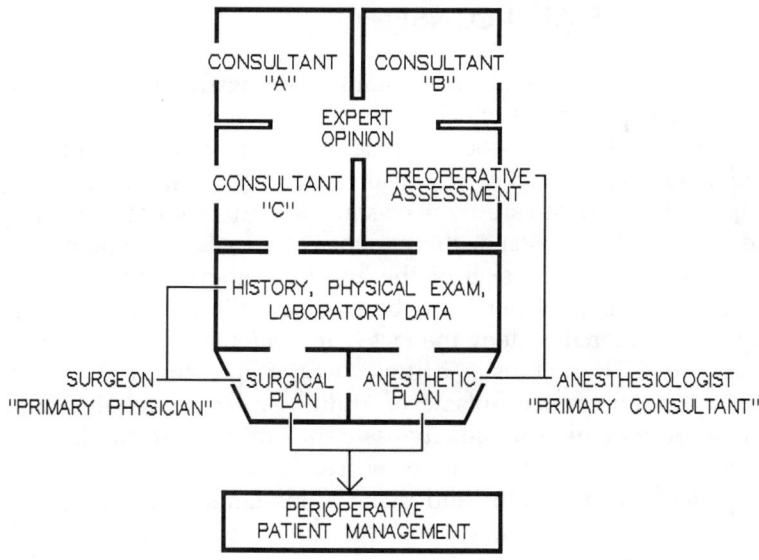

FIG 11–5.
Flow of information and decision making involved in determination of the anesthetic plan and the details of perioperative patient management. The anesthesiologist functions as a "primary consultant," since he fulfills the consultant's role by providing expert opinion and, simultaneously, the actions of the primary physician in providing directly a major aspect of patient care and autonomous decision making for critical choices.

Rather, during the short but intense period of time associated with anesthetic administration and immediate postoperative recovery, he assumes independent and comprehensive responsibility for most aspects of patient care.

Therefore, in one sense, the anesthesiologist might be best described as a "primary consultant." His duties and responsibilities require both the expertise normally attributed to the traditional consultant and the broad knowledge required for management of all aspects of patient care, a burden generally assumed by the primary physician. In the operating room the anesthesiologist is, in effect, a primary physician functioning in parallel with the continuing role of the surgeon. Each has specific responsibilities for those issues that fall clearly within their areas of expertise, but each is also required to share the authority needed to manage a patient during the critical events associated with anesthesia and surgery. Surgeon and anesthesiologist function as independent physician "co-contractors," accountable not to each other, but each accountable directly to the patient.[98]

EXPECTATIONS AND CONSENT

In his role as a primary consultant, the anesthesiologist must be aware of the expectations of each patient, as well as those of society at large, in regard to anesthetic outcome. The patient's expectations are rarely limited to the practice of anesthesia at a level that represents an acceptable standard of care by a reasonable and prudent practitioner, as the law specifies. Instead, the patient is typically more demanding. His implied trust in the skill of the anesthesiologist expresses an assumption that his anesthetic will be free of complications or risk, although it is irrational to deny the fact that accidents and errors can and will occur in environments as complex as the operating room. In contemporary practice, mechanisms of audit[99] and peer group comparisons may provide internal quality assurance to increase the likelihood of an uncomplicated perioperative course.[100]

A patient's expectations and those of his family are complexly intertwined with their own emotions regarding illness and surgery. As a primary consultant, the anesthesiologist should provide a logical, detailed, and thoughtful perspective on the frequency and nature of adverse outcomes associated with the anesthetic needed for the proposed surgical procedure. His views can be focused appropriately on the needs of the patient and expressed realistically in terms of general risk and benefit.

The concept of informed consent does not require recitation of exhaustive and macabre lists of anesthesia-related morbidity and mortality. Instead, the process of informed consent can represent a fair balance between the patient's right to be informed and to hear information needed to make rational choices, a reasonable yet practical dialogue concerning the likelihood of untoward events. The process of informed consent should be realistic without being unnecessarily alarming. In addition, because the anesthetic plan will be implemented under his direct supervision, the anesthesiologist should provide special insight as to how the details of anesthetic management will be conducted.

Also implied in the concept of the anesthesiologist as a primary consultant is receptiveness to new or evolving standards of anesthetic and postoperative care. The anesthetic plan formulated by a consultant in anesthesiology should reflect not only contemporary minimum standards of care, but also those advances that occur naturally as techniques are improved, concepts are clarified, and personal experience permits. As a full-time occupant of the operating room, the anesthesiologist is in a unique position to exercise authority and to accept responsibility for many of the details of patient traffic flow, intraoperative patient safety and positioning, the monitoring of vital functions, and the general adequacy of the operating room as a working environment and patient care facility. As such, he may play a greater role in determining perioperative morbidity and mortality than has been generally assumed.

SUMMARY

Some adverse perioperative outcome reflects random human error in the administration and management of anesthesia and systematic errors in judgment that can occur in this complex setting. The primary cause of catastrophic, anesthesia-related injury is nervous system hypoxia due to hypoventilation, airway mismanagement, or mechanical malfunction of the ventilator or the breathing circuit. Some simple incidents contribute to anesthetic morbidity or mortality because of inadequate monitoring practices or surveillance errors. However, much anesthesia-related injury is the inevitable consequence of technical deficiency or judgmental error, in particular a failure to anticipate patients in whom ventilation or tracheal intubation will be difficult.[101] Recent advances in continuous monitoring of oxygenation and ventilation and improved familiarity and facility with invasive cardiovascular monitoring may be reducing anesthesia-related morbidity and mortality dramatically in contemporary anesthetic practice.

Patients for whom there is objective evidence of a significantly increased risk of perioperative complications include those with preexisting cardiac or pulmonary disease that is severe enough to limit daily activity, patients who are morbidly obese, other patients at risk because of abnormal airway anatomy, or those with an increased risk of reflux and aspiration of gastric contents. Patients who have upper abdominal or thoracic surgery and those who require emergency surgery of any kind also appear to be part of a surgical subpopulation that experiences anesthetic complications at a rate higher than that seen after elective surgery outside of major body cavities. Age itself appears to be a risk factor primarily to the extent that it is associated with a high prevalence of age-related disease.

The anesthesiologist may function at times in a manner analogous to the primary physician, assuming almost total responsibility for the patient's welfare, yet at other times he may be required to give highly specialized assessments because of his expertise as a consultant. As a "primary consultant," the anesthesiologist exercises authority independently of the surgeon with regard to the moment-to-moment details of life support and vital functions. However, he shares the responsibility for the creation and implementation of an intraoperative and postoperative environment that is compatible with the needs of the patient and the surgeon and the expectations associated with accepted standards of anesthetic practice.

REFERENCES

1. Goldstein A Jr, Keats AS: The risk of anesthesia. *Anesthesiology* 1970; 33:130–142.
2. Keats AS: What do we know about anesthetic mortality? *Anesthesiology* 1979; 50:387–392.
3. Bendixen HH, Duberman SM: The concept of fail-safe monitoring. *Semin Anesth* 1986; 5:153–157.
4. David DA: An analysis of anesthetic mishaps from medical liability claims. *Int Anesthesiol Clin* 1984; 22:31–42.
5. Siker ES: The 1981 Rovenstein Lecture: A measure of worth. *Anesthesiology* 1982; 57:219–225.
6. Bishop HF: Operating room deaths. *Anesthesiology* 1946; 7:651–662.
7. Edwards G, Morton HJV, Pask EA, et al: Deaths associated with anaesthesia: A report on 1,000 cases. *Anaesthesia* 1956; 11:194–220.
8. Dinnick OP: Deaths associated with anaesthesia: Observations on 600 cases. *Anaesthesia* 1964; 19:536–556.

9. Brown DL: Anesthesia risk: A historical perspective, in Brown DL (ed): *Risk and Outcome in Anesthesia.* Philadelphia, JB Lippincott, 1988, pp 1–29.

10. Eichhorn JH: Prevention of intraoperative anesthesia accidents and related severe injury through safety monitoring. *Anesthesiology* 1989; 70:572–577.

11. Cooper JB: Towards prevention of anesthesia mishaps. *Int Anesthesiol Clin* 1984; 22:167–183.

12. Cooper JB, Newbower RS, Long CD, et al: Preventable anesthesia mishaps: A study of human factors. *Anesthesiology* 1978; 49:399–406.

13. Gaba DM, Maxwell M, DeAnda A: Anesthetic mishaps: Breaking the chain of accident evolution. *Anesthesiology* 1987; 66:670–676.

14. Cooper JB, Newbower RS, Kitz RJ: An analysis of major errors and equipment failures in anesthesia management: Considerations for prevention and detection. *Anesthesiology* 1984; 60:34–42.

15. Hyman WA, Drinker PA: Design of medical device alarm systems. *Med Instrum* 1983; 17:103–106.

16. Stafford TJ: Whither monitoring? *Crit Care Med* 1982; 10:792–795.

17. Rennels GD, Miller PL: Artificial intelligence research in anesthesia and intensive care. *J Clin Monit* 1988; 4:274–289.

18. Meyers RR, Kalichman MW, Reisner LS, et al: Neurotoxicity of local anesthetics: Altered perineural permeability, edema, and nerve fiber injury. *Anesthesiology* 1986; 64:29–35.

19. Whitcher C, Ream AK, Parsons D, et al: Anesthetic mishaps and the cost of monitoring: A proposed standard for monitoring equipment. *J Clin Monit* 1988; 4:5–15.

20. Caplan RA, Ward RJ, Posner K, et al: Unexpected cardiac arrest during spinal anesthesia: A closed claims analysis of predisposing factors. *Anesthesiology* 1988; 68:5–11.

21. Muravchick S: The aging patient and age-related disease, in Barash PG (ed): *Refresher Courses in Anesthesiology,* vol 16. Philadelphia, JB Lippincott, 1988, pp 145–153.

22. Marx GF, Mateo CV, Orkin LR: Computer analysis of postanesthestic deaths. *Anesthesiology* 1973; 39:54–58.

23. Atrash HK, Cheek TG, Hogue CJR: Legal abortion mortality and general anesthesia. *Am J Obstet Gynecol* 1988; 158:420–424.

24. Taylor G, Larson P, Prestwich R: Unexpected cardiac arrest during anesthesia and surgery. *JAMA* 1976; 236:2758–2760.

25. Harrison GG: Death attributable to anaesthesia. *Br J Anaesth* 1978; 50:1041–1046.

26. Utting JE, Gray TC, Shelley FC: Human misadventure in anaesthesia. *Can Anaesth Soc J* 1979; 26:472–478.

27. Holland R: Anesthetic-related mortality in Australia. *Int Anesthesiol Clin* 1984; 22:61–71.

28. Salem MR, Bennet EJ, Schweiss JF, et al: Cardiac arrest related to anesthesia: Contributing factors in infants and children. *JAMA* 1975; 233:238–241.

29. Samsoon GLT, Young JRB: Difficult tracheal intubation: A retrospective study. *Anaesthesia* 1987; 42:487–490.
30. Rosenberg H, Rosenberg H: Airway obstruction and causes of difficult intubation, in Orkin F, Cooperman LH (eds): *Complications in Anesthesiology*. Philadelphia, JB Lippincott, 1983, pp 125–143.
31. Safar P, Escarrage LA, Chang F: Upper airway obstruction in the unconscious patient. *J Appl Physiol* 1959; 14:760–764.
32. Deweese EL, Sullivan TY: Effects of upper airway anesthesia on pharyngeal patency during sleep. *J Appl Physiol* 1988; 64:1346–1353.
33. Walsh RE, Michaelson ED, Harkleroad LE: Upper airway obstruction in obese patients with sleep disturbance and somnolence. *Ann Intern Med* 1972; 76:185–192.
34. Sackner MA, Landa J, Forrest T, et al: Periodic sleep apnea: Chronic sleep deprivation related to intermittent upper airway obstruction and central nervous system disturbance. *Chest* 1975; 67:164–171.
35. White A, Kander PL: Anatomic factors in difficult direct laryngoscopy. *Br J Anaesth* 1975; 47:468–474.
36. Watson CB: Fiberoptic bronchoscopy for anesthesia. *Anesthesiol Rev* 1982; 9:17–26.
37. Fund D, Raymon F: Rheumatoid arthritis of the cricoarytenoid joints: An airway hazard. *Anesth Analg* 1975; 54:742–745.
38. Bannister FB, Macbeth RG: Direct laryngoscopy and tracheal intubation. *Lancet* 1944; 2:651–654.
39. Mallampati SR, Gatt SP, Gugino LD, et al: A clinical sign to predict difficult tracheal intubation. *Can Anaesth Soc J* 1985; 32:429–434.
40. Kopman AJ, Wollman SB, Ross K, et al: Awake endotracheal intubation: A review of 267 cases. *Anesth Analg* 1975; 54:323–327.
41. Stiles CM, Stiles PR, Denson JS: A flexible fiberoptic laryngoscope. *JAMA* 1972; 221:1246–1247.
42. Taylor PA, Towey RM: The bronchofiberscope as an aid to endotracheal intubation. *Br J Anaesth* 1972; 44:611–612.
43. Stewart R, Ellis D: Lighted stylet and endotracheal intubation (letter). *Anesthesiology* 1987; 66:851.
44. Barriot P, Riou B: Retrograde technique for tracheal intubation with trauma patients. *Crit Care Med* 1988; 16:712–713.
45. Magill IW: Blind nasal intubation. *Anaesthesia* 1975; 30:476–479.
46. Frumin MJ, Epstein RM, Cohen G: Apneic oxygenation in man. *Anesthesiology* 1959; 20:789–798.
47. Gold MI, Muravchick S: Arterial oxygenation during laryngoscopy and intubation. *Anesth Analg* 1981; 60:316–318.
48. Drummond GB, Park GR: Arterial oxygen saturation before intubation of the trachea. *Br J Anaesth* 1984; 56:987–992.
49. Fraioli RL, Sheffer LA, Steffenson JL: Pulmonary and cardiovascular effects of apneic oxygenation. *Anesthesiology* 1973; 39:588–596.
50. Hall AW, Moussa AR, Clark J, et al: The effects of premedication drugs on the lower oesophageal high pressure zone and reflux status of rhesus monkeys and man. *Gut* 1975; 16:347–352.

51. Fisher A, Waterhouse TD, Adams AP: Obesity: Its relation to anaesthesia. *Anaesthesia* 1975; 30:633–647.
52. Snow RG: The muscle relaxants and the cardia, including the clinical management of patients likely to vomit and regurgitate. *Br J Anaesth* 1963; 35:541–545.
53. Rex MAE: A review of the structural and functional basis of laryngospasm and a discussion of the nerve pathways involved in the reflex and its clinical significance in man and animals. *Br J Anaesth* 1970; 42:891–899.
54. Brahams D: Death of a patient participating in a trial of oral morphine for relief of postoperative pain. *Lancet* 1984; 1:1083.
55. Snow RG, Nunn JF: Induction of anaesthesia in the foot-down position for patients with a full stomach. *Br J Anaesth* 1959; 31:493–497.
56. Cotton BR, Smith G: The lower oesophageal sphincter and anaesthesia. *Br J Anaesth* 1984; 56:37–46.
57. Keats AS: The ASA classification of physical status—a recapitulation (editorial). *Anesthesiology* 1978; 49:233–236.
58. Goldman L: Cardiac risks and complications of noncardiac surgery. *Ann Intern Med* 1983; 98:504–513.
59. Gage AA, Bhayana JN, Balu V, et al: Assessment of cardiac risk in surgical patients. *Arch Surg* 1977; 112:1488–1492.
60. Swan HJC, Ganz W, Forrester J, et al: Catheterization of the heart in man with use of a flow-directed balloon-tipped catheter. *N Engl J Med* 1970; 283:447–451.
61. Gerson MC, Hurst JM, Hertzberg VS, et al: Cardiac prognosis in noncardiac geriatric surgery. *Ann Intern Med* 1985; 103:832–837.
62. Mangano DT: Monitoring pulmonary arterial pressure in coronary artery disease. *Anesthesiology* 1980; 53:364–370.
63. Lazor L, Russell JC, DaSilva J, et al: Use of multiple uptake gated acquisition scan for the preoperative assessment of cardiac risk. *Surg Gynecol Obstet* 1988; 167:234–238.
64. Moorman JR, Hlatky MA, Eddy DM, et al: The yield of the routine admission electrocardiogram. *Ann Intern Med* 1985; 103:590–595.
65. Charlson ME, MacKenzie CR, Ales K, et al: Surveillance for postoperative myocardial infarction after non-cardiac operations. *Surg Gynecol Obstet* 1988; 167:407–414.
66. Del Guercio LRM, Cohn JD: Monitoring operative risk in the elderly. *JAMA* 1980; 243:1350–1355.
67. MacKenzie CR, Charlson ME: Assessment of perioperative risk in the patient with diabetes mellitus. *Surg Gynecol Obstet* 1988; 167:293–299.
68. Eagle KA, Coley CM, Newell JB, et al: Combining clinical and thallium data optimizes preoperative assessment of cardiac risk before major vascular surgery. *Ann Intern Med* 1989; 110:859–866.
69. Steen PA, Tinker JH, Tarhan S: Myocardial reinfarction after anesthesia and surgery. *JAMA* 1978; 239:2566–2570.
70. Rao TLK, Jacobs KH, El-Etr AA: Reinfarction following anesthesia in patients with myocardial infarction. *Anesthesiology* 1983; 59:499–505.

71. Rao TLK: Cardiac monitoring for the noncardiac surgical patient. *Semin Anesth* 1983; 2:241–250.
72. Shibutani K, Del Guercio LRM: Preoperative hemodynamic assessment of the high-risk patient. *Semin Anesth* 1983; 2:231–240.
73. Marshall WK, Bedford RF: Use of a pulmonary-artery catheter for detection and treatment of venous air embolism. *Anesthesiology* 1980; 52:131–134.
74. Waller J, Kaplan J, Bauman D, et al: Clinical evaluation of a new fiberoptic catheter oximeter during cardiac surgery. *Anesth Analg* 1982; 61:676–679.
75. Lappas D, Lell WA, Gabel JC, et al: Indirect measurement of left-atrial pressure in surgical patients—pulmonary capillary wedge and pulmonary artery diastolic pressures compared with left atrial pressure. *Anesthesiology* 1973; 38:77–80.
76. Rao TL, Wong AY, Salem MR: A new approach to percutaneous catheterization of the internal jugular vein. *Anesthesiology* 1977; 46:362–364.
77. McDaniel DD, Stone JG, Faltas AN, et al: Catheter-induced pulmonary artery hemorrhage. *J Thorac Cardiovasc Surg* 1981; 82:1–4.
78. Jobes DR, Schwartz AJ, Greenhow DE, et al: Safer jugular vein cannulation: Recognition of arterial puncture and preferential use of the external jugular route. *Anesthesiology* 1983; 59:353–355.
79. Geha DG, Davis NJ, Lappas DG: Persistent atrial arrhythmias associated with placement of a Swan-Ganz catheter. *Anesthesiology* 1973; 39:651–653.
80. Bedford RF, Wollman H: Complications of radial artery cannulation: An objective prospective study. *Anesthesiology* 1973; 38:228–236.
81. Slogoff S, Keats AS, Arlund C: On the safety of radial artery cannulation. *Anesthesiology* 1983; 59:42–47.
82. Gaensler EA, Weisel RD: The risks in abdominal and thoracic surgery in COPD. *Postgrad Med* 1973; 54:183–191.
83. Norlander O, Hallen B: Anaesthetic mortality and pulmonary function, in Vickers MD, Lunn JN (eds): *Mortality in Anaesthesia*. Berlin, Springer-Verlag, 1983, pp 59–68.
84. Williams CD, Brenowitz JB: Prohibitive lung function and major surgical procedures. *Am J Surg* 1976; 132:763–766.
85. Tarhan S, Moffitt EA, Sessler AD, et al: Risk of anesthesia and surgery in patients with chronic bronchitis and chronic obstructive pulmonary disease. *Surgery* 1973; 74:720–726.
86. Stein M, Koota GM, Simon M, et al: Pulmonary evaluation of surgical patients. *JAMA* 1962; 181:765–770.
87. Latimer RG, Dickman M, Day WC, et al: Ventilatory patterns and pulmonary complications after upper abdominal surgery determined by preoperative and postoperative computerized spirometry and blood gas analysis. *Am J Surg* 1971; 122:622–632.
88. Gracey DR, Divertie MB, Didier EP: Preoperative pulmonary preparation

of patients with chronic obstructive pulmonary disease. *Chest* 1979; 76:123–129.

89. Cain H, Stevens PM, Adaniya R: Preoperative pulmonary function and complications after cardiovascular surgery. *Chest* 1979; 76:130–135.
90. Milledge JS, Nunn JF: Criteria of fitness for anesthesia in patients with chronic obstructive lung disease. *Br Med J* 1975; 3:670–673.
91. Carp D, Hines R: Routine preoperative pulmonary function tests: Numbers without benefit. *Anesthesiology* 1985; 63:A75.
92. Wahba WM, Don HF, Craig DB: Postoperative epidural anesthesia: Effect on lung volumes. *Can Anaesth Soc J* 1975; 22:519–527.
93. Egan TM, Herman SJ, Doucette EJ, et al: A randomized, controlled trial to determine the effectiveness of fascial infiltration of bupivacaine in preventing respiratory complications after elective abdominal surgery. *Surgery* 1988; 104:734–740.
94. Kingston HGC, Hirshman CA: Perioperative management of the patient with asthma. *Anesth Analg* 1984; 63:844–855.
95. Lee KWT, Downes JJ: Pulmonary edema secondary to laryngospasm in children. *Anesthesiology* 1983; 59:347–349.
96. Oswalt CE, Gates GA, Holmstrom FMG: Pulmonary edema as a complication of acute airway obstruction. *JAMA* 1977; 238:1833–1835.
97. Weissman C, Damask MC, Yang J: Noncardiogenic pulmonary edema following laryngeal obstruction. *Anesthesiology* 1984; 60:163–165.
98. Dornette WHL: Who's liable? Medicine and the law of agency, in Artusio JF (ed): *Legal Aspects of Anesthesia.* Philadelphia, FA Davis, 1972. pp 419–436.
99. Brown EM: Quality assurance in anesthesiology—the problem-oriented audit. *Anesth Analg* 1984; 63:611–615.
100. Vitez TS: *The Las Vegas Model for Quality Assessment in Anesthesiology.* Las Vegas, Nev. 1988.
101. Keenan RL: Anesthesia disasters: Incidence, causes, and preventability. *Semin Anesth* 1986; 5:175–179.
102. Otto CW: Tracheal intubation, in Nunn JF, Utting JE, Brown BR Jr (eds): *General Anaesthesia,* ed 5. London, Butterworth, 1989, pp 512–539.

Index